Artificial Intelligence in Oral Health

Artificial Intelligence in Oral Health

Editor

Jae-Hong Lee

MDPI • Basel • Beijing • Wuhan • Barcelona • Belgrade • Manchester • Tokyo • Cluj • Tianjin

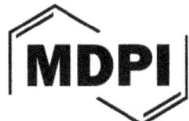

Editor
Jae-Hong Lee
Periodontology
Wonkwang University
College of Dentistry
Daejeon
Korea, South

Editorial Office
MDPI
St. Alban-Anlage 66
4052 Basel, Switzerland

This is a reprint of articles from the Special Issue published online in the open access journal *Diagnostics* (ISSN 2075-4418) (available at: www.mdpi.com/journal/diagnostics/special_issues/Dentistry_Oral_Health).

For citation purposes, cite each article independently as indicated on the article page online and as indicated below:

LastName, A.A.; LastName, B.B.; LastName, C.C. Article Title. *Journal Name* **Year**, *Volume Number*, Page Range.

ISBN 978-3-0365-5144-9 (Hbk)
ISBN 978-3-0365-5143-2 (PDF)

© 2022 by the authors. Articles in this book are Open Access and distributed under the Creative Commons Attribution (CC BY) license, which allows users to download, copy and build upon published articles, as long as the author and publisher are properly credited, which ensures maximum dissemination and a wider impact of our publications.

The book as a whole is distributed by MDPI under the terms and conditions of the Creative Commons license CC BY-NC-ND.

Contents

Preface to "Artificial Intelligence in Oral Health" vii

Jae-Hong Lee
Special Issue "Artificial Intelligence in Oral Health"
Reprinted from: *Diagnostics* **2022**, *12*, 1866, doi:10.3390/diagnostics12081866 1

Andreas Vollmer, Babak Saravi, Michael Vollmer, Gernot Michael Lang, Anton Straub and Roman C. Brands et al.
Artificial Intelligence-Based Prediction of Oroantral Communication after Tooth Extraction Utilizing Preoperative Panoramic Radiography
Reprinted from: *Diagnostics* **2022**, *12*, 1406, doi:10.3390/diagnostics12061406 3

Xiujiao Lin, Dengwei Hong, Dong Zhang, Mingyi Huang and Hao Yu
Detecting Proximal Caries on Periapical Radiographs Using Convolutional Neural Networks with Different Training Strategies on Small Datasets
Reprinted from: *Diagnostics* **2022**, *12*, 1047, doi:10.3390/diagnostics12051047 17

Mahmut Emin Celik
Deep Learning Based Detection Tool for Impacted Mandibular Third Molar Teeth
Reprinted from: *Diagnostics* **2022**, *12*, 942, doi:10.3390/diagnostics12040942 31

Ariya Chantaramanee, Kazuharu Nakagawa, Kanako Yoshimi, Ayako Nakane, Kohei Yamaguchi and Haruka Tohara
Comparison of Tongue Characteristics Classified According to Ultrasonographic Features Using a K-Means Clustering Algorithm
Reprinted from: *Diagnostics* **2022**, *12*, 264, doi:10.3390/diagnostics12020264 45

Łukasz Zadrożny, Piotr Regulski, Katarzyna Brus-Sawczuk, Marta Czajkowska, Laszlo Parkanyi and Scott Ganz et al.
Artificial Intelligence Application in Assessment of Panoramic Radiographs
Reprinted from: *Diagnostics* **2022**, *12*, 224, doi:10.3390/diagnostics12010224 57

Roopa S. Rao, Divya B. Shivanna, Kirti S. Mahadevpur, Sinchana G. Shivaramegowda, Spoorthi Prakash and Surendra Lakshminarayana et al.
Deep Learning-Based Microscopic Diagnosis of Odontogenic Keratocysts and Non-Keratocysts in Haematoxylin and Eosin-Stained Incisional Biopsies
Reprinted from: *Diagnostics* **2021**, *11*, 2184, doi:10.3390/diagnostics11122184 69

Rong Wang, Aparna Naidu and Yong Wang
Oral Cancer Discrimination and Novel Oral Epithelial Dysplasia Stratification Using FTIR Imaging and Machine Learning
Reprinted from: *Diagnostics* **2021**, *11*, 2133, doi:10.3390/diagnostics11112133 85

Luya Lian, Tianer Zhu, Fudong Zhu and Haihua Zhu
Deep Learning for Caries Detection and Classification
Reprinted from: *Diagnostics* **2021**, *11*, 1672, doi:10.3390/diagnostics11091672 101

Tianer Zhu, Daqian Chen, Fuli Wu, Fudong Zhu and Haihua Zhu
Artificial Intelligence Model to Detect Real Contact Relationship between Mandibular Third Molars and Inferior Alveolar Nerve Based on Panoramic Radiographs
Reprinted from: *Diagnostics* **2021**, *11*, 1664, doi:10.3390/diagnostics11091664 113

Anne Schlickenrieder, Ole Meyer, Jule Schönewolf, Paula Engels, Reinhard Hickel and Volker Gruhn et al.
Automatized Detection and Categorization of Fissure Sealants from Intraoral Digital Photographs Using Artificial Intelligence
Reprinted from: *Diagnostics* **2021**, *11*, 1608, doi:10.3390/diagnostics11091608 . . . . **123**

Sanjeev B. Khanagar, Sachin Naik, Abdulaziz Abdullah Al Kheraif, Satish Vishwanathaiah, Prabhadevi C. Maganur and Yaser Alhazmi et al.
Application and Performance of Artificial Intelligence Technology in Oral Cancer Diagnosis and Prediction of Prognosis: A Systematic Review
Reprinted from: *Diagnostics* **2021**, *11*, 1004, doi:10.3390/diagnostics11061004 . . . . **133**

Esther Alia-García, Manuel Ponce-Alonso, Claudia Saralegui, Ana Halperin, Marta Paz Cortés and María Rosario Baquero et al.
Machine Learning Study in Caries Markers in Oral Microbiota from Monozygotic Twin Children
Reprinted from: *Diagnostics* **2021**, *11*, 835, doi:10.3390/diagnostics11050835 . . . . **145**

Seok-Ki Jung, Ho-Kyung Lim, Seungjun Lee, Yongwon Cho and In-Seok Song
Deep Active Learning for Automatic Segmentation of Maxillary Sinus Lesions Using a Convolutional Neural Network
Reprinted from: *Diagnostics* **2021**, *11*, 688, doi:10.3390/diagnostics11040688 . . . . **157**

Seung Hyun Jeong, Jong Pil Yun, Han-Gyeol Yeom, Hwi Kang Kim and Bong Chul Kim
Deep-Learning-Based Detection of Cranio-Spinal Differences between Skeletal Classification Using Cephalometric Radiography
Reprinted from: *Diagnostics* **2021**, *11*, 591, doi:10.3390/diagnostics11040591 . . . . **169**

Preface to "Artificial Intelligence in Oral Health"

Artificial intelligence (AI), including deep learning and machine learning, is undergoing rapid development and has garnered substantial public attention in recent years. In particular, AI is positioned to become one of the most transformative technologies for medical applications and demonstrates great potential and useful properties for improving the analysis of various medical imaging datasets such as plain radiographs or three-dimensional imaging modalities. Several AI-based deep learning architectures have already been approved by the FDA and are being applied in clinical practice. In the dental field, the usefulness of AI has been assessed for the detection, classification, and segmentation of anatomical variables for orthodontic landmarks, dental caries, periodontal disease, and osteoporosis; however, these applications are still in very preliminary stages.

Jae-Hong Lee
Editor

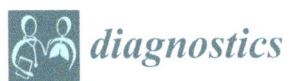

Editorial

Special Issue "Artificial Intelligence in Oral Health"

Jae-Hong Lee

Department of Periodontology, Daejeon Dental Hospital, Institute of Wonkwang Dental Research, Wonkwang University College of Dentistry, Daejeon 35233, Korea; ljaehong@gmail.com

Citation: Lee, J.-H. Special Issue "Artificial Intelligence in Oral Health". *Diagnostics* 2022, *12*, 1866. https://doi.org/10.3390/diagnostics12081866

Received: 26 July 2022
Accepted: 30 July 2022
Published: 2 August 2022

Publisher's Note: MDPI stays neutral with regard to jurisdictional claims in published maps and institutional affiliations.

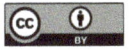

Copyright: © 2022 by the author. Licensee MDPI, Basel, Switzerland. This article is an open access article distributed under the terms and conditions of the Creative Commons Attribution (CC BY) license (https://creativecommons.org/licenses/by/4.0/).

I thank all authors, reviewers and the editorial staff who contributed to this Special Issue. In recent years, an increasing body of evidence has shown a direct or indirect correlation between oral health and chronic systemic diseases, including diabetes mellitus, atherosclerosis, rheumatoid arthritis, cancer, cardiovascular disease, and other non-communicable chronic diseases, although these findings remain controversial [1,2]. Typical oral disease parameters are evaluated and assessed by dental professionals using common clinical and radiographic tools including periodontal probe, dental mirror, dental explorer, and panoramic, periapical, and bitewing radiographic images, as well as cone beam computed tomography scans in some cases [3,4]. However, these conventional methods are inherently subjective, time-consuming, and expensive and may result in the under- or overestimation of diagnostic accuracy and performance [5,6]. Despite several attempts to overcome these limitations, they remain challenging and do not provide practical benefits over conventional diagnostic methods with regard to time, cost-effectiveness, and standardization.

Artificial intelligence (AI) refers to the ability of a machine that possesses its own form of intelligence to perform tasks that require human cognition. AI-based technology has emerged as a promising approach in the healthcare domain since the 2000s [7,8]. AI and machine learning based on the digitized big data archives and computing infrastructure are revolutionizing medical practice [9]. AI assists in clinical decision making through rapid and reliable data interpretation, the automation of administrative workflows to reduce non-patient-care-related activities, and direct patient participation in monitoring their health to improve health literacy [10]. AI has led to a paradigm shift in dental science, including in restorative dentistry, oral and maxillofacial surgery, prosthodontics, orthodontics, endodontics, and periodontics [11]. In particular, AI has significantly transformed dentistry and is viewed as a promising tool to revolutionize clinical diagnosis and management of oral disease. However, the exact role of AI in the prevention, diagnosis, and management of oral disease remains controversial.

AI-based algorithms will facilitate rapid, accurate, and reliable diagnosis of oral diseases and adoption of preventive strategies, as well as prompt intervention for improved treatment outcomes. Therefore, AI scores over traditional analytics and clinical decision making techniques through unbiased, consistent, and good-quality diagnosis and treatment in clinical and epidemiological scenarios. AI is particularly useful for standardized diagnosis and treatment of oral disease, which will benefit dental professionals in clinical practice. Several AI-based deep learning architectures have already been approved by the FDA and are being applied in clinical practice. In the dental field, the usefulness of AI has been assessed for the detection, classification, and segmentation of anatomical variables for orthodontic landmarks, dental caries, periodontal disease, and osteoporosis; however, these applications are still in very preliminary stages. This Special Issue is intended to lay the foundation of AI applications focusing on oral health, including general dentistry, periodontology, implantology, oral surgery, oral radiology, orthodontics, and prosthodontics, among others.

Funding: This study was supported by a National Research Foundation of Korea (NRF) grant funded by the Korean government (MSIT) (No. 2019R1A2C1083978).

Conflicts of Interest: The author declares no conflict of interest.

References

1. Lee, J.H.; Choi, J.K.; Jeong, S.N.; Choi, S.H. Charlson comorbidity index as a predictor of periodontal disease in elderly participants. *J. Periodontal Implant Sci.* **2018**, *48*, 92–102. [CrossRef] [PubMed]
2. Beck, J.D.; Papapanou, P.N.; Philips, K.H.; Offenbacher, S. Periodontal medicine: 100 years of progress. *J. Dent. Res.* **2019**, *98*, 1053–1062. [CrossRef] [PubMed]
3. Preshaw, P.M. Detection and diagnosis of periodontal conditions amenable to prevention. *BMC Oral Health* **2015**, *15* (Suppl 1), S5. [CrossRef] [PubMed]
4. Woelber, J.P.; Fleiner, J.; Rau, J.; Ratka-Kruger, P.; Hannig, C. Accuracy and usefulness of cbct in periodontology: A systematic review of the literature. *Int. J. Periodontics Restor. Dent.* **2018**, *38*, 289–297. [CrossRef] [PubMed]
5. Christiaens, V.; De Bruyn, H.; Thevissen, E.; Koole, S.; Dierens, M.; Cosyn, J. Assessment of periodontal bone level revisited: A controlled study on the diagnostic accuracy of clinical evaluation methods and intra-oral radiography. *Clin. Oral Investig.* **2018**, *22*, 425–431. [CrossRef] [PubMed]
6. Haas, L.F.; Zimmermann, G.S.; De Luca Canto, G.; Flores-Mir, C.; Correa, M. Precision of cone beam ct to assess periodontal bone defects: A systematic review and meta-analysis. *Dentomaxillofac. Radiol.* **2018**, *47*, 20170084. [CrossRef] [PubMed]
7. Ghahramani, Z. Probabilistic machine learning and artificial intelligence. *Nature* **2015**, *521*, 452–459. [CrossRef] [PubMed]
8. Jiang, F.; Jiang, Y.; Zhi, H.; Dong, Y.; Li, H.; Ma, S.; Wang, Y.; Dong, Q.; Shen, H.; Wang, Y. Artificial intelligence in healthcare: Past, present and future. *Stroke Vasc. Neurol.* **2017**, *2*, 230–243. [CrossRef] [PubMed]
9. Yu, K.H.; Beam, A.L.; Kohane, I.S. Artificial intelligence in healthcare. *Nat. Biomed. Eng.* **2018**, *2*, 719–731. [CrossRef] [PubMed]
10. Topol, E.J. High-performance medicine: The convergence of human and artificial intelligence. *Nat. Med.* **2019**, *25*, 44–56. [CrossRef] [PubMed]
11. Khanagar, S.B.; Al-Ehaideb, A.; Maganur, P.C.; Vishwanathaiah, S.; Patil, S.; Baeshen, H.A.; Sarode, S.C.; Bhandi, S. Developments, application, and performance of artificial intelligence in dentistry—A systematic review. *J. Dent. Sci.* **2021**, *16*, 508–522. [CrossRef] [PubMed]

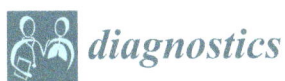

Article

Artificial Intelligence-Based Prediction of Oroantral Communication after Tooth Extraction Utilizing Preoperative Panoramic Radiography

Andreas Vollmer [1,*], Babak Saravi [2], Michael Vollmer [3], Gernot Michael Lang [2], Anton Straub [1], Roman C. Brands [1], Alexander Kübler [1], Sebastian Gubik [1] and Stefan Hartmann [1]

[1] Department of Oral and Maxillofacial Plastic Surgery, University Hospital of Würzburg, 97070 Würzburg, Germany; straub_a@ukw.de (A.S.); brands_r@ukw.de (R.C.B.); kuebler_a@ukw.de (A.K.); gubik_s@ukw.de (S.G.); hartmann_s2@ukw.de (S.H.)

[2] Department of Orthopedics and Trauma Surgery, Medical Centre-Albert-Ludwigs-University of Freiburg, Faculty of Medicine, Albert-Ludwigs-University of Freiburg, 79106 Freiburg, Germany; babak.saravi@jupiter.uni-freiburg.de (B.S.); gernot.michael.lang@uniklinik-freiburg.de (G.M.L.)

[3] Department of Oral and Maxillofacial Surgery, Tuebingen University Hospital, Osianderstrasse 2-8, 72076 Tuebingen, Germany; michael.vollmer@med.uni-tuebingen.de

* Correspondence: vollmer_a@ukw.de

Abstract: Oroantral communication (OAC) is a common complication after tooth extraction of upper molars. Profound preoperative panoramic radiography analysis might potentially help predict OAC following tooth extraction. In this exploratory study, we evaluated n = 300 consecutive cases (100 OAC and 200 controls) and trained five machine learning algorithms (VGG16, InceptionV3, MobileNetV2, EfficientNet, and ResNet50) to predict OAC versus non-OAC (binary classification task) from the input images. Further, four oral and maxillofacial experts evaluated the respective panoramic radiography and determined performance metrics (accuracy, area under the curve (AUC), precision, recall, F1-score, and receiver operating characteristics curve) of all diagnostic approaches. Cohen's kappa was used to evaluate the agreement between expert evaluations. The deep learning algorithms reached high specificity (highest specificity 100% for InceptionV3) but low sensitivity (highest sensitivity 42.86% for MobileNetV2). The AUCs from VGG16, InceptionV3, MobileNetV2, EfficientNet, and ResNet50 were 0.53, 0.60, 0.67, 0.51, and 0.56, respectively. Expert 1–4 reached an AUC of 0.550, 0.629, 0.500, and 0.579, respectively. The specificity of the expert evaluations ranged from 51.74% to 95.02%, whereas sensitivity ranged from 14.14% to 59.60%. Cohen's kappa revealed a poor agreement for the oral and maxillofacial expert evaluations (Cohen's kappa: 0.1285). Overall, present data indicate that OAC cannot be sufficiently predicted from preoperative panoramic radiography. The false-negative rate, i.e., the rate of positive cases (OAC) missed by the deep learning algorithms, ranged from 57.14% to 95.24%. Surgeons should not solely rely on panoramic radiography when evaluating the probability of OAC occurrence. Clinical testing of OAC is warranted after each upper-molar tooth extraction.

Keywords: artificial intelligence; deep learning; X-ray; tooth extraction; oroantral fistula; operative planning

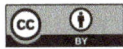

1. Introduction

When teeth are surgically removed in the maxilla, the opening of the maxillary sinus is a relevant complication, especially in the posterior region. Recent studies indicate that surgical removal of the upper third molar in the maxilla may cause maxillary sinus opening in up to 13% of cases, whereas completely displaced teeth may further increase the prevalence to up to 25% [1]. Usually, primary treatments cannot prevent oroantral communication (OAC). More invasive surgical interventions than novel, less invasive ones, for example, are associated with a higher likelihood of complications [2,3]. An illustration of the relationship between upper molars and the oroantral region is shown in Figure 1. The maxillary sinus can have variable anatomy due to maxillary sinus septa, temporary mucosal swelling, previous operations (Caldwell–Luc operation), or tumors [4]. Two-dimensional radiographic imaging is the standard imaging for routine extraction of maxillary teeth [5]. Panoramic radiography is the most widely used imaging modality for common oral surgical procedures. In addition to the general overview of the maxilla and mandible in a 2D X-ray/panoramic radiography, it is also characterized by its high availability, low radiation exposure, and low cost compared to 3D cone beam computer tomography [6,7]. Surgical intervention is required when the mucosal perforation exceeds 3 mm [5]. To be able to treat this complication, preoperative planning is necessary, such as planning the incision to be able to form a possible mucoperiosteal flap [8]. Simple closures with a single suture are possible but carry a high risk of complications [9]. Preoperative risk stratification algorithms could help lower the possible postoperative complications associated with OAC by utilizing them in alert-like systems for patients at risk in clinics.

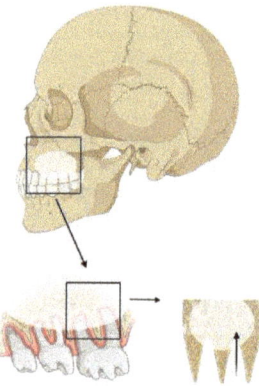

Figure 1. Illustration of the relationship between upper molars and the oroantral regions. Upper molar tooth extraction can lead to a perforation of the maxillary sinus floor and subsequent communication of the oral cavity with the maxillary sinus.

In 1978, mathematician Richard Bellman defined artificial intelligence (AI) as the automation of activities associated with human thinking skills, such as learning, decision making, and problem solving [10]. A clinical decision-support system is a computer algorithm developed to support clinical decision making in healthcare systems. This process involves processing a wide variety of medical data points necessary or valuable for interpretation [11,12]. As a branch of artificial intelligence, machine learning uses statistical learning algorithms to create systems that learn and enhance on their own without being explicitly programmed. The concept of "deep learning" is an applied machine learning method based on how the human brain filters information and learns from examples. Filtering input data through layers enables a computer model to anticipate and classify information. The term "convolutional neural networks" refers to artificial neural networks commonly applied to medical image prediction and classification. Essentially, it is a deep learning algorithm that takes an image as input and assigns weights/biases to specific characteristics and objects in the image in order to distinguish between them. CNNs are composed of many hidden layers, such as convolutional layers, pooling layers, fully connected layers, and normalizing layers. A ConvNet is designed to mimic the organization of the visual cortex and the pattern of connectivity of the neurons in the human brain [13]. In dentistry, interest in this area of research has increased significantly in recent years [14]. In a systematic review by Khanagar et al. (2021), many areas of application of AI in dentistry have already been identified [14]. The studies included in this systematic review were mainly concerned with the application of AI for the detection and diagnosis of dental caries and other oral pathologies. Here, the algorithms reached satisfying diagnostic accuracy.

A high predictive probability for sinusitis of the maxillary sinus has already been described [15]. As compared with experienced clinicians, at least a comparable level of sensitivity and specificity has been achieved [16]. Artificial intelligence is a beneficial tool to provide adequate guidance to the practitioner in case no other three-dimensional imaging is available. To the best of our knowledge, the AI-based predictive accuracy of panoramic radiography for maxillary sinus perforation after tooth extraction has not yet been described. Thus, we sought to evaluate several deep learning models for the prediction of OAC after tooth extraction utilizing preoperative panoramic radiography and compare the diagnostic accuracy with the accuracy obtained from human experts' evaluations. The overall aim of this exploratory study is to evaluate whether the anatomical situation found in panoramic radiography can predict OAC reliably after tooth extractions. Generally, we aimed to (1) assess the feasibility of OAC prediction from preoperative panoramic radiography utilizing multiple deep learning algorithms; (2) evaluate the feasibility of OAC prediction from expert evaluations; and (3) assess whether there are differences in diagnostic metrics for expert evaluations and deep learning algorithms regarding the OAC predictions.

2. Materials and Methods

2.1. Study Design

The examination is conducted in accordance with the Declaration of Helsinki and the Professional Code of Conduct for Physicians of the Bavarian Medical Association in the respective current versions. Although informed consent is regarded as a requirement for research purposes according to the Declaration of Helsinki and the Professional Code of Conduct for Physicians of the Bavarian Medical Association in the respective current versions, the ethics committee waived the need for informed consent in the present study due to the anonymization of X-ray data. All consecutive patients examined from 2010 through 2020 at the University Hospital Würzburg with indications of tooth extraction in the posterior region of the upper jaw were included in this study. Exclusion criteria were malignant diseases in the surgical area, fractures in the surgical site, syndromal anatomical variants, inflammation process on the root tip, and chronic/pre-existing OAC. In total, 300 patients with extracted teeth were included consecutively. The study was reviewed by the Ethics Committee of the University of Würzburg and approved under the authentication number 2022011702.

The data were acquired in the data management system of the University Hospital of Würzburg. Patients who had a tooth extraction in the maxillary posterior region between 2010 and 2020 were screened. These patients were explicitly selected based on ICD codes. The respective operation report was reviewed in detail for the group of patients who had an OAC after tooth extraction. The preoperative panoramic radiography was extracted only in the case that OAC could be determined clinically with various examinations. The panoramic radiography was extracted as a completely anonymized image file. For the control group, patients who had an extraction in the maxillary posterior region were searched and allocated to the control group after reviewing the surgical report, in which OAC was excluded and/or not diagnosed. The extraction of the radiograph was performed in the same way as described above. Overall, 100 consecutive cases with similar image and positioning quality in the OAC group (from 2010 to 2020) and 200 cases in the control group were collected for data analysis.

2.2. Expert Evaluations

In order to evaluate and compare the results of the deep learning algorithms, a comparative analysis was carried out by four oral and maxillofacial clinicians. A sequence of a total of 300 randomly arranged panoramic radiography images was produced. This sequence included a total of 100 images with a postoperative OAC and 200 images without this complication. The examiners were asked to decide from the preoperative panoramic radiography whether or not postoperative OAC occurs after the extraction of teeth in the maxillary posterior region (binary code: 1 for OAC and 0 for non-OAC). The diagnostic performance was determined for the respective practitioners and compared with the results of the deep learning algorithms.

2.3. Convolutional Neural Networks

The original images were taken utilizing multiple panoramic imaging devices. Images were randomly split into a train, test, and validation sets (60%, 20%, 20%). The validation data comprised the dataset used during training to check the outcome and adopt the model structure/hyperparameters. The test data comprised the hold-out dataset that was not used until the training process was finished to evaluate metrics. Then, we rescaled (224 × 224) all dataset images and pre-processed the train dataset images by applying data augmentation techniques (rotation range of ±30 degrees, horizontal flipping, brightness of 20–80%). Image augmentation was used to reduce overfitting and improve generalization. The region of interest was set manually by one surgeon to define the maxilla and the sinus area. We then utilized multiple supervised pre-trained deep learning models to classify the two study classes OAC versus non-OAC. For this, we applied five deep learning models (VGG16, ResNet50, Inceptionv3, EfficientNet, and MobileNetV2) to solve the classification problem. The algorithms' structure and the code are available in the data availability section. The models were frozen in the way that we used the basic models and made changes to the final layer only, as these models were designed to handle multiple classes, whereas we needed to solve a binary classification problem. For this, we made the layer non-trainable and built a last fully connected layer. Overall, we flattened the output of our base model to one dimension, added a fully connected layer with hidden units and ReLU activation, used a dropout rate, and added a final fully connected sigmoid layer. The specific characteristics of the models, including each layer, are shown in the code available in the data availability section. We used the RMSProp Optimizer (VGG16, InceptionV2, EfficientNet), SGD optimizer (ResNet50), or Adam optimizer (MobileNetV2) with a learning rate of 0.0001 and binary cross-entropy for loss evaluation. Steps per epoch were calculated as the sample size for the training set divided (using the integer division operator) by the batch size, where the batch size was 10. Models were trained for 10 epochs. We did not use a grid search, random search, or Bayesian optimization for hyperparameter tuning but used a manual search to adjust the parameters until the best metrics were obtained. Grid search and manual search are the most widely used strategies for hyper-parameter optimization [17]. Hyperparameter tuning using fine-tuning algorithms was intended to be applied to improve models more precisely in the case where an AUC over 0.75 could be reached for any model. In case no evidence was found that models were suitable to reach higher accuracies, we decided not to perform further hyperparameter tunings in a resource-oriented way, as these fine-tuning techniques are more intended to build precise models to classification tasks than to explore the feasibility/exploratory approach of whether a reliable classification is possible or not.

To evaluate each model's performance, accuracy, precision, recall, F1 score, and AUC were calculated. Accuracy is a metric used in classification problems to determine the percentage of accurate predictions. Precision is the ratio of true positives to true positives and false positives. The recall consists of the proportion of true positives to true positives and false negatives. An F1 score is derived by dividing precision and recall by (2 × precision + recall)/(precision + recall), while the AUC represents the area under the receiver operating characteristics (ROC) curve. To evaluate the clinical usability of AI, the results of panoramic radiography reads by AI and four oral and maxillofacial surgery specialists were compared. The diagnostic performance was assessed using the AUC, sensitivity, and specificity metrics. Agreement for expert evaluations was assessed with Cohen's kappa statistics. Algorithms were built and evaluated in Python using the OpenCV,

NumPy, Pillow, Seaborn, Matplotlib, TensorFlow, Keras, and scikit-learn libraries. The hardware and software environment specifications were as follows:
- CPU: AMD Ryzen 9 5950X 16-Core Processor;
- RAM: 64 GB;
- GPU: NVIDIA Geforce RTX 3090 (24 GB GDDR6X RAM);
- Python version: 3.10.4 (64-bit);
- OS: Windows 10.

Statistical analyses were conducted in Python, Stata Statistical Software Release 15 (StataCorp. 2011, College Station, TX, USA), and SPSS v26 (IBM, Armonk, NY, USA). Figure 1 was created with BioRender.com software (BioRender, Toronto, ON, Canada).

3. Results

3.1. Convolutional Neural Network Performance

According to the accuracy and area under the curve (AUC) measure, the best-performing models were MobileNetV2 and IncepionV3. The accuracy, AUC, precision, recall, and F1 score for the MobileNetV2 model were 0.74, 0.67, 0.75, 0.43, and 0.55, respectively (Table 1). The accuracy, AUC, precision, recall, and F1 score for the InceptionV3 model were 0.70, 0.60, 1.00, 0.19, and 0.32, respectively.

Table 1. Model performance of the convolutional neural networks. Values show the metrics for the independent test dataset (hold-out dataset).

Algorithm	Accuracy	AUC	Precision	Recall	F1-Score
VGG16	0.63	0.53	0.50	0.14	0.22
MobileNetV2	0.74	0.67	0.75	0.43	0.55
InceptionV3	0.70	0.60	1.00	0.19	0.32
ResNet50	0.56	0.45	0.17	0.05	0.07
EfficientNet	0.63	0.51	0.50	0.05	0.09

Precision, TP/(TP + FP); Recall, TP/(TP + FN); F1 score, 2 × (recall × precision)/(recall + precision); AUC, area under the curve; Accuracy, (TP + TN)/(TP + TN + FP + FN).

The confusion matrices and metrics of each model performed on the hold-out dataset (validation dataset) can be found in the data availability section. The specificity ranged from 0.8611 to 1.0000, with the highest specificity reached by the InceptionV3 model. The sensitivity ranged from 0.0476 to 0.4286, with the highest sensitivity reached by the MobileNetV2 model. The sensitivities from the EfficientNet, InceptionV3, MobileNetV2, ResNet50, and VGG16 were 0.0476, 0.1905, 0.4286, 0.0476, and 0.1429, respectively. The specificities from the EfficientNet, InceptionV3, MobileNetV2, ResNet50, and VGG16 were 0.9722, 1.0000, 0.9167, 0.8611, and 0.9167, respectively. The false-negative rate, i.e., the rate of true-positive cases (OAC) that were missed by the algorithms, ranged from 57.14% (MobileNetV2) to 95.24% (EfficientNet and ResNet50).

3.2. Expert Evaluations

Table 2 shows the performance metrics for each of the four expert evaluations. The area under the curve (AUC) ranged from 0.5458 to 0.7059. The specificity ranged from 51.74% to 95.02%, whereas the sensitivity ranged from 14.14% to 59.60%. Cohen's kappa exhibited a poor agreement for the oral and maxillofacial expert evaluations (Cohen's kappa: 0.1285).

The comparison of all ROC curves and AUC is shown in Figure 2 The deep learning model MobileNetV2 reached the highest AUC (AUC: 0.673), followed by a human expert (expert 2; AUC: 0.629).

Table 2. Detailed report of examiners (n = 300). AUC: area under the receiver operating characteristic (ROC) curve.

Observer	Sensitivity	Specificity	Correctly Classified	AUC
1	14.14	95.02	68.33	0.5458
2	59.60	81.59	74.33	0.7059
3	34.69	76.12	62.54	0.5541
4	68.69	51.74	57.33	0.6021

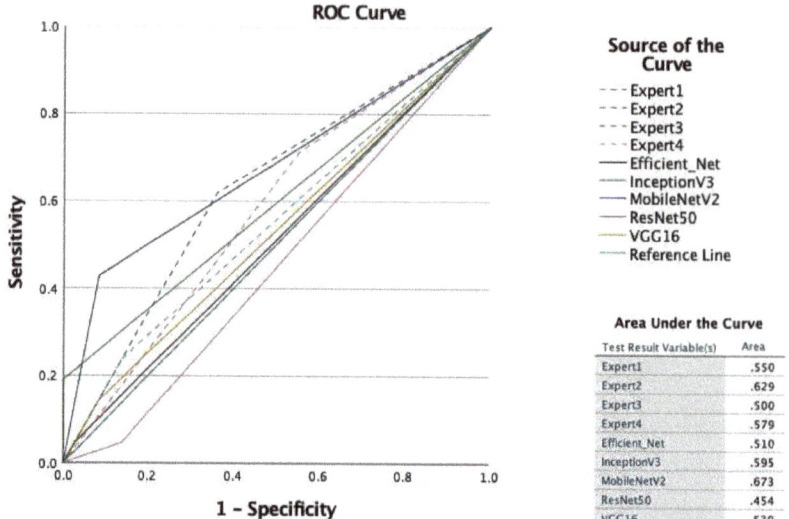

Figure 2. Receiver operating characteristic (ROC) curves and area under the ROC curves for all deep learning models and examiners.

4. Discussion

The present study sought to evaluate the feasibility of OAC prediction after upper-molar tooth extraction utilizing preoperative panoramic radiography. The results showed that although the MobileNetV2 algorithm and one expert reached an AUC of 0.673 and 0.629, respectively, the overall predictability of OAC from panoramic radiography was low. The false-negative rate, i.e., the rate of positive cases (OAC) missed by the deep learning algorithms, ranged from 57.14% to 95.24%. Further, there was a poor agreement for the oral and maxillofacial expert evaluations (Cohen's kappa: 0.1285).

Due to the fact that there are no comparable predictive studies currently available, it is not possible to compare our diagnostic metrics with others for the prediction of OAC after upper-molar tooth extraction. Using two data sets, one study compared AI-based and human examiner-based evaluations of inflammatory processes in the maxillary sinus from panoramic radiography [16]. The AI-based models achieved an AUC of 0.93 and 0.88 compared to the radiologist with 0.83 and 0.89. For predicting the postoperative injury of the inferior alveolar nerve from panoramic radiography, a systematic review of current evidence showed that sensitivity ranges from 0.06 to 0.49, and specificity ranges from 0.42 to 0.89, which is in accordance with our deep learning results for OAC [6]. These findings were also comparable to our expert evaluations for OAC although the agreement between the experts was low. We could not find a general superiority of the AI-based algorithms compared to the expert evaluations, as described before for panoramic radiography predictions; however, one deep learning algorithm reached the highest AUC [6,16]. This finding may be due to the fact that the information available in panoramic radiography was not sufficient to detect patterns on the basis of which an AI would be able to predict

OAC reliably. One systematic review evaluated several risk assessment studies assessing the risk of OAC based on clinical data, panoramic radiography, or cone-beam computer tomography (CBCT) utilizing statistical models. The authors concluded that panoramic radiographies are not reliable for assessing risk factors for OAC compared to CBCT based on current evidence [5]. We could confirm this finding by applying multiple deep-learning algorithms and letting experts evaluate the preoperative panoramic radiography.

Two-dimensional images (panoramic radiography) are not able to reflect the three-dimensional anatomical situation of molar roots. Bouquet et al. were able to show that in panoramic radiography, the root of the tooth appeared to protrude into the maxillary sinus, whereas in three-dimensional imaging (CBCT), there was no contact and thus no anatomical relationship [18]. Teeth can appear more inclined than they are in panoramic radiography [18]. This finding can be explained by the fact that deformations can occur when projecting a volume onto a flat surface. Such deformations are not expected in a 3D image [18]. It must also be borne in mind that in the majority of cases, the spatial development of the maxillary sinus is buccal to the roots of the maxillary molars [18,19]. For this reason, the analysis of the more palatal/distal tooth part seems to be less relevant for the chosen question of perforation of the maxillary sinus. Furthermore, no information is available regarding the number of roots. Iwata et al. showed that single-rooted teeth had a higher incidence of oroantral connections than multi-rooted teeth [20].

Using a defined classification (Archer classification, inclination, and root sinus classification), it has been shown that the positional relationship of maxillary molars to the maxillary sinus or their neighboring teeth can predict the probability of OAC [20]. In addition, other factors such as treatment components (incision, bone removal, maxillary tuber fractures, and extensive bleeding) correlate significantly with the likelihood of OAC [20]. The multifactorial genesis makes a prediction using 2D imaging difficult even with reliable classification systems. If the positional relationship or number of roots is unclear, 3D imaging is a helpful tool [18]. For AI-based prediction models, it is therefore difficult to reliably predict the occurrence of OAC based only on 2D imaging. It remains to be verified whether prediction with 3D imaging, for example, 3D magnet resonance tomography for soft tissue illustrations, can produce better results because of the additional information processed with an AI approach in specific classification tasks [21]. In the expert evaluations, we also showed that only low agreement could be identified between experts, indicating that 2D imaging is also not sufficient to predict OAC from the clinical perspective.

At present, deep learning methods are still being developed. An important advantage of convolutional neural networks is their ability to rapidly develop a feature extraction model, which is not overly concerned with the effectiveness of some features. It is, however, difficult to compare and explain performance. MobileNetV2 is one of the most popular deep learning methods that are widely used today since it has one of the most lightweight network architectures. This model showed the best performance in our study. MobileNetV1 introduced depth-wise separable convolution, which dramatically reduced the network's complexity costs and model size, making it suitable for low-processing devices, such as smartphones. In MobileNetV2, a better module with the inverted residual structure, is introduced. It eliminates non-linearities in narrow layers. In addition to achieving state-of-the-art performances for feature extraction, MobileNetV2 also achieves advanced results for object detection and semantic segmentation [22]. In general, MobileNetV2 is very similar to the original MobileNet, with the exception that it uses a novel layer module called the inverted residual with linear bottleneck, which reduces the memory requirement for processing since it has fewer parameters than the original MobileNet. As a result, the MobileNet V2 is less prone to overfitting. The proposed method uses MobileNetV2 as the basis for the transfer learning process. Due to the lightweight network architecture, the developed model can be implemented more quickly in clinical settings or mobile devices, making it more practical for use in clinical settings. Additionally, we included MobileNetV2 because a recent study showed that it is possible to perform classification tasks from panoramic radiographs with MobileNetV2 achieving higher accuracy than has been seen in the past, for instance, in classifying caries in the third molars [23]. Apostolopoulos et al. used VGG19 and MobileNetV2 to perform feature extraction on X-ray images and found that MobileNetV2 performed better than VGG19 in terms of specificity [24]. As a result, they believe that MobileNetV2 is the most robust model for specific classification tasks and data samples. In general, more research needs to be undertaken in order to evaluate why MobileNetV2 outperforms other methods in various settings. Notably, there might also be other image classification algorithms that could outperform the included models, such as artificial neural networks based on the successive geometric transformations model (SGTM) [25]. Several studies involving CNN in orthopedics, oncology, ophthalmology, and neurosurgery have been cited in the *PubMed* database since 2013. In 2017, Miki et al. published one of the first reports using CNNs with cone-beam computed tomography in the dental field [26]. CNN has been used in recent publications in cariology, periodontology, and endodontics as well as practical applications in clinics that are to be exploited in the near future [27–29]. Recent research describes a method to identify teeth using orthopantomography and registering them using simple CNNs that can help dentists in filling out dental charts more quickly and efficiently [30]. Other researchers developed a method of calculating age utilizing global fuzzy segmentation and local feature extraction based upon a projection-based feature transformation with a deep CNN model designed for molar classification [31]. In a scoping study on CNN applications in dental image diagnostics, it was observed that CNNs could be utilized in diagnostic-assistance systems in the dental arena [32]. At present, the implementation of CNN technology is challenging for dentists. It is expected that the generalization of such technology will be made easier through the development of improved algorithms. Previously, discriminant handcrafted features (e.g., histograms of oriented gradients features or local binary patterns features) dominated digital image analysis, but recent advances in deep learning algorithms have displaced the handcrafted approach, allowing automated image analysis. Convolutional neural networks are a type of deep learning algorithm that has become a workhorse. In recent data challenges for medical image analysis, all of the top-ranked teams used CNN. Except for one team, the top ten ranked solutions in the CAMELYON17 challenge used CNN for automatic detection and classification [33]. Shi et al. showed that the characteristics recovered via deep learning are superior to those extracted from handmade approaches [34]. In practice, however, deep learning algorithms such as CNN require a considerable quantity of training data under ideal conditions, resulting in a data-scarcity problem. A number of obstacles, such as the scarcity of expert-annotated data sets and the small size of medical cohorts, are well-known. Several studies have attempted to solve this problem by utilizing transfer learning or domain adaptation [35]. These approaches try to produce a high performance on target activities by applying knowledge learned from source tasks. Recent studies of transfer learning approaches from a data and model perspective were reviewed in 2020 by Zhuang et al. [36]. Researchers are increasingly interested in unsupervised transfer learning, an emerging academic subject. In their review of unsupervised deep domain adaptations, Wilson and Cook [37] examined a large number of articles. The use of generative adversarial networks-based frameworks has gained momentum recently [38], with Domain Adversarial Neural Network (DANN) being particularly promising [39]. A number of other methods have also been utilized for unsupervised transfer learning, including multiple kernel active learning [40] and collaborative unsupervised methods [41].

The study is associated with strengths and limitations. To the best of our knowledge, it is the first study evaluating the prediction of OAC utilizing both AI-based and expert-based evaluations of preoperative panoramic radiography. Thus, it contributes to the existing evidence, which solely applied statistical modeling (i.e., regression models) to evaluate risk factors for OAC. Further, the presented algorithms and dataset can be used to expand the methodology, compare diagnostic metrics with 3D assessment metrics, and perform external validations. However, there are also limitations associated with the present study. Unknown confounding factors due to the nature of retrospective analysis must be considered. In retrospective studies, it must be taken into account that small OAC may have occurred and were not documented in the patient information system, as this did not result in any additional need for intervention. Hence, although we accurately checked the available surgical reports to ensure whether OAC occurred or not, there might be misallocations. Thus, it should be noted that the control group included cases that were not assigned to the intervention group due to the lack of documentation in cases of low clinical suspicion, small OAC not worthy of treatment, or OAC that had occurred but were not documented. This might bias the allocation process. A more precise allocation would be possible with a prospective study design with standardized clinical testing algorithms for OAC. Overall, external validation utilizing prospective datasets is warranted. Another limitation is the determination of the ROI in our study. We decided to include a rather larger ROI to evaluate whether shapes of the sinus or adjacent structures are related to OAC. This was based on a previous study showing that the Archer and Root Sinus classification of teeth impaction is significantly associated with OAC [20]. As both classifications focus not only on the extracted teeth but also on adjacent structures, we decided to include a larger ROI. In our subsequent study, including larger sample size, we limited the ROI to the sinus area to evaluate whether the automatized classification of Archer and RS classes would be possible (unpublished data). In addition, here, we did not find evidence that panoramic radiography is feasible for this classification task, which is also in accordance with the expert evaluations. Although we included an extensive period to extract all images in our institution, the number of OAC cases might still be small, limiting the capabilities of deep learning algorithms to reliably learn the features from the dataset that can predict OAC, potentially reflecting the low sensitivity obtained from our algorithms. Sample size calculations for image classifications are known to require more than 1000 images per class for accurate predictions. However, this is often not possible in monocentric studies coming from surgical departments, as also shown in a recent systematic review assessing whether studies to date have performed sample size calculations for deep learning purposes in the literature [42]. These sample-size calculations might be more beneficial if there is evidence in an initial dataset analysis showing that classification is accurate and feasible from the dataset. A subsequent sample-size calculation can further improve future research models to a specific degree although studies have shown that sample size also affects the robustness of neural networks [43]. Another common mistake is to use the same data sets for validation and training. To avoid this bias, we separated the dataset into a training, testing, and validation sets, limiting the size of the training dataset further [44,45]. Nevertheless, the present study was the first feasibility study to evaluate whether multi-center studies would be beneficial in assessing the study question. As we did not find convincing evidence that panoramic radiography can predict OAC, our approach might have saved research resources associated with multi-center evaluations. Notably, the predictions of the algorithms are exclusively based on panoramic radiography. In this case, the practitioner's clinical decision-making process, which is carried out by considering all additional clinical data (i.e., clinical examinations, the extent of surgical invasiveness), cannot be fully simulated by the AI algorithms [46]. In addition, binary classification by human experts might not be as accurate as Likert-like scales or visual analogue scales, where expert decisions might be better reflected. This approach would also be more comparable with the algorithms that provide the probability metrics. Notably, we used the whole dataset for expert evaluations, which might be a discussion point, as this strategy limit the comparability with the metrics obtained from the hold-out dataset of the deep learning models. For metrics evaluations in deep learning, we used the metrics of the test dataset (hold-out dataset) because the same dataset to evaluate the model metrics should not be used as the dataset used to train (train dataset) and fine-tune the model (validation dataset). This approach was not necessary for the expert evaluations, thus justifying the use of the whole dataset for the evaluation process to evaluate whether experts are able to detect OAC from the dataset. Furthermore, the comparison of metrics between institutions may be limited due to different radiography protocols [44]. In addition, the surgical approach and the individual experience of the practitioner (i.e., learning curves) cannot be fully considered in prediction studies trying to predict OAC from panoramic radiography. Although prospective studies could adjust their study designs to evaluate data from solely one surgeon with a single technique extracting wisdom teeth, this seems not feasible considering that large datasets are required for deep learning evaluations. It is an inherent limitation of artificial intelligence-based algorithms based on only one data modality to lack multi-perspectivity when predicting images. Multi-input-mixed data hybrid models could help to improve the predictive capacities in the future [12]. In summary, the decision making based on AI algorithms remains complex and is beyond the practitioner's control [47,48]. Thus, clinical applicability may be limited. However, our primary aim was not to evaluate the algorithms as potential alert-like systems in clinics that can help to screen patients at risk for OAC but to generally evaluate the feasibility of OAC prediction based on preoperative panoramic radiography. Although such alert-like systems may be interesting in clinics, the authors recommend testing clinically whether an OAC has occurred after each extraction. Various options have been established for clinical testing. Starting with the least invasive test, the Valsalva test puts pressure on the maxillary sinus and, therefore, a possible OAC. The escaping air can be detected by air bubbles, a whistling sound, or a fogging mirror. However, this test can be falsely negative if mucous membranes are obstructed. Blunt probing and the insertion of objects impermeable to X-rays are not recommended because of their invasiveness and the possibility of germs spreading into the maxillary sinus [49]. Although the aforementioned clinical tests have limitations, they might be the easiest, fastest, and most accurate option currently available when considering the available evidence and our results.

Final clinical decisions should be made considering all aspects that potentially affect patients and can only be made by the practitioner. Supporting this decision-making process with the objective perspective of an AI-based approach may improve the quality of treatment. However, in the context of the present results, both experts and deep learning algorithms were not able to predict OAC reliably from patients' panoramic radiography.

5. Conclusions

Whether preoperative panoramic radiography information can help predict OAC after a tooth extraction is currently unknown. The results showed that although the MobileNetV2 algorithm and one expert reached an AUC of 0.673 and 0.629, respectively, the overall feasibility of OAC prediction from panoramic radiography was low. The false-negative rate, i.e., the rate of positive cases (OAC) missed by the deep learning algorithms, ranged from 57.14% to 95.24%. Further, there was a poor agreement for the oral and maxillofacial expert evaluations (Cohen's kappa: 0.1285). AI approaches utilized in the present work seem to be not feasible in predicting OAC based on the results shown. However, larger sample sizes, modification of the region of interest, and the inclusion of other algorithms could help to improve the knowledge presented with the work. Surgeons should not solely rely on panoramic radiography when evaluating the probability of OAC occurrence. Clinical testing of OAC is warranted after each upper-molar tooth extraction.

Supplementary Materials: The following supporting information can be downloaded at: https://www.mdpi.com/article/10.3390/diagnostics12061406/s1, Figure S1: Confusion matrix, model performance measures, and receiver operating characteristic (ROC) curve for the EfficientNet algorithm. Precision: TP/(TP + FN); Recall: TP/(TP + FN); F1 score: 2*(recall*precision)/(recall + precision); support: actual occurrence of the class in the dataset. Values are showing the metrics for the independent test dataset (hold-out dataset); Figure S2: Confusion matrix, model performance measures and receiver operating characteristic (ROC) curve for the InceptionV3 algorithm. Precision: TP/(TP + FN); Recall: TP/(TP + FN); F1 score: 2*(recall*precision)/(recall + precision); support: actual occurrence of the class in the dataset. Values are showing the metrics for the independent test dataset (hold-out dataset); Figure S3: Confusion matrix, model performance measures and receiver operating characteristic (ROC) curve for the MobileNetV2 algorithm. Precision: TP/(TP + FN); Recall: TP/(TP + FN); F1 score: 2*(recall*precision)/(recall + precision); support: actual occurrence of the class in the dataset. Values are showing the metrics for the independent test dataset (hold-out dataset); Figure S4: Confusion matrix, model performance measures and receiver operating characteristic (ROC) curve for the ResNet50 algorithm. Precision: TP/(TP + FN); Recall: TP/(TP + FN); F1 score: 2*(recall*precision)/(recall + precision); support: actual occurrence of the class in the dataset. Values are showing the metrics for the independent test dataset (hold-out dataset); Figure S5: Confusion matrix, model performance measures, and receiver operating characteristic (ROC) curve for the VGG16 algorithm. Precision: TP/(TP + FN); Recall: TP/(TP + FN); F1 score: 2*(recall*precision)/(recall + precision); support: actual occurrence of the class in the dataset. Values are showing the metrics for the independent test dataset (hold-out dataset); Figure S6: Example images from the whole data set.

Author Contributions: Data curation, A.V.; investigation, A.V.; methodology, A.V. and B.S.; project administration, A.V.; resources, A.V.; software, B.S.; supervision, R.C.B., A.K. and S.H.; validation, A.V., B.S., M.V. and S.G.; visualization, A.V.; writing—original draft, A.V. and B.S.; writing—review and editing, M.V., G.M.L., A.S., R.C.B., A.K. and S.H. All authors have read and agreed to the published version of the manuscript.

Funding: This research received no external funding.

Institutional Review Board Statement: The study was conducted in accordance with the Declaration of Helsinki and approved by the Institutional Review Board (or Ethics Committee) of the Ethics Committee of the Faculty of Medicine University of Wuerzburg (2022011702 and date of approval; Würzburg 17 February 2022).

Informed Consent Statement: Patient consent was waived due to the anonymization of X-ray data.

Data Availability Statement: Algorithm metrics are provided in Supplementary File S1. The raw images are anonymized and available from the corresponding author on reasonable request. Example images for pre-processing are shown in Supplementary File S2. The python code and deep learning algorithm structures are available from: https://github.com/Freiburg-AI-Research (accessed on 6 January 2022).

Conflicts of Interest: The authors declare no conflict of interest.

References

1. Rothamel, D.; Wahl, G.; D'Hoedt, B.; Nentwig, G.-H.; Schwarz, F.; Becker, J. Incidence and predictive factors for perforation of the maxillary antrum in operations to remove upper wisdom teeth: Prospective multicentre study. *Br. J. Oral Maxillofac. Surg.* **2007**, *45*, 387–391. [CrossRef] [PubMed]
2. Thereza-Bussolaro, C.; Galván, J.G.; Pachêco-Pereira, C.; Flores-Mir, C. Maxillary osteotomy complications in piezoelectric surgery compared to conventional surgical techniques: A systematic review. *Int. J. Oral Maxillofac. Surg.* **2019**, *48*, 720–731. [CrossRef] [PubMed]
3. Moore, R.; Miller, R.; Henderson, S. Risk management in oral surgery. *Br. Dent. J.* **2019**, *227*, 1035–1040. [CrossRef] [PubMed]
4. Van Den Bergh, J.P.A.; Ten Bruggenkate, C.M.; Disch, F.J.M.; Tuinzing, D.B. Anatomical aspects of sinus floor elevations. *Clin. Oral Implant. Res.* **2000**, *11*, 256–265. [CrossRef]
5. Lewusz-Butkiewicz, K.; Kaczor, K.; Nowicka, A. Risk factors in oroantral communication while extracting the upper third molar: Systematic review. *Dent. Med. Probl.* **2018**, *55*, 69–74. [CrossRef]
6. Su, N.; van Wijk, A.; Berkhout, E.; Sanderink, G.; De Lange, J.; Wang, H.; van der Heijden, G.J. Predictive Value of Panoramic Radiography for Injury of Inferior Alveolar Nerve After Mandibular Third Molar Surgery. *J. Oral Maxillofac. Surg.* **2017**, *75*, 663–679. [CrossRef] [PubMed]
7. Suomalainen, A.; Esmaeili, E.P.; Robinson, S. Dentomaxillofacial imaging with panoramic views and cone beam CT. *Insights Imaging* **2015**, *6*, 1–16. [CrossRef]
8. Visscher, S.H.; van Roon, M.R.; Sluiter, W.J.; van Minnen, B.; Bos, R.R. Retrospective Study on the Treatment Outcome of Surgical Closure of Oroantral Communications. *J. Oral Maxillofac. Surg.* **2011**, *69*, 2956–2961. [CrossRef] [PubMed]
9. Wowern, N. Frequency of oro-antral fistulae after perforation to the maxillary sinus. *Eur. J. Oral Sci.* **1970**, *78*, 394–396. [CrossRef] [PubMed]
10. Bellman, R. *Artificial Intelligence: Can Computers Think?* Course Technology: Boston, MA, USA, 1978; ISBN 0-87835-149-3.
11. Shortliffe, E.H. Testing Reality: The Introduction of Decision-Support Technologies for Physicians. *Methods Inf. Med.* **1989**, *28*, 1–5. [CrossRef] [PubMed]
12. Saravi, B.; Hassel, F.; Ülkümen, S.; Zink, A.; Shavlokhova, V.; Couillard-Despres, S.; Boeker, M.; Obid, P.; Lang, G.M. Artificial Intelligence-Driven Prediction Modeling and Decision Making in Spine Surgery Using Hybrid Machine Learning Models. *J. Pers. Med.* **2022**, *12*, 509. [CrossRef] [PubMed]

13. Shavlokhova, V.; Sandhu, S.; Flechtenmacher, C.; Koveshazi, I.; Neumeier, F.; Padrón-Laso, V.; Jonke, Ž.; Saravi, B.; Vollmer, M.; Vollmer, A.; et al. Deep Learning on Oral Squamous Cell Carcinoma Ex Vivo Fluorescent Confocal Microscopy Data: A Feasibility Study. *J. Clin. Med.* **2021**, *10*, 5326. [CrossRef]
14. Khanagar, S.B.; Al-Ehaideb, A.; Maganur, P.C.; Vishwanathaiah, S.; Patil, S.; Baeshen, H.A.; Sarode, S.C.; Bhandi, S. Developments, application, and performance of artificial intelligence in dentistry—A systematic review. *J. Dent. Sci.* **2020**, *16*, 508–522. [CrossRef]
15. Murata, M.; Ariji, Y.; Ohashi, Y.; Kawai, T.; Fukuda, M.; Funakoshi, T.; Kise, Y.; Nozawa, M.; Katsumata, A.; Fujita, H.; et al. Deep-learning classification using convolutional neural network for evaluation of maxillary sinusitis on panoramic radiography. *Oral Radiol.* **2018**, *35*, 301–307. [CrossRef]
16. Kim, Y.; Lee, K.J.; Sunwoo, L.; Choi, D.; Nam, C.-M.; Cho, J.; Kim, J.; Bae, Y.J.; Yoo, R.-E.; Choi, B.S.; et al. Deep Learning in Diagnosis of Maxillary Sinusitis Using Conventional Radiography. *Investig. Radiol.* **2019**, *54*, 7–15. [CrossRef]
17. Bergstra, J.; Bengio, Y. Random Search for Hyper-Parameter Optimization. *J. Mach. Learn. Res.* **2012**, *13*, 281–305.
18. Bouquet, A.; Coudert, J.-L.; Bourgeois, D.; Mazoyer, J.-F.; Bossard, D. Contributions of reformatted computed tomography and panoramic radiography in the localization of third molars relative to the maxillary sinus. *Oral Surg. Oral Med. Oral Pathol. Oral Radiol. Endodontol.* **2004**, *98*, 342–347. [CrossRef]
19. Jung, Y.-H.; Cho, B.-H. Assessment of maxillary third molars with panoramic radiography and cone-beam computed tomography. *Imaging Sci. Dent.* **2015**, *45*, 233–240. [CrossRef] [PubMed]
20. Iwata, E.; Hasegawa, T.; Kobayashi, M.; Tachibana, A.; Takata, N.; Oko, T.; Takeda, D.; Ishida, Y.; Fujita, T.; Goto, I.; et al. Can CT predict the development of oroantral fistula in patients undergoing maxillary third molar removal? *Oral Maxillofac. Surg.* **2020**, *25*, 7–17. [CrossRef]
21. Tesfai, A.S.; Vollmer, A.; Özen, A.C.; Braig, M.; Semper-Hogg, W.; Altenburger, M.J.; Ludwig, U.; Bock, M. Inductively Coupled Intraoral Flexible Coil for Increased Visibility of Dental Root Canals in Magnetic Resonance Imaging. *Investig. Radiol.* **2021**, *57*, 163–170. [CrossRef]
22. Sandler, M.; Howard, A.; Zhu, M.; Zhmoginov, A.; Chen, L.-C. MobileNetV2: Inverted Residuals and Linear Bottlenecks. In Proceedings of the 2018 IEEE/CVF Conference on Computer Vision and Pattern Recognition, Salt Lake City, UT, USA, 18–23 June 2018; pp. 4510–4520.
23. Vinayahalingam, S.; Kempers, S.; Limon, L.; Deibel, D.; Maal, T.; Hanisch, M.; Bergé, S.; Xi, T. Classification of caries in third molars on panoramic radiographs using deep learning. *Sci. Rep.* **2021**, *11*, 12609. [CrossRef]
24. Apostolopoulos, I.D.; Mpesiana, T.A. COVID-19: Automatic detection from X-ray images utilizing transfer learning with convolutional neural networks. *Phys. Eng. Sci. Med.* **2020**, *43*, 635–640. [CrossRef] [PubMed]
25. Khavalko, V.; Tsmots, I.G.; Kostyniuk, A.K.; Strauss, C. Classification and Recognition of Medical Images Based on the SGTM Neuroparadigm. *IDDM* **2019**, *2488*, 234–245.
26. Miki, Y.; Muramatsu, C.; Hayashi, T.; Zhou, X.; Hara, T.; Katsumata, A.; Fujita, H. Classification of teeth in cone-beam CT using deep convolutional neural network. *Comput. Biol. Med.* **2016**, *80*, 24–29. [CrossRef] [PubMed]
27. Lee, J.-H.; Kim, D.-H.; Jeong, S.-N.; Choi, S.-H. Detection and diagnosis of dental caries using a deep learning-based convolutional neural network algorithm. *J. Dent.* **2018**, *77*, 106–111. [CrossRef]
28. Krois, J.; Ekert, T.; Meinhold, L.; Golla, T.; Kharbot, B.; Wittemeier, A.; Dörfer, C.; Schwendicke, F. Deep Learning for the Radiographic Detection of Periodontal Bone Loss. *Sci. Rep.* **2019**, *9*, 8495. [CrossRef]
29. Ekert, T.; Krois, J.; Meinhold, L.; Elhennawy, K.; Emara, R.; Golla, T.; Schwendicke, F. Deep Learning for the Radiographic Detection of Apical Lesions. *J. Endod.* **2019**, *45*, 917–922. [CrossRef]
30. Tuzoff, D.V.; Tuzova, L.N.; Bornstein, M.M.; Krasnov, A.S.; Kharchenko, M.A.; Nikolenko, S.I.; Sveshnikov, M.M.; Bednenko, G.B. Tooth detection and numbering in panoramic radiographs using convolutional neural networks. *Dentomaxillofac. Radiol.* **2019**, *48*, 20180051. [CrossRef] [PubMed]
31. Kahaki, S.M.M.; Nordin, M.J.; Ahmad, N.S.; Arzoky, M.; Ismail, W. Deep convolutional neural network designed for age assessment based on orthopantomography data. *Neural Comput. Appl.* **2019**, *32*, 9357–9368. [CrossRef]
32. Schwendicke, G.; Dreher, K.J. Convolutional Neural Networks for Dental Image Diagnostics: A Scoping Review. *J. Dent.* **2019**, *91*, 103226. [CrossRef] [PubMed]
33. CAMELYON17—Grand Challenge. Grand-Challenge.Org. Available online: https://Camelyon17.Grand-Challenge.Org/Evaluation/Challenge/Leaderboard/ (accessed on 18 May 2022).
34. Shi, B.; Grimm, L.; Mazurowski, M.A.; Baker, J.A.; Marks, J.R.; King, L.M.; Maley, C.C.; Hwang, E.S.; Lo, J.Y. Prediction of Occult Invasive Disease in Ductal Carcinoma in Situ Using Deep Learning Features. *J. Am. Coll. Radiol.* **2018**, *15*, 527–534. [CrossRef]
35. Wang, Z.; Du, B.; Guo, Y. Domain Adaptation with Neural Embedding Matching. *IEEE Trans. Neural Netw. Learn. Syst.* **2019**, *31*, 2387–2397. [CrossRef] [PubMed]
36. Zhuang, F.; Qi, Z.; Duan, K.; Xi, D.; Zhu, Y.; Zhu, H.; Xiong, H.; He, Q. A Comprehensive Survey on Transfer Learning. *Proc. IEEE* **2021**, *109*, 43–76. [CrossRef]
37. Wilson, G.; Cook, D.J. A Survey of Unsupervised Deep Domain Adaptation. *ACM Trans. Intell. Syst. Technol.* **2020**, *11*, 1–46. [CrossRef] [PubMed]
38. Zhang, T.; Cheng, J.; Fu, H.; Gu, Z.; Xiao, Y.; Zhou, K.; Gao, S.; Zheng, R.; Liu, J. Noise Adaptation Generative Adversarial Network for Medical Image Analysis. *IEEE Trans. Med. Imaging* **2019**, *39*, 1149–1159. [CrossRef]

39. Ganin, Y.; Ustinova, E.; Ajakan, H.; Germain, P.; Larochelle, H.; Laviolette, F.; Marchand, M.; Lempitsky, V. Domain-Adversarial Training of Neural Networks. In *Domain Adaptation in Computer Vision Applications*; Advances in Computer Vision and Pattern Recognition book series; Springer: Cham, Switzerland, 2017; pp. 189–209. [CrossRef]
40. Wang, Z.; Du, B.; Tu, W.; Zhang, L.; Tao, D. Incorporating Distribution Matching into Uncertainty for Multiple Kernel Active Learning. *IEEE Trans. Knowl. Data Eng.* **2019**, *33*, 128–142. [CrossRef]
41. Zhang, Y.; Wei, Y.; Wu, Q.; Zhao, P.; Niu, S.; Huang, J.; Tan, M. Collaborative Unsupervised Domain Adaptation for Medical Image Diagnosis. *IEEE Trans. Image Process.* **2020**, *29*, 7834–7844. [CrossRef]
42. Balki, I.; Amirabadi, A.; Levman, J.; Martel, A.L.; Emersic, Z.; Meden, B.; Garcia-Pedrero, A.; Ramirez, S.C.; Kong, D.; Moody, A.R.; et al. Sample-Size Determination Methodologies for Machine Learning in Medical Imaging Research: A Systematic Review. *Can. Assoc. Radiol. J.* **2019**, *70*, 344–353. [CrossRef] [PubMed]
43. Lei, S.; Zhang, H.; Wang, K.; Su, Z. How Training Data Affect the Accuracy and Robustness of Neural Networks for Image Classification. In Proceedings of the International Conference on Learning Representations, New Orleans, LA, USA, 6–9 May 2019.
44. Gianfrancesco, M.A.; Tamang, S.; Yazdany, J.; Schmajuk, G. Potential Biases in Machine Learning Algorithms Using Electronic Health Record Data. *JAMA Intern. Med.* **2018**, *178*, 1544–1547. [CrossRef]
45. England, J.R.; Cheng, P. Artificial Intelligence for Medical Image Analysis: A Guide for Authors and Reviewers. *Am. J. Roentgenol.* **2019**, *212*, 513–519. [CrossRef]
46. Schwendicke, F.; Samek, W.; Krois, J. Artificial Intelligence in Dentistry: Chances and Challenges. *J. Dent. Res.* **2020**, *99*, 769–774. [CrossRef] [PubMed]
47. Shan, T.; Tay, F.; Gu, L. Application of Artificial Intelligence in Dentistry. *J. Dent. Res.* **2020**, *100*, 232–244. [CrossRef] [PubMed]
48. Magrabi, F.; Ammenwerth, E.; McNair, J.B.; De Keizer, N.F.; Hyppönen, H.; Nykänen, P.; Rigby, M.; Scott, P.J.; Vehko, T.; Wong, Z.S.-Y.; et al. Artificial Intelligence in Clinical Decision Support: Challenges for Evaluating AI and Practical Implications. *Yearb. Med. Inform.* **2019**, *28*, 128–134. [CrossRef] [PubMed]
49. Pauly, G.; Kashyap, R.; Shetty, R.; Kini, R.; Rao, P.; Giridh, R. Oro-Antral Fistula: Radio-diagnostic lessons from a rare case. *Am. J. Diagn. Imaging* **2017**, *4*, 21. [CrossRef]

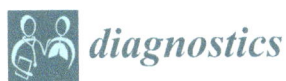

Article

Detecting Proximal Caries on Periapical Radiographs Using Convolutional Neural Networks with Different Training Strategies on Small Datasets

Xiujiao Lin [1,2], Dengwei Hong [1,2], Dong Zhang [3], Mingyi Huang [3] and Hao Yu [1,2,4,*]

1. Fujian Provincial Engineering Research Center of Oral Biomaterial, School and Hospital of Stomatology, Fujian Medical University, Fuzhou 350005, China; cherishlin686@gmail.com (X.L.); denthdw@163.com (D.H.)
2. Department of Prosthodontics, School and Hospital of Stomatology, Fujian Medical University, Fuzhou 350005, China
3. College of Computer and Data Science, Fuzhou University, Fuzhou 350025, China; zhangdong@fzu.edu.cn (D.Z.); hmy9029@163.com (M.H.)
4. Department of Applied Prosthodontics, Graduate School of Biomedical Sciences, Nagasaki University, Nagasaki 852-8521, Japan
* Correspondence: haoyu-cn@hotmail.com

Abstract: The present study aimed to evaluate the performance of convolutional neural networks (CNNs) that were trained with small datasets using different strategies in the detection of proximal caries at different levels of severity on periapical radiographs. Small datasets containing 800 periapical radiographs were randomly categorized into a training and validation dataset ($n = 600$) and a test dataset ($n = 200$). A pretrained Cifar-10Net CNN was used in the present study. Different training strategies were used to train the CNN model independently; these strategies were defined as image recognition (IR), edge extraction (EE), and image segmentation (IS). Different metrics, such as sensitivity and area under the receiver operating characteristic curve (AUC), for the trained CNN and human observers were analysed to evaluate the performance in detecting proximal caries. IR, EE, and IS recognition modes and human eyes achieved AUCs of 0.805, 0.860, 0.549, and 0.767, respectively, with the EE recognition mode having the highest values (p all < 0.05). The EE recognition mode was significantly more sensitive in detecting both enamel and dentin caries than human eyes (p all < 0.05). The CNN trained with the EE strategy, the best performer in the present study, showed potential utility in detecting proximal caries on periapical radiographs when using small datasets.

Keywords: neural networks; proximal caries; training strategy; small dataset; periapical radiograph

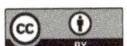

1. Introduction

Globally, dental caries is the most common oral disease, with 2.3 billion people suffering from caries of permanent teeth and more than 530 million children suffering from caries of deciduous teeth [1]. In China, an increasing caries prevalence is observed in line with the fourth national oral health epidemiological survey, with results demonstrating a prevalence of 38.5% in permanent teeth and 71.9% in deciduous teeth, respectively [2–4]. Dental caries occurs when plaque-associated bacteria produce acid that demineralizes the tooth. Controlling oral microbial biofilms is crucial for preventing dental caries. However, dental caries develops despite the use of antibiotics since bacterial resistance occurs due to excessive antibiotic use [5]. Generally, tooth loss is mainly attributed to dental caries [6], which is related to detrimental dietary changes and may lead to gastrointestinal disorders, even increasing the risk of Alzheimer's disease [7,8]. To manage dental caries, especially early caries lesions, precise detection is required before non-invasive or invasive treatment [9,10]. In particular, initial caries lesions occurring on the proximal surface in premolars and molars usually require auxiliary examination [11] since initial proximal caries lesions are difficult to detect by clinical examination unless the disease is advanced [12].

Intraoral radiographs, including bitewing radiographs and periapical radiographs, are commonly used to assist the diagnosis of proximal caries [13,14]. Akarslan et al. [15] compared the diagnostic accuracy of bitewing radiographs, periapical radiographs, and panoramic radiographs for proximal caries detection in posterior teeth. Both bitewing and periapical radiographs demonstrated a mean area under the receiver operating characteristic curve (AUC) that was higher than 0.9, indicating excellent performance. However, the performance of bitewing radiographs in detecting early caries lesions was somewhat contradictory, as they have been reported to have higher sensitivity than periapical radiographs [16] and a low diagnostic yield [17]. According to previous studies, only approximately 60% of proximal caries lesions were detected on bitewing radiographs [18,19]. Notably, bitewing radiographs are limited in their ability to offer information that allows cavitated and non-cavitated lesions to be distinguished from one another in the initial stages of progression [20]. In terms of periapical radiographs, a systematic review including 117 studies revealed that a low sensitivity of 42% was found for the detection of proximal caries [21]. Regrettably, a noteworthy limitation of periapical radiographs is that 40% of the tooth tissue has been demineralized when caries is successfully diagnosed by human eyes [12,22]. Thus, seeking a method to improve the diagnostic accuracy of dental caries on intraoral radiographs is of great significance.

Recently, convolutional neural networks (CNNs), a class of deep learning algorithms, have been widely applied in dentistry [23,24]. For example, CNNs have been applied to evaluate dental caries in bitewing and periapical radiographs [9] and periodontal bone loss in periapical or panoramic radiographs [25]. Lee et al. [9] explored the performance of CNNs in detecting dental caries lesions in periapical radiographs, obtaining an accuracy of 82.0% with a dataset of 3000 periapical images. According to a recent review, at least 1000 CT training datasets were required to obtain 98.0% validation accuracy with deep learning; also, 4092 CT training datasets were required to reach the desired accuracy of 99.5% [24]. CNNs are far more data hungry due to the millions of learnable parameters that they estimate [23]. Collecting data and making ground truth labels are essential to establish a successful deep learning project since these labels are used to train and test a model [23]. However, acquiring high-quality labelled data can be costly and time-consuming [23]. Notably, it is difficult to secure a large medical dataset due to patient privacy and security policies [26]. Therefore, strategies to improve the accuracy of CNNs trained with small datasets should be explored [27].

In general, the procedure used to carry out the learning process is called the training strategy; this strategy is applied to the neural network to obtain the best possible loss and increase accuracy [28]. In previous studies, different training strategies, such as different preprocessing strategies (e.g., contrast enhancement and average subtraction) and data augmentation were conducted to improve the performance of CNNs [29]. GoogLeNet achieved the best performance (96.69% accuracy) with the original images, while AlexNet performed better (94.33% accuracy) by using average subtraction [29]. Interestingly, Khojasteh et al. [30] introduced a novel layer in CNNs in which a preprocessing layer (e.g., contrast enhancement) was embedded followed by the first convolutional layer; this approach increased the accuracy of CNNs from 81.4% to 87.6%. Different strategies may work for different networks. Based on the current evidence, it should be considered that if small datasets (fewer than 1000 units per group [24]) of periapical radiographs were obtained, different training strategies, such as image preprocessing before training, could be adopted to improve diagnostic accuracy [27,29,31]. However, limited studies have focused on the recognition differences in neural networks with different training strategies (e.g., different preprocessing strategies) in dentistry, especially using small datasets. In addition, information regarding the performance in detecting dental caries at different levels of severity (different levels of caries progression) is scarce. Therefore, the present study aimed to evaluate the performance of a deep learning-based CNN in detecting proximal caries at different levels of progression on periapical radiographs, in which the CNN was trained with small datasets using different strategies. The following null hypotheses were tested: (1) no differences would be found in the performance of the trained CNN; and (2) the trained CNN would be more sufficient and accurate than human eyes in detecting proximal caries.

2. Materials and Methods

The research was performed following the principles of the Declaration of Helsinki and received approval from the Research Ethics Committee at the School and Hospital of Stomatology, Fujian Medical University (approval no.: 2018Y0029; approval date: 20 June 2018). The current study followed the guidelines of the Standards for Reporting of Diagnostics Accuracy Studies (STARD).

2.1. Study Design

In the present study, in which the CNN was trained with small datasets using different strategies, the performances of human observers and a deep learning-based CNN in evaluating proximal caries at different levels of severity on periapical radiographs were compared.

In this study, a pretrained Cifar-10Net CNN network was used as a classification model to distinguish caries from non-caries. Cifar-10Net was applied for its better efficiency object recognition [32]. Cifar-10Net is the basic network model used to classify the Cifar-10 dataset and is frequently used in image recognition [32]. As a subset of the larger dataset of 80 million tiny images, Cifar-10 included 60,000 colour images that contained 10 object classes [33].

According to previous study, different metrics were deployed to assess the classification performance of human observers and the CNN, including the diagnostic accuracy, sensitivity, specificity, positive predictive value (PPV), negative predictive value (NPV), receiver operating characteristic (ROC) curve, AUC, a precision-recall (P-R) curve, and the F1-score (F1-score = 2 × precision × recall/(precision + recall)).

2.2. Reference Dataset

Anonymous periapical radiographs were collected from patients who visited the Hospital of Stomatology, Fujian Medical University, from 2019 to 2020, following the randomization principle. All the periapical radiographs were taken by radiologists applying the paralleling technique [34]. Periapical radiographs obtained from the patient archiving and communication system (PACS) (Infinitt PACS, Infinitt Healthcare Co. Ltd., Seoul, Korea) were downloaded and saved in a bitmap image (BMP) file format [9]. The metadata, e.g., age, sex, and image creation date, were also obtained. Periapical radiographs with proximal caries limited to the crown or integral proximal surface were selected, excluding those with restorations and with severe noise, haziness, distortion, and shadows [9]. Periapical radiographs were cropped into images containing two posterior teeth to meet the training requirements; for inclusion, one tooth suffered from proximal caries (caries occurred in 1 or 2 proximal surfaces) and the other tooth was intact. All images were clearly revalidated, and proximal caries (including enamel and dentin caries of permanent teeth) were distinguished from non-proximal caries by 3 endodontists independently. No clinical records were acquired or evaluated in the procedure [35]. The 3 examiners all had more than 5 years of clinical experience [35]. For a single image, a consensus of the 3 examiners was required to identify the dental caries. Discussion was carried out when inconsistent evaluations arose. Periapical radiographs were excluded when disputes remained unsolved. To reduce the diagnostic bias which that might be caused by image cropping, original periapical radiographs were also provided to 3 the examiners for further needs. Consequently, small datasets of 800 periapical radiographs matching the training requirements were generated from 3165 periapical radiographs. The included radiographs were from 385 men and 415 women (mean age: 45.3 years). All 800 periapical radiographs were given a random number by using the RAND function and were randomly assigned to the training or test dataset by using the data sorting function in Microsoft Excel (Microsoft office 2016, Microsoft, Redmond, WA, USA). Subsequently, a training and validation dataset ($n = 600$) and a test dataset ($n = 200$) were randomly generated. Original datasets were then converted to grayscale images using uniform parameters, which was called the normalization of images.

2.3. Data Processing

2.3.1. Image Preprocessing

The training dataset of 600 periapical radiographs was preprocessed in MATLAB (MATLAB 2016b, MathWorks, Natick, MA, USA). Three preprocessing strategies of image recognition (without image preprocessing, IR), image segmentation (IS) [36] and edge extraction (EE) [31] were employed; IR and EE images were then overlaid into the original periapical radiographs. IS was performed based on a marked watershed segmentation algorithm [36]. The Canny operator was used when the image was preprocessed by means of EE [31]. An alpha transparency blending algorithm was utilized in the process of image superposition.

2.3.2. Image Labelled in MATLAB

The training dataset of 600 periapical radiographs was uploaded to the app in MATLAB used to label the images; caries lesions were marked using a training image labeler (TIL) based on the agreement among the 3 examiners and shown as the region of interest (ROI). According to the ROI, the level of caries severity was then evaluated. Caries progression was evaluated based on the following criteria [37]: level 0, non-proximal caries; level 1, proximal caries limited to the outer half of the enamel; level 2, proximal caries limited to the inner half of the enamel; level 3, proximal caries limited to the dento–enamel junction (DEJ); level 4, proximal caries limited to the outer half of the dentin; and level 5, proximal caries limited to the inner half of the dentin.

2.4. Training the CNN

A pretrained Cifar-10Net CNN network was used in the present study, which consists of an input layer, convolutional layer, rectified linear unit (ReLU) layer, pooling layer, fully connected layer, SoftMax layer, and output layer [33,38]. The convolutional, ReLU, and pooling layer form the core building blocks of the CNN. Specifically, the convolutional layer was responsible for updating filter weights during the data training; the ReLU layer mapped image pixels to the semantic content of the image; the pooling layer down sampled the data flowing through the network [33]. Before the output layer, the SoftMax layer, which acted as a classifier [39], received a two-dimensional vector from the fully connected layer and subsequently decided on the caries. Transfer learning was used to train the data to prevent overfitting, in which some parameters of the pretrained Cifar-10Net CNN network were transferred to the targeted Cifar-10Net CNN network [40]. Taking the loss value as the evaluation metric, a base learning rate of 0.0001 was set, and 400 epochs were run. Fine-tuning was conducted during transfer learning to improve diagnostic accuracy [9]. No standardized grayscale thresholding was used in the present CNN because the Cifar-10Net CNN is a nonlinear network instead of a regressor that needs a threshold [33,41]. Different training strategies implementing IR, IS, and EE were used to train the CNN independently [29], consequently generating three kinds of training models.

2.5. Test

The test process was carried out on the recognition model using a test dataset with no labels. Different recognition modes were established based on the training models, which were correspondingly distinguished as IR, IS, and EE. Finally, the detection of dental caries was conducted through the CNN algorithm that was trained, in which original images were pre-processed with IR, IS, EE and then analysed. Image superposition was performed between the original and preprocessed images when IS and EE strategies were used to detect proximal caries lesions. The diagnostic process of different recognition modes is shown in Figure 1. In addition, the workflow process of the CNN is exhibited in Figure 2.

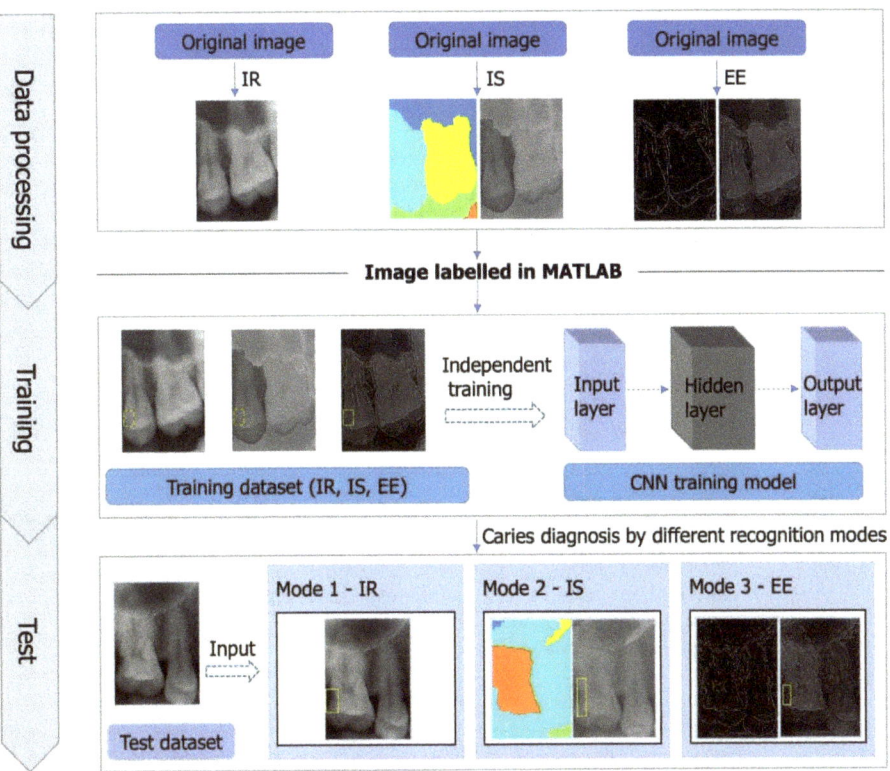

Figure 1. Proximal caries detection on periapical radiographs using deep learning with different recognition modes.

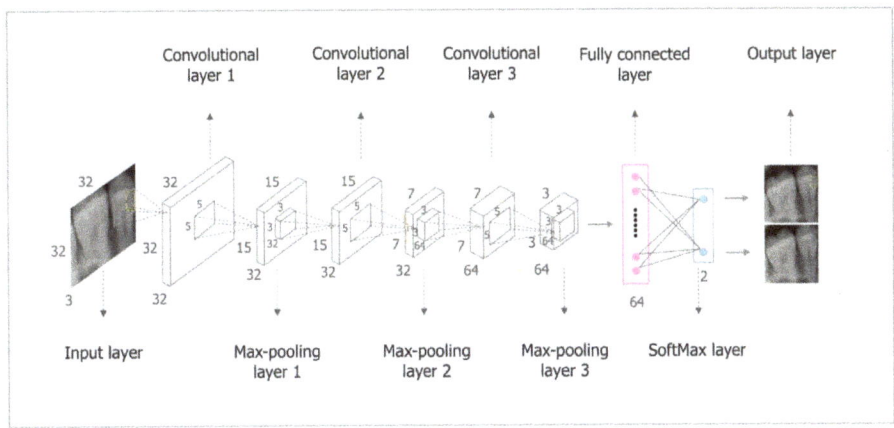

Figure 2. The workflow process of the CNN.

The main functions of relevant codes and some parameters in Data processing and Training were conducted as follows: IS, function imgf = fenge(rgb); EE, function img-Canny = edge_canny(I,gaussDim,sigma,percentOfPixelsNotEdges,thresholdRatio); Image superposition, function C = diejia(pic_1,pic_2); Training, function training = trainRCNNObjectDetector (Unnamed, mylayers, options, . . . 'NegativeOverlapRange', [0 0.3]).

2.6. Human Observers

Proximal caries on original periapical radiographs from the test dataset with no label was also assessed by the other 3 endodontists who had 3 to 10 years of clinical experience [35]. These images served as a comparator group that was used to gauge the performance of different recognition modes against that of human eyes [35]. Consensus should be achieved among 3 human observers when diagnosing proximal caries.

The test dataset was evaluated according to the evaluation criteria mentioned above and was used as the gold standard to compare the performance of IR, IS, EE and human observers.

2.7. Statistical Analysis

For different recognition modes and human eyes, the metrics to evaluate the performances were compared using the chi-square test and Z test. The p value was set at 0.05, and the 95% confidence interval (CI) was assessed.

3. Results

Consistency among examiners was checked before the revalidation, and Kendall's W coefficient of 0.830 ($p < 0.001$) showed strong consistency. The caries occurrences in proximal surfaces in the reference dataset, that is, the evaluation from the three examiners, are depicted in Table 1. The diagnostic accuracy, sensitivity, specificity, PPV, and NPV, including the 95% CI, for the detection of proximal caries using different recognition modes and human eyes are shown in Table 2.

Table 1. Caries occurrences in proximal surfaces in the reference dataset.

Dataset	Level 0	Level 1	Level 2	Level 3	Level 4	Level 5
Training dataset	1289	53	139	78	336	505
Test dataset	465	15	55	35	83	147
Overall	1754	68	194	113	419	652

Table 2. Accuracy, sensitivity, specificity, PPV, and NPV for the detection of proximal caries using different recognition modes and human eyes.

Recognition Mode	Accuracy (%, 95% CI)	Sensitivity (%, 95% CI)	Specificity (%, 95% CI)	PPV (%, 95% CI)	NPV (%, 95% CI)
IR	82.1 (79.5~84.8) [a,b]	70.1 (65.2~75.1) [a]	90.8 (88.1~93.4) [a]	84.5 (80.3~88.8) [a]	80.8 (77.5~84.2) [a]
EE	85.9 (83.5~88.3) [a]	86.9 (83.2~90.5) [b]	85.2 (81.9~88.4) [a,b]	80.8 (76.8~84.9) [a]	90.0 (87.2~92.8) [b]
IS	60.6 (57.2~64.0) [c]	19.4 (15.2~23.7) [c]	90.3 (87.6~93.0) [a]	59.1 (49.8~68.4) [b]	60.9 (57.2~64.5) [c]
Human eyes	78.0 (75.1~80.1) [b]	69.0 (64.0~73.9) [a]	84.5 (81.2~87.8) [b]	76.2 (71.4~81.1) [a]	79.1 (75.5~82.7) [a]

Different lowercase letters in a column indicate significant differences in different recognition modes and in human eyes.

A comparison of the ROC curves and P-R curves are shown in Figures 3 and 4, respectively, for both different recognition modes and human eyes. For the IR recognition mode, the AUC was 0.805 (95% CI 0.771~0.838). In the case of the EE recognition mode, the AUC was 0.860 (95% CI 0.832~0.888). Regarding the IS recognition mode, the AUC was 0.549 (95% CI 0.508~0.589). In the case of human eyes, the AUC was 0.767 (95% CI 0.732~0.802). The AUCs of IR and EE recognition modes were both significantly greater than that of the IS recognition mode (p all < 0.001). The AUC of the EE recognition mode was significantly higher than that of the IR recognition mode ($p = 0.013$). Compared to human eyes, only the AUC of the EE recognition mode was significantly higher ($p < 0.001$). The IR, EE, and IS recognition modes and human eyes achieved F1-scores of 0.766, 0.837, 0.292 and 0.724, respectively.

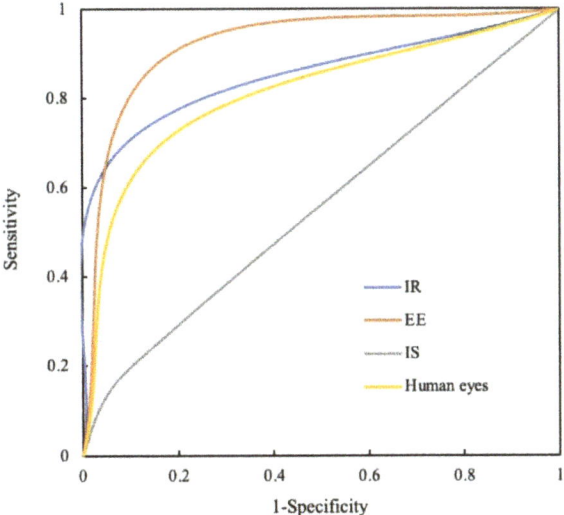

Figure 3. The ROC curves of different recognition modes and human eyes.

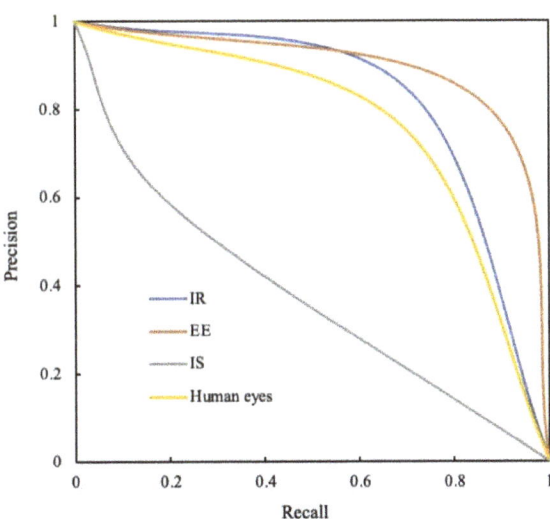

Figure 4. The P-R curves of different recognition modes and human eyes.

ROC = receiver operating characteristic; IR = image recognition; EE = edge extraction; IS = image segmentation.

P-R = precision-recall; IR = image recognition; EE = edge extraction; IS = image segmentation.

A comparison of the performance of IR, EE, and IS recognition modes and human eyes in detecting proximal caries at different levels of severity is demonstrated in Table 3. A comparison of the performance of IR, EE, and IS recognition modes and human eyes in detecting proximal caries at the enamel and dentin levels is exhibited in Table 4.

Table 3. A comparison of the performance of IR, EE, and IS recognition modes and human eyes in detecting proximal caries at different levels of severity.

Recognition Mode	Level 0 (Sample, %)	Level 1 (Sample, %)	Level 2 (Sample, %)	Level 3 (Sample, %)	Level 4 (Sample, %)	Level 5 (Sample, %)
IR	422/465 (90.8%) [a]	8/15 (53.3%) [a,b]	33/55 (60.0%) [a,b]	18/35 (51.4%) [a]	49/83 (59.0%) [a]	127/147 (86.4%) [a]
EE	396/465 (85.2%) [a,b]	10/15 (66.7%) [a]	42/55 (76.4%) [a]	28/35 (80.0%) [a]	70/83 (84.3%) [b]	141/147 (95.9%) [b]
IS	420/465 (90.3%) [a]	3/15 (20.0%) [a,b]	8/55 (14.5%) [c]	5/35 (14.3%) [b]	14/83 (16.9%) [c]	35/147 (23.8%) [c]
Human eyes	393/465 (84.5%) [b]	2/15 (13.3%) [b]	28/55 (50.9%) [b]	19/35 (54.3%) [a]	53/83 (63.9%) [a]	129/147 (87.8%) [a,b]

Different lowercase letters in a column indicate significant differences in different recognition modes and in human eyes.

Table 4. A comparison of the performance of IR, EE, and IS recognition modes and human eyes in detecting proximal caries at the enamel and dentin levels.

Recognition Mode	Enamel (Sample, %)	Dentin (Sample, %)
IR	41/70 (58.6%) [a,b]	194/265 (73.2%) [a]
EE	52/70 (74.3%) [a]	239/265 (90.2%) [b]
IS	11/70 (15.7%) [c]	54/265 (20.4%) [c]
Human eyes	30/70 (42.9%) [b]	201/265 (75.8%) [a]

Different lowercase letters in a column indicate significant differences in different recognition modes and in human eyes.

4. Discussion

Based on the present findings, the null hypotheses that no differences would be found in the performance of the trained CNN and that the trained CNN would be more sufficient and accurate than human eyes in the detection of proximal caries were partially accepted. In particular, the CNN trained with EE and IR strategies performed better than that with the IS strategy; and the CNN trained with the EE strategy achieved higher accuracy and sensitivity than human eyes in the detection of proximal caries.

Early intervention can remineralize softened enamel, which can block or reverse the process of dental caries [42]. Thus, finding an approach to detect initial caries, especially proximal caries, efficiently is of great significance [35]. Various diagnostic technologies have been developed to overcome the limitations of clinical and radiographic diagnosis and to improve the accuracy of caries detection [9]. Deep-learning-based CNNs are a class of artificial neural networks that are attracting interest across various fields, including radiology [23]. Compared to natural images, medical images are thought to have unique characteristics and are well fitted to deep learning [26]. Recently, using deep learning to detect dental caries lesions on periapical radiographs [9] and bitewing radiographs [35] has been studied. Compared to human eyes, deep-learning-based CNNs showed a satisfying discerning ability in detecting dental caries on periapical radiographs or bitewings [35]. A recent study revealed that approximately half of proximal caries lesions that reached the outer half of dentin were cavitated [43]. Moreover, it was suggested that restorations should be restricted to cavitated lesions [20], advising infiltration and sealing to manage non-cavitated proximal lesions as well as proximal lesions limited to one third of the outer dentin [20,44]. Thus, distinguishing proximal caries into different levels of severity is important for its guiding significance in dental treatment [43]. However, the performance of CNNs in detecting proximal caries at different levels of severity has not yet been reported. Notably, considering the difficulty in obtaining massive amounts of labelled medical data and patient security and confidentiality, different training strategies, such as image preprocessing, were conducted to search for the solution [23,26,27,29]. Pertinently, the present study first trained the CNN with small datasets (fewer than 1000 units per group) using different training strategies; that is, the CNN was trained with IR, IS, and EE strategies, which correspondingly resulted in different trained neural networks. Importantly, periapical radiographs were selected because of their clinical usage [45]. The AUCs of different trained neural networks (referred to as different recognition modes) were ultimately calculated and compared because of their significance in diagnostic performance [46].

Mandrekar et al. [46] suggested that an AUC of 0.8 to 0.9 is considered excellent in diagnostic performance. Accordingly, the recognition modes of IR and EE performed exceptionally in detecting proximal caries in the present study, with AUCs of 0.805 and 0.860, respectively. However, the IS recognition mode, with an AUC of 0.549, showed no discrimination in detecting proximal caries [46]. The EE recognition mode showed the greatest accuracy and achieved significantly higher accuracy than the human eye; thus, it was proposed that the EE recognition mode should be considered for small datasets. Edges are produced by the transition between various areas in the image, which is one of the most basic feature signals in the image signal [31]. For periapical radiographs, the changes in greyscale partly produce image edges. Pertinently, image edge extraction plays an important role in image recognition and processing [31]. In the present study, CNNs performed better than those in a previous study, which may be due to the Canny operator used in [31]. The use of the Canny operator strengthened the edge feature, which enabled CNNs to detect edges more efficiently [31]. The poor performance of the IS recognition mode may be attributed to excessive extrema and noise [36]. Furthermore, Lee et al. [9] reported that an AUC of 0.845 was achieved on both premolar and molar models based on a CNN. The EE recognition mode achieved an AUC of 0.860. Given the suggestions from Lee et al. [9], fine-tuning and transfer learning technology were used in the present study, which may account for the minor differences.

Based on the present findings, the highest sensitivity was obtained by the EE recognition mode, which might be due to the use of the Canny operator [31]. More specifically, the EE recognition mode was more sensitive than the IS recognition mode for the detection of enamel and dentin caries. However, the EE recognition mode did not demonstrate its superiority until level 4 caries detection (proximal caries limited to the outer half of dentin) and level 5 detection (proximal caries limited to the inner half of dentin) compared with the IR recognition mode. This contradictory phenomenon may result from the limited sample size. The EE, IR, and IS recognition modes all showed satisfying specificity, which could not be ignored when high sensitivity was achieved [9].

Based on the present results, the EE recognition mode was significantly more sensitive than human eyes for the detection of enamel and dentin caries. In terms of level 1 (proximal caries limited to the outer half of enamel), the EE recognition mode achieved higher sensitivity than the human eye, which was consistent with a previous report that enamel caries on periapical radiographs could be detected by human observers only after caries lesions advanced into the outer half of enamel [9]. It was probable that the EE recognition mode combined the greyscale changes and the features of caries edges, making this approach more capable of detecting initial caries even when learning on small datasets [31].

In addition, the P-R curve was observed, and the F1-score was calculated to assess the performance of the recognition model in cases where the dataset was unbalanced (e.g., the number of caries samples and non-caries samples differed extremely in quantity) [47]. The P-R curve was established by plotting data with precision (PPV) on the y-axis and recall (sensitivity) on the x-axis [48]. The F1-score was the harmonic of the precision and recall, which represents agreement with truth [48]. In the present study, the EE recognition mode achieved a precision score of 0.808, a recall score of 0.869, and the highest

F1-score of 0.837. These scores were higher than those reported in the study performed by Srivastava et al. [48], which achieved a precision score of 0.615, a recall score of 0.805, and an F1-score of 0.700 for the detection of tooth caries in bitewing radiographs using deep learning. The high recall of our recognition model showed that the model missed only a few proximal caries from the ground teeth [48]. More importantly, the high precision indicated that few false positives occurred based on the high sensitivity [48].

According to previous studies, GoogLeNet and U-Net were used to detect dental caries on periapical radiographs and bitewings, respectively [9,35]. Compared to the approaches utilizing GoogLeNet and U-Net, different models equipped with different loss functions and combinations of the parameters contributed to the main differences among existing approaches and the present proposal [9,35]. GoogLeNet, using a dataset of 3000 periapical radiographs, showed a sensitivity of 81.0%, a specificity of 83.0%, a PPV of 82.7% and an NPV of 81.4% [9]. U-Net, utilizing a dataset of 3686 bitewings, obtained a sensitivity of 75.0%, a specificity of 83.0%, a PPV of 70.0% and an NPV of 86.0% [35]. Notably, the present EE results were a sensitivity of 86.9%, a specificity of 85.2%, a PPV of 80.8% and an NPV of 90.0% based on the small dataset of 800 periapical radiographs; thus, a better performance was found in the present CNN compared to that of GoogLeNet. Differences between the present CNN and U-Net may be due to the different training strategies and detection objects [49]. Therefore, a preprocessing strategy that is common but well suited to medical images, such as EE strategy, was proposed to preprocess periapical radiographs that are commonly used in clinical practice [45].

Fine-tuning, one way to utilize a pretrained network [23], was the method selected to pretrain Cifar-10Net in the present study. Transfer learning was applied since this approach allowed generic features learned on a sufficiently large dataset to be shared with seemly disparate datasets [23]. Compared to other networks, such as AlexNet [50], Cifar-10Net has fewer layers and faster recognition speed, which partly reduces the recognition rate.

Several limitations should be considered in the present study. First, radiological dosage standardization was lacking since changes in the applied radiological dosage may occur for individual oral conditions, for example, soft tissue conditions [51]. Establishing a record of the applied dosage when taking periapical radiographs could be considered for obtaining standard images, which should be accomplished in cooperation with radiologists. Second, in the absence of a "hard" reference test, only radiographical evaluations were conducted, lacking clinical evaluations [9,35]. Furthermore, inconsistent with the CNN trained with EE and IR strategies that performed well, the CNN trained with IS strategy, namely, the IS recognition mode, behaved indiscriminately in detecting proximal caries and showed a poorer performance than that achieved by human eyes. Moreover, the sample size was unbalanced at different levels of caries severity, which may have impacted the present findings. A larger sample size and balanced dataset (different levels of caries severity) could be considered to enhance the generalizability of the present approach and exploring the impact of using the network on treatment decisions. Additionally, the recognition rate was partly sacrificed to increase the training and recognition speed [38]. The number of network layers should be increased to improve the recognition rate in future studies. Last, a further clinical comparison group (such as combining the clinical records when caries evaluations are conducted) to indicate the false-positive and false-negative rates of the calibrated examiners and the Cifar-10Net CNN process could be considered to further verify the current findings.

5. Conclusions

Within the limitations of a lack of standardization of the radiological dosage and a small sample size, we prudently concluded that the deep-learning-based CNN trained with the EE strategy performed excellently in detecting proximal caries on periapical radiographs; different training strategies, such as image preprocessing, could be considered to improve the accuracy of the CNN model, especially when a small dataset was used. Pertinently, the present proposed method should be regarded as a computer-aided caries detection system in clinical practice, in which clinical evaluations should be combined and not discarded. However, the challenges of how the proposed method could be generalized and applied to treatment decisions should be considered. Additionally, regarding the limitation of only conducting the radiographical evaluations, a further clinical comparison group to indicate the false-positive and false-negative rates of the calibrated examiners and the Cifar-10Net CNN process could be considered to further verify the current findings.

Author Contributions: Conceptualization, H.Y. and D.Z.; methodology, X.L., H.Y. and D.Z.; software, M.H. and D.H.; validation, D.H. and M.H.; formal analysis, X.L.; investigation, X.L. and D.H.; resources, X.L. and D.H.; data curation, M.H.; writing—original draft preparation, X.L.; writing—review and editing, H.Y.; supervision, H.Y.; project administration, H.Y. and D.Z. All authors have read and agreed to the published version of the manuscript.

Funding: This research was funded by the Guiding Project of Science and Technology Plan of Fujian Province, grant number 2018Y0029.

Institutional Review Board Statement: The study was conducted in accordance with the Declaration of Helsinki and approved by the Ethics Committee of the School and Hospital of Stomatology, Fujian Medical University (approval no.: 2018Y0029; approval date: 20 June 2018).

Informed Consent Statement: Patient consent was waived due to the use of anonymous patient data.

Data Availability Statement: The data presented in this study are available on request from the corresponding author. The data are not publicly available because of privacy restrictions.

Acknowledgments: The authors want to thank the Radiology Department for its cooperation and help.

Conflicts of Interest: The authors declare no conflict of interest.

References

1. Vos, T.; Lim, S.S.; Abbafati, C.; Abbas, K.M.; Abbasi, M.; Abbasifard, M.; Abbasi-Kangevari, M.; Abbastabar, H.; Abd-Allah, F.; Abdelalim, A.; et al. Global burden of 369 diseases and injuries in 204 countries and territories, 1990–2019: A systematic analysis for the Global Burden of Disease Study 2019. *Lancet* **2020**, *396*, 1204–1222. [CrossRef]
2. Du, M.Q.; Li, Z.; Jiang, H.; Wang, X.; Feng, X.P.; Hu, Y.; Lin, H.C.; Wang, B.; Si, Y.; Wang, C.X.; et al. Dental caries status and its associated factors among 3- to 5-year-old children in China: A national survey. *Chin. J. Dent. Res.* **2018**, *21*, 167–179. [CrossRef] [PubMed]
3. Quan, J.K.; Wang, X.Z.; Sun, X.Y.; Yuan, C.; Liu, X.N.; Wang, X.; Feng, X.P.; Tai, B.J.; Hu, Y.; Lin, H.C.; et al. Permanent teeth caries status of 12- to 15-year-olds in China: Findings from the 4th National Oral Health Survey. *Chin. J. Dent. Res.* **2018**, *21*, 181–193. [CrossRef] [PubMed]
4. Gao, Y.B.; Hu, T.; Zhou, X.D.; Shao, R.; Cheng, R.; Wang, G.S.; Yang, Y.M.; Li, X.; Yuan, B.; Xu, T.; et al. Dental caries in Chinese elderly people: Findings from the 4th National Oral Health Survey. *Chin. J. Dent. Res.* **2018**, *21*, 213–220. [CrossRef]
5. Niu, J.Y.; Yin, I.X.; Wu, W.K.K.; Li, Q.L.; Mei, M.L.; Chu, C.H. Antimicrobial peptides for the prevention and treatment of dental caries: A concise review. *Arch. Oral Biol.* **2021**, *122*, 105022. [CrossRef]
6. Frencken, J.E.; Sharma, P.; Stenhouse, L.; Green, D.; Laverty, D.; Dietrich, T. Global epidemiology of dental caries and severe periodontitis—A comprehensive review. *J. Clin. Periodontol.* **2017**, *44* (Suppl. 18), S94–S105. [CrossRef]
7. Harding, A.; Gonder, U.; Robinson, S.J.; Crean, S.; Singhrao, S.K. Exploring the association between Alzheimer's disease, oral health, Microbial Endocrinology and Nutrition. *Front. Aging Neurosci.* **2017**, *9*, 398. [CrossRef]
8. Stein, P.S.; Desrosiers, M.; Donegan, S.J.; Yepes, J.F.; Kryscio, R.J. Tooth loss, dementia and neuropathology in the Nun study. *J. Am. Dent. Assoc.* **2007**, *138*, 1314–1322, quiz 1381–1312. [CrossRef]
9. Lee, J.H.; Kim, D.H.; Jeong, S.N.; Choi, S.H. Detection and diagnosis of dental caries using a deep learning-based convolutional neural network algorithm. *J. Dent.* **2018**, *77*, 106–111. [CrossRef]
10. Innes, N.P.T.; Chu, C.H.; Fontana, M.; Lo, E.C.M.; Thomson, W.M.; Uribe, S.; Heiland, M.; Jepsen, S.; Schwendicke, F. A century of change towards prevention and minimal intervention in Cariology. *J. Dent. Res.* **2019**, *98*, 611–617. [CrossRef]
11. Gimenez, T.; Piovesan, C.; Braga, M.M.; Raggio, D.P.; Deery, C.; Ricketts, D.N.; Ekstrand, K.R.; Mendes, F.M. Visual inspection for caries detection: A systematic review and meta-analysis. *J. Dent. Res.* **2015**, *94*, 895–904. [CrossRef] [PubMed]
12. Schwendicke, F.; Elhennawy, K.; Paris, S.; Friebertshäuser, P.; Krois, J. Deep learning for caries lesion detection in near-infrared light transillumination images: A pilot study. *J. Dent.* **2020**, *92*, 103260. [CrossRef] [PubMed]
13. Schwendicke, F.; Rossi, J.G.; Göstemeyer, G.; Elhennawy, K.; Cantu, A.G.; Gaudin, R.; Chaurasia, A.; Gehrung, S.; Krois, J. Cost-effectiveness of artificial intelligence for proximal caries detection. *J. Dent. Res.* **2021**, *100*, 369–376. [CrossRef]

14. Şeker, O.; Kamburoğlu, K.; Şahin, C.; Eratam, N.; Çakmak, E.E.; Sönmez, G.; Özen, D. In vitro comparison of high-definition US, CBCT and periapical radiography in the diagnosis of proximal and recurrent caries. *Dentomaxillofacial Radiol.* **2021**, *50*, 20210026. [CrossRef]
15. Akarslan, Z.Z.; Akdevelioğlu, M.; Güngör, K.; Erten, H. A comparison of the diagnostic accuracy of bitewing, periapical, unfiltered and filtered digital panoramic images for approximal caries detection in posterior teeth. *Dentomaxillofacial Radiol.* **2008**, *37*, 458–463. [CrossRef]
16. Takahashi, N.; Lee, C.; Da Silva, J.D.; Ohyama, H.; Roppongi, M.; Kihara, H.; Hatakeyama, W.; Ishikawa-Nagai, S.; Izumisawa, M. A comparison of diagnosis of early stage interproximal caries with bitewing radiographs and periapical images using consensus reference. *Dentomaxillofacial Radiol.* **2019**, *48*, 20170450. [CrossRef]
17. Vaarkamp, J.; Ten Bosch, J.J.; Verdonschot, E.H.; Bronkhoorst, E.M. The real performance of bitewing radiography and fiber-optic transillumination in approximal caries diagnosis. *J. Dent. Res.* **2000**, *79*, 1747–1751. [CrossRef]
18. Chan, M.; Dadul, T.; Langlais, R.; Russell, D.; Ahmad, M. Accuracy of extraoral bite-wing radiography in detecting proximal caries and crestal bone loss. *J. Am. Dent. Assoc.* **2018**, *149*, 51–58. [CrossRef]
19. Gaalaas, L.; Tyndall, D.; Mol, A.; Everett, E.T.; Bangdiwala, A. Ex vivo evaluation of new 2D and 3D dental radiographic technology for detecting caries. *Dentomaxillofacial Radiol.* **2016**, *45*, 20150281. [CrossRef]
20. Ammari, M.M.; Soviero, V.M.; Da Silva Fidalgo, T.K.; Lenzi, M.; Ferreira, D.M.; Mattos, C.T.; de Souza, I.P.; Maia, L.C. Is non-cavitated proximal lesion sealing an effective method for caries control in primary and permanent teeth? A systematic review and meta-analysis. *J. Dent.* **2014**, *42*, 1217–1227. [CrossRef]
21. Schwendicke, F.; Tzschoppe, M.; Paris, S. Radiographic caries detection: A systematic review and meta-analysis. *J. Dent.* **2015**, *43*, 924–933. [CrossRef]
22. Onem, E.; Baksi, B.G.; Sen, B.H.; Söğüt, Ö.; Mert, A. Diagnostic accuracy of proximal enamel subsurface demineralization and its relationship with calcium loss and lesion depth. *Dentomaxillofacial Radiol.* **2012**, *41*, 285–293. [CrossRef]
23. Yamashita, R.; Nishio, M.; Do, R.K.G.; Togashi, K. Convolutional neural networks: An overview and application in radiology. *Insights Imaging* **2018**, *9*, 611–629. [CrossRef]
24. Hwang, J.J.; Jung, Y.H.; Cho, B.H.; Heo, M.S. An overview of deep learning in the field of dentistry. *Imaging Sci. Dent.* **2019**, *49*, 1–7. [CrossRef]
25. Lee, J.H.; Kim, D.H.; Jeong, S.N.; Choi, S.H. Diagnosis and prediction of periodontally compromised teeth using a deep learning-based convolutional neural network algorithm. *J. Periodontal Implant Sci.* **2018**, *48*, 114–123. [CrossRef]
26. Cho, J.; Lee, K.; Shin, E.; Choy, G.; Do, S. How much data is needed to train a medical image deep learning system to achieve necessary high accuracy. *arXiv* **2015**, arXiv:1511.06348.
27. Kokol, P.; Kokol, M.; Zagoranski, S. Machine learning on small size samples: A synthetic knowledge synthesis. *Sci. Prog.* **2022**, *105*, 368504211029777. [CrossRef]
28. Rađenović, Ž.; Krstić, B.; Marković, M. Smart farming in agricultural industry: Mobile technology perspective. *Ekon. Poljopr.* **2020**, *67*, 925–938. [CrossRef]
29. Rodrigues, L.F.; Naldi, M.C.; Mari, J.F. Comparing convolutional neural networks and preprocessing techniques for HEp-2 cell classification in immunofluorescence images. *Comput. Biol. Med.* **2020**, *116*, 103542. [CrossRef]
30. Khojasteh, P.; Aliahmad, B.; Arjunan, S.P.; Kumar, D.K. Introducing a novel layer in convolutional neural network for automatic identification of diabetic Retinopathy. In Proceedings of the 2018 40th Annual International Conference of the IEEE Engineering in Medicine and Biology Society (EMBC), Honolulu, HI, USA, 17–21 July 2018.
31. Kanchanatripop, P.; Zhang, D. Adaptive image edge extraction based on discrete algorithm and classical Canny operator. *Symmetry* **2020**, *12*, 1749. [CrossRef]
32. Patalas-Maliszewska, J.; Halikowski, D. A deep learning-based model for the automated assessment of the activity of a single worker. *Sensors* **2020**, *20*, 2571. [CrossRef]
33. Mathworks. Available online: https://www.mathworks.com/help/vision/examples/object-detection-using-deep-learning.html (accessed on 10 April 2020).
34. Patel, S.; Wilson, R.; Dawood, A.; Mannocci, F. The detection of periapical pathosis using periapical radiography and cone beam computed tomography—Part 1: Pre-operative status. *Int. Endod. J.* **2012**, *45*, 702–710. [CrossRef]
35. Cantu, A.G.; Gehrung, S.; Krois, J.; Chaurasia, A.; Rossi, J.G.; Gaudin, R.; Elhennawy, K.; Schwendicke, F. Detecting caries lesions of different radiographic extension on bitewings using deep learning. *J. Dent.* **2020**, *100*, 103425. [CrossRef]
36. Zhang, M.; Xue, Y.; Ge, Y.; Zhao, J. Watershed Segmentation Algorithm Based on Luv Color Space Region Merging for Extracting Slope Hazard Boundaries. *ISPRS Int. J. Geo-Inf.* **2020**, *9*, 246. [CrossRef]
37. Cheng, J.G.; Zhang, Z.L.; Wang, X.Y.; Zhang, Z.Y.; Ma, X.C.; Li, G. Detection accuracy of proximal caries by phosphor plate and cone-beam computerized tomography images scanned with different resolutions. *Clin. Oral Investig.* **2012**, *16*, 1015–1021. [CrossRef]
38. Xu, Q.; Pan, G. SparseConnect: Regularising CNNs on fully connected layers. *Electron. Lett.* **2017**, *53*, 1246–1248. [CrossRef]
39. Cho, C.; Choi, W.; Kim, T. Leveraging uncertainties in Softmax decision-making models for low-power IoT devices. *Sensors* **2020**, *20*, 4603. [CrossRef]
40. Lian, L.; Zhu, T.; Zhu, F.; Zhu, H. Deep Learning for caries detection and classification. *Diagnostics* **2021**, *11*, 1672. [CrossRef]

41. Fong, Y.; Huang, Y.; Gilbert, P.B.; Permar, S.R. Chngpt: Threshold regression model estimation and inference. *BMC Bioinform.* **2017**, *18*, 454. [CrossRef]
42. Gomez, J.; Tellez, M.; Pretty, I.A.; Ellwood, R.P.; Ismail, A.I. Non-cavitated carious lesions detection methods: A systematic review. *Community Dent. Oral Epidemiol.* **2013**, *41*, 54–66. [CrossRef]
43. Schwendicke, F.; Göstemeyer, G. Conventional bitewing radiographs. In *Detection and Assessment of Dental Caries: A Clinical Guide*, 1st ed.; Ferreira Zandona, A., Longbottom, C., Eds.; Springer International Publishing: Cham, Switzerland, 2019; pp. 109–117, ISBN 978-3-030-16967-1.
44. Chen, Y.; Chen, D.; Lin, H. Infiltration and sealing for managing non-cavitated proximal lesions: A systematic review and meta-analysis. *BMC Oral Health* **2021**, *21*, 13. [CrossRef] [PubMed]
45. Antony, D.P.; Thomas, T.; Nivedhitha, M.S. Two-dimensional periapical, panoramic radiography versus three-dimensional cone-beam computed tomography in the detection of periapical lesion after endodontic treatment: A systematic review. *Cureus* **2020**, *12*, e7736. [CrossRef] [PubMed]
46. Mandrekar, J.N. Receiver operating characteristic curve in diagnostic test assessment. *J. Thorac. Oncol.* **2010**, *5*, 1315–1316. [CrossRef]
47. Chicco, D.; Jurman, G. The advantages of the Matthews correlation coefficient (MCC) over F1 score and accuracy in binary classification evaluation. *BMC Genom.* **2020**, *21*, 6. [CrossRef]
48. Srivastava, M.; Kumar, P.; Pradhan, L.; Varadarajan, S. Detection of tooth caries in bitewing radiographs using deep learning. In Proceedings of the NIPS Workshop on Machine Learning for Health (NIPS ML4H 2017), Long Beach, CA, USA, 8 December 2017.
49. Ronneberger, O.; Fischer, P.; Brox, T. U-Net: Convolutional networks for biomedical image segmentation. In Proceedings of the Medical Image Computing and Computer Assisted Intervention (MICCAI 2015), Munich, Germany, 5–9 October 2015.
50. Miki, Y.; Muramatsu, C.; Hayashi, T.; Zhou, X.; Hara, T.; Katsumata, A.; Fujita, H. Classification of teeth in cone-beam CT using deep convolutional neural network. *Comput. Biol. Med.* **2017**, *80*, 24–29. [CrossRef]
51. Shin, H.S.; Nam, K.C.; Park, H.; Choi, H.U.; Kim, H.Y.; Park, C.S. Effective doses from panoramic radiography and CBCT (cone beam CT) using dose area product (DAP) in dentistry. *Dentomaxillofacial Radiol.* **2014**, *43*, 20130439. [CrossRef]

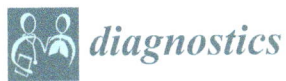

Article

Deep Learning Based Detection Tool for Impacted Mandibular Third Molar Teeth

Mahmut Emin Celik

Department of Electrical Electronics Engineering, Faculty of Engineering, Gazi University, Eti mah. Yukselis sk. No: 5 Maltepe, Ankara 06570, Turkey; mahmutemincelik@gazi.edu.tr

Abstract: Third molar impacted teeth are a common issue with all ages, possibly causing tooth decay, root resorption, and pain. This study was aimed at developing a computer-assisted detection system based on deep convolutional neural networks for the detection of third molar impacted teeth using different architectures and to evaluate the potential usefulness and accuracy of the proposed solutions on panoramic radiographs. A total of 440 panoramic radiographs from 300 patients were randomly divided. As a two-stage technique, Faster RCNN with ResNet50, AlexNet, and VGG16 as a backbone and one-stage technique YOLOv3 were used. The Faster-RCNN, as a detector, yielded a mAP@0.5 rate of 0.91 with ResNet50 backbone while VGG16 and AlexNet showed slightly lower performances: 0.87 and 0.86, respectively. The other detector, YOLO v3, provided the highest detection efficacy with a mAP@0.5 of 0.96. Recall and precision were 0.93 and 0.88, respectively, which supported its high performance. Considering the findings from different architectures, it was seen that the proposed one-stage detector YOLOv3 had excellent performance for impacted mandibular third molar tooth detection on panoramic radiographs. Promising results showed that diagnostic tools based on state-ofthe-art deep learning models were reliable and robust for clinical decision-making.

Keywords: impacted; tooth; detection; deep learning; panoramic radiograph; machine learning; dentistry

Citation: Celik, M.E. Deep Learning Based Detection Tool for Impacted Mandibular Third Molar Teeth. *Diagnostics* 2022, 12, 942. https://doi.org/10.3390/diagnostics12040942

Academic Editor: Jae-Hong Lee

Received: 13 February 2022
Accepted: 8 April 2022
Published: 9 April 2022

Publisher's Note: MDPI stays neutral with regard to jurisdictional claims in published maps and institutional affiliations.

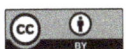

Copyright: © 2022 by the author. Licensee MDPI, Basel, Switzerland. This article is an open access article distributed under the terms and conditions of the Creative Commons Attribution (CC BY) license (https://creativecommons.org/licenses/by/4.0/).

1. Introduction

Dental clinics frequently use different types of radiography with distinct properties. They visualize different regions of interest for diagnosis and further treatment planning [1]. Panoramic radiographs were initially one of the most common visualization techniques in dentistry that scans a wide area with a significantly lower radiation dose [2]. They enable a variety of anomalies, conditions, and lesions to be diagnosed by experts [1–3]. However, complex anatomical structures, pathologies, and imaging distortions can make detecting a case or interpreting a critical condition difficult. Computer-assisted diagnostic systems can help clinicians in decision-making [4]. Recently, the introduction of artificial intelligence-based approaches has efficiently overcome the limitations of traditional methods. Automatically identifying the optimal representations, learning features from raw data are used instead of hand-crafted features [5].

Artificial intelligence (AI) refers to systems and devices designed to address real-life problems as creative as human beings treat them by mimicking natural human intelligence and behavior [6–8]. Machine learning (ML) is a subset of AI and consists of algorithms to learn from a large set of data that enables computers to learn how to solve a problem by performing a specific task [9,10]. They improve as they experience more data at the task [11]. Deep learning (DL) is a subset of ML and consists of algorithms inspired by structural and functional properties of the human brain, called artificial neural networks [12,13]. They train themselves to learn to perform specific tasks. More extensive neural networks and training them with more data scales the performance up for real-life tasks such as classification, object detection, segmentation, and object recognition [14–16]. Convolutional neural networks (CNNs) are a version of the neural networks that include convolution operations in at least one of the layers.

In recent years, DL models have been intensively applied to many fields, including healthcare, which covers a wide range of applications related to medical diagnosis purposes. There has been a growing interest in artificial intelligence-based systems in dentistry. The use of deep learning in dentistry, including orthodontics, periodontology, endodontics, dental radiology, and forensic medicine, has shown promising results in classification, segmentation, and detection tasks [17,18]. Applications are based on teeth, oral structures, pathologies, cephalometric landmarks, bone loss, periodontal inflammation, and root morphology [19–27]. According to the number of published research, a smaller number of several initiatives in dental care develop software and digital dental approaches to diagnostic tools [28]. Some of them are CranioCatch, Digital Smile Design (DSD), 3Shape software (3Shape Design Studio and 3Shape Implant Studio), Exocad, and Bellus 3D.

Object detection task refers to determining the coordinates of a specific object in the input data, while classification refers to automatically assigning the objects into pre-determined categories. When the artificial intelligence-based computer-aided systems are engaged in the field, they can:

support clinicians and physicians who are busy all day to avoid misdiagnosis;
help populations with a shortage of radiologists or screening modalities;
help radiologists manage their workloads in large hospitals;
create reports about pathologic or anatomical conditions in panoramic radiographs, which results in saving time;
provide a focus on the education of observers and new graduates in clinics.

Partially or entirely impacted third molars are the most common developmental conditions affecting humans and require surgical intervention [29–31]. Tooth position, adjacent tooth, alveolar bone, and surrounding mucosal soft tissue usually cause failed eruption [32]. They may cause pain, tooth decay, swelling, and root resorption for various reasons, while they might asymptomatically indicate other pathologies, like caries, periodontal diseases, cysts, or tumors, around the second or third molar [32–34]. Removal of the third molar for severe cases alleviates symptoms and helps the patients' oral health [32,35,36]. It is one of the most common surgical procedures performed in secondary care in the UK [37].

This work aimed to develop a decision support system that will help dentists. It presents a state-of-the-art artificial intelligence-based detection solution, including deep learning algorithms with multiple convolutional neural networks to mandibular third molar impacted teeth problems in panoramic radiographs. Two different detectors were used, namely Faster RCNN and YOLOv3. While the YOLOv3 was a single-step technique, the Faster RCNN was a two-stage method in which different backbones were needed to finalize the detection process. Three different backbones, ResNet50, AlexNet, and VGG16, were combined with Faster RCNN. The detection performance was evaluated by mean average precision (mAP), recall, and precision. Classification accuracy was also calculated for each model.

Related Works

It is intended to explore studies directly related to a detection task for third molars on panoramic radiographs.

Faure et al. (2021) proposed an approach to automatically diagnosing impacted teeth with 530 panoramic radiographs. They implemented only one model using Faster-RCNN with ResNet101, identifying impacted teeth with performances between 51.7% and 88.9% [38]. Kuwada et al. (2020) used deep learning models on panoramic radiographs to detect and classify the presence of impacted supernumerary teeth in the anterior maxillary area [4]. It was reported that DetectNet showed the highest accuracy value of 0.96. Zhang et al. (2018) predicted postoperative facial swelling following impacted mandibular third molars extraction using 15 factors related to patients [39]. Orhan et al. (2021) performed a segmentation task to detect third molar teeth using Cone-Beam Computed Tomography [40]. One hundred twelve teeth are used. A precision value of 0.77 was reported. Basaran et al. (2021) developed a diagnostic charting for ten dental situations, including impacted teeth [41]. Faster R-CNN Inception v2 was implemented using 1084 panoramic radiographs. The precision value for the impacted tooth was 0.779.

Other studies performed detection tasks that aimed to recognize automatically and number teeth [19–21,42]. Panoramic, periapical, and dental bitewing radiographs were used. Their results were presented for all teeth together instead of a separate analysis for impacted third molars. Moreover, previous works did not include categorization for angulation concerning adjacent teeth.

2. Materials and Methods

The Ethical Review Board approved this study at Ankara Yildirim Beyazit University (approval number 2021-69). It was performed following the ethical standards of the Helsinki Declaration.

Panoramic radiographs of 300 patients older than 18 with at least one impacted tooth in the third-molar region were randomly selected from the image database from January 2018 and January 2020. Panoramic radiographs (PRs) with complete or incomplete impacted tooths with complete root formations for patients older than 18 years old were included, while PRs with artifacts, movement, and position-based distortions and incomplete root formations were excluded.

The Winter classification approach was used to categorize mandibular third molar teeth into mesioangular, horizontal positions for both sides [43,44]. The idea was based on the angle between the long axes of the third molar and second molar tooth. While the mesioangular position indicated an angle from 11° to 79°, the horizontal position referred angle from 80° to 100°, as shown schematically in Figure 1.

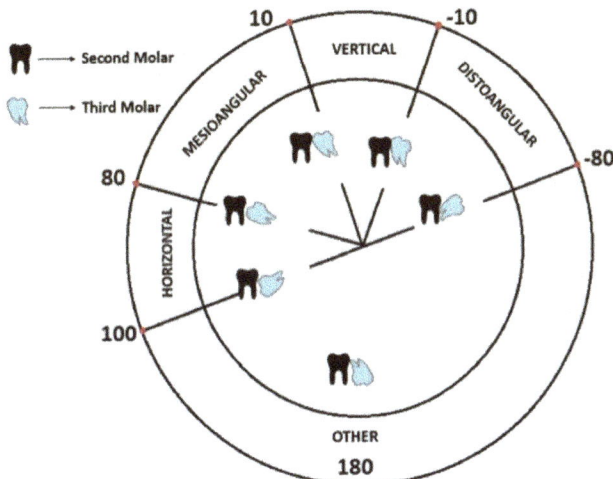

Figure 1. Winter's mandibular third molar teeth classification scheme [34].

The original files had DCM format with a resolution of 2943 × 1435. They first converted to PNG using MATLAB, then resized to 640 × 640 before passing to the models. The PyTorch library was used for developing the models. The dataset was analyzed and labeled by an oral and maxillofacial radiologist with more than five years of experience in the field using labelImg [45]. Rectangular bounding boxes enclosing the crown and root of the interested tooth were used. Experiments were performed using k-fold cross-validation (k = 5) instead of a single standard split. It ensures that models were tested on all kinds of potentially tricky cases. The best performance of each fold is determined.

Previous studies on the prevalence of impacted third molars showed that they were twice more likely to be seen in the mandible than in the maxilla [46–54]. Almost half of the angulation of incidences was mesioangular. There was no statistically significant difference between the right and left sides. In the light of the preceding findings and the available dataset, mandibular third molars with four classes were chosen to be analyzed. Four classes were defining mandibular third molar teeth that t1, t4, t5, and t8 indicated mesioangular left, horizontal left, mesioangular right and horizontal right impacted teeth respectively. Class distributions were balanced. The total number of impacted third molars was 588 from 440 panoramic radiographs. To keep the dataset balanced for experiments, the number of each class for t1, t4, t5, and t8 was determined as 155, 134, 169, and 130 respectively in the design phase of the work. Figure 2 demonstrates four panoramic radiographs with impacted teeth used as inputs for the proposed detection solution. Figure 2a has only a mesioangular tooth on the left, class t1. Figure 2b has two mesioangular teeth on both sides, classes of t1 and t5. Figure 2c,d has two horizontal teeth on both sides, classes t4 and t8.

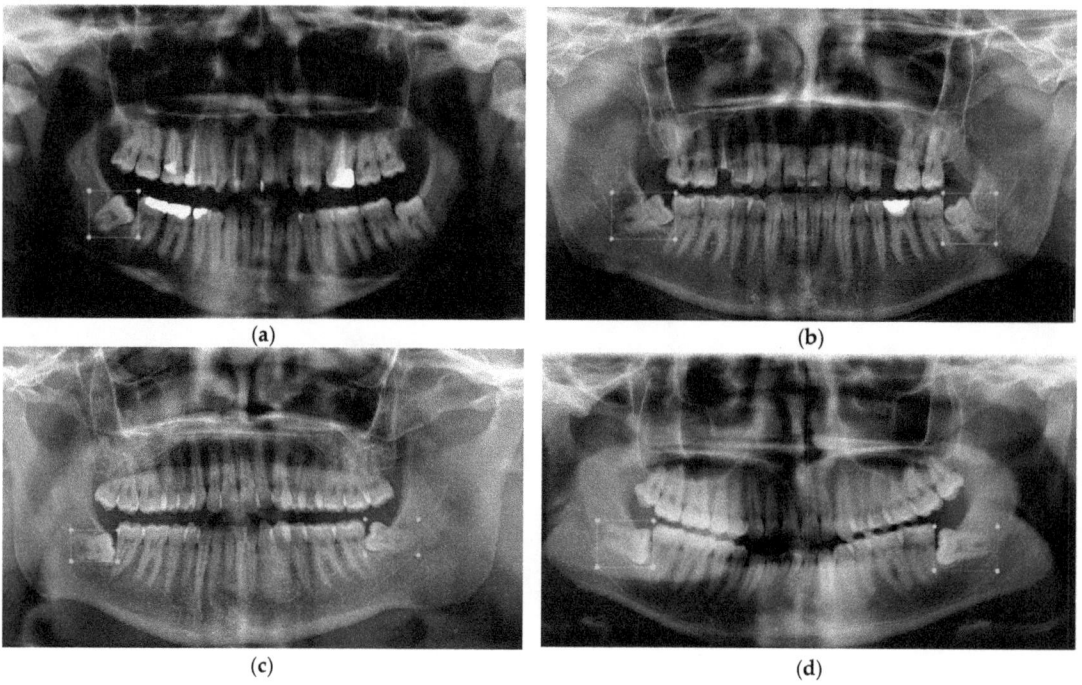

Figure 2. Examples of panoramic radiographs with bounding boxes. (**a**) One impacted tooth—mesioangular left, (**b**) two impacted teeth—mesioangular left and right, (**c**,**d**) horizontal left and right.

To date, the state-of-the-art object detectors are categorized into two classes, namely two-stage methods and one-stage methods [55,56]. Two-stage detectors have proposal-driven mechanisms that first candidate object locations, bounding boxes, are firstly proposed, and then each candidate location is assigned to classes using a convolutional neural network [57]. In contrast, one-stage detectors, with the advantage of being simpler, makes use of anchor boxes to localize and restrict the region and the shape of an object to be detected in the image; in other words, they find bounding boxes in a single step without using region proposals [58–60].

The AI-based model development phase includes two detectors, namely Faster RCNN and YOLOv3 [57,58]. YOLOv3 performs the detection in a single-phase, although Faster RCNN is a two-stage technique that needs a backbone as a feature extractor. So, ResNet50, AlexNet, and VGG16 are also used as a backbone and Faster RCNN one at a time.

AlexNet consists of 5 convolutional and three fully connected layers. It features Rectified Linear Units to model a neuron's output, and provides training on multiple GPUs and overlapping pooling, making the process faster [61]. VGG16 is a convolutional neural network model with 13 convolutional and five pooling layers. Large kernel filters used in AlexNet are replaced with 3 × 3 kernel-sized filters in VGG16 architecture for better performance with ease of implementation [62]. After AlexNet and VGG16, architectures begin to become deeper; however, it makes the back-propagated gradient extremely small sometimes, resulting in saturated or decreased performance. Residual Networks, ResNet50, solves this issue by suggesting identity shortcut connections that skip one or more layers and perform identity mappings [63]. It has a depth of up to 152 layers and reduces the number of parameters needed for a deep network.

YOLO, You Only Look Once, is an object detector that uses features learned by a deep convolutional neural network to detect objects [58]. The architecture of YOLO v3 includes 106 layer fully convolutional layers. It makes predictions of bounding boxes at three scales by downsampling the dimensions of the input image at different layers and extracting features from them. Darknet-53 performs feature extraction that is more powerful and efficient. Up-sampled layers help hold fine features, making it better at detecting small objects. Class predictions for each bounding box are made using cross-entropy loss and logistic regression instead of softmax. The network architecture of the model is shown in Figure 3.

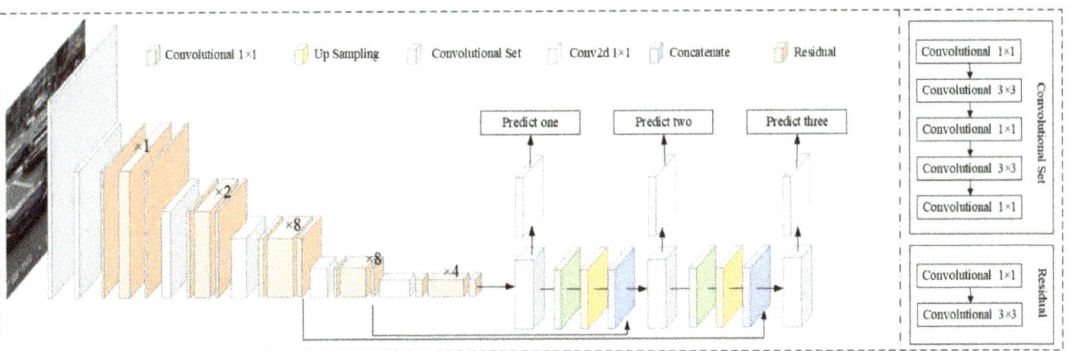

Figure 3. YOLOv3 network architecture that predicts at three scales [64].

Faster R-CNN uses Region Proposal Networks, a fully convolutional network that simultaneously predicts object bounds and objectness scores, to create potential bounding boxes and afterward runs a classifier on these proposed boxes instead of using Selective Search as a region proposal technique. Classification is followed by a post-processing phase that refines bounding boxes, excluding duplications and score bounding boxes again [65]. Figure 4 summarizes how it proceeds from beginning to end.

Adam optimizer was used with a learning rate of 0.0001. The model was run on Windows OS with NVIDIA GeForce RTX 3080 graphics processor unit. Object detection models give outputs bounding box and class of the objects in input images. The detection performance is evaluated by mean average precision (mAP), recall, and precision metrics. The mAP is also used for Pattern Analysis, Statistical modeling and Computational Learning (PASCAL) Visual Object Classes (VOC) Challenge [66]. It can briefly be described step by step as follows.

Intersection Over Union (IOU) defines how the bounding box is predicted correctly. It is calculated as a ratio of overlap between the predicted bounding box area and the ground truth area. It takes values between 0 and 1, indicating no overlap and exact overlap, respectively, as shown in Equation (1) [6,9,13].

$$IoU = \frac{area(ground\ truth\ \cap\ predicted)}{area(ground\ truth\ \cup\ predicted)} \quad (1)$$

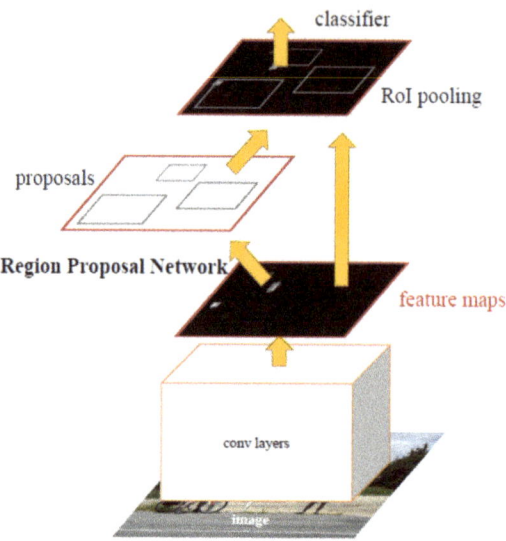

Figure 4. Faster R-CNN system for object detection with RPN [57].

Precision refers to how exactly the model identifies relevant objects, while recall measures the model's ability to propose correct detections among all ground truths, which are given in Equations (2) and (3) [6,9,13]. While comparing two models, a model with high precision and recall value are considered better performance.

$$\text{precision} = \frac{\text{number of correct regions detected}}{\text{number of correct regions detected} + \text{number of false regions detected}} \quad (2)$$

$$\text{recall} = \frac{\text{number of correct regions detected}}{\text{number of all regions}} \quad (3)$$

Average Precision represents the area under the precision-recall curve that is evaluated at an IoU threshold. It is defined in Equation (4) [6,9,13].

$$\text{AP@threshold} = \int_0^1 p(r)dr \quad (4)$$

The notation of AP@threshold indicates that AP is calculated at a given IoU threshold. For most models, it is considered 0.5 and shown by AP@0.5. AP is calculated for each class in the data, resulting in n-different AP values for n-classes. When these values are averaged, mean Average Precision (mAP) is obtained for n classes with Equation (5) [6,9,13].

$$\text{mAP@threshold} = \frac{1}{n}\sum_{i=1}^{n} AP_i \quad (5)$$

Accuracy is a metric used to evaluate classification performance. It refers to the percentage of the correct predictions for the test dataset, as shown in Equation (6). It describes how the model performs for all classes [6,9,13].

$$\text{accuracy} = \frac{\text{number of correct predictions}}{\text{number of all predictions}} \quad (6)$$

Object detection algorithms make predictions with a bounding box and a class label. For each object, the predicted bounding box and ground truth are measured by intersection over union (IoU) [67]. If the IoU value of the prediction is bigger than the IoU threshold, the object is classified as true positive (TP). Precision and Recall are calculated based on the measured IoU and IoU threshold. Average precision (AP) is the area under the Precision-Recall curve. The mean average precision (mAP) is calculated by considering the mean AP over all classes [68].

While mAP@0.5 refers to the mAP when the IoU threshold is 0.5, mAP@0.5–0.95 means the average mAP over different IoU thresholds from 0.5 to 0.95 [69]. Many algorithms, including Faster RCNN, YOLO, use mAP to evaluate the model performance [57,58].

3. Results

Findings were categorized into two groups of one-stage and two-stage detectors in structural design. Detection performances of four different architectures were presented based on mAP with thresholds values of 0.5 and 0.5–0.95, which are given in Table 1.

Table 1. Detection performances of two detectors, one with three different backbones.

	Fold	mAP@0.5	mAP@0.5:0.95
One-stage technique			
YOLOv3	1	0.941	0.751
	2	0.979	0.783
	3	0.936	0.746
	4	0.981	0.761
	5	0.98	0.771
	Avg	0.96	0.76
Two-stage technique			
Faster RCNN–ResNet50	1	0.912	0.628
	2	0.904	0.673
	3	0.86	0.646
	4	0.944	0.71
	5	0.953	0.713
	Avg	0.91	0.71
Faster RCNN–AlexNet	1	0.814	0.433
	2	0.878	0.518
	3	0.773	0.47
	4	0.916	0.52
	5	0.923	0.513
	Avg	0.86	0.49
Faster RCNN–VGG16	1	0.838	0.464
	2	0.89	0.486
	3	0.802	0.423
	4	0.898	0.484
	5	0.937	0.583
	Avg	0.87	0.49

As a two-stage technique, Faster RCNN was used as a detector together with three different backbones, ResNet50, AlexNet, and VGG16. They produced mAP@0.5 value of 0.91, 0.86 and 0.87 while mAP@0.5:0.95 value of 0.71, 0.49 and 0.49 respectively. ResNet50 produced the highest mAP performance, while the other two gave a slightly lower rate. On the other hand, YOLOv3 provided the highest rate among all, with a mAP@0.5 value of 0.96 and mAP@0.5:0.95 value of 0.76. The precision and recall were 0.88 and 0.93. Train and validation loss for YOLOv3 were given in Figure 5. Training and validation losses were from a single fold with the best performance.

YOLOv3 outperforms ResNet ($p = 0.042$), AlexNet ($p = 0.011$) and VGG16 ($p = 0.015$). It was not seen that there was a significant difference between ResNet and AlexNet ($p = 0.158$)–VGG16 ($p = 0.193$). Accuracy is calculated for each model and used for statistical analysis. It was presented in Table 2.

Table 2. Classification accuracies.

Fold	YOLOv3	Faster RCNN–ResNet50	Faster RCNN–AlexNet	Faster RCNN–VGG16
1	0.824	0.814	0.636	0.674
2	0.86	0.727	0.68	0.693
3	0.834	0.713	0.529	0.653
4	0.897	0.856	0.76	0.736
5	0.891	0.854	0.81	0.792
Avg	0.86	0.79	0.68	0.7

YOLOv3 performed better than AlexNet ($p = 0.016$) and VGG16 ($p = 0.001$) in classification accuracy, but there was not a statistically significant difference between the classification accuracies of YOLOv3 and ResNet ($p = 0.079$). Among backbones used in Faster RCNN, a statistically significant difference was not seen between ResNet and AlexNet ($p = 0.085$)–VGG16 ($p = 0.068$).

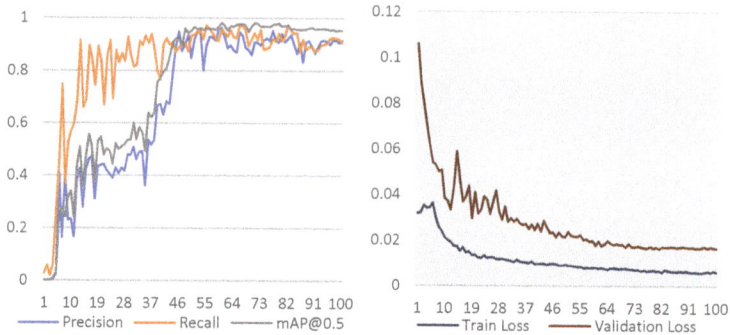

Figure 5. Change of performance metrics and losses for YOLOv3.

Findings were also shown on panoramic radiographs with annotations and predictions together. Figure 6 demonstrates how accurately they were detected. Figure 6a–c showed ground truth annotations for the impacted teeth, b-d showed corresponding predictions from the proposed solution using YOLOv3. They were detected and assigned to the proper classes. Figure 6e–g demonstrates random detection result samples from ResNet, AlexNet, and VGG16.

The detection performance for each class was also investigated. It was seen that t1, t4, t5 and t8 showed the mAP@0.5 rate of 0.96, 0.98, 0.984, 0.995 and AP@0.5:0.95 rate of 0.774, 0.775, 0.793, 0.791 respectively. Table 3 shows the performance metrics of each class for the solution with YOLOv3.

Table 3. Inter-class detection performances for the solution with YOLOv3.

Class	AP@0.5	AP@0.5:0.95	Precision	Recall
t1—mesioangular left	0.96	0.774	0.849	0.95
t4—horizontal left	0.98	0.775	0.96	0.833
t5—mesioangular right	0.984	0.793	0.908	0.987
t8—horizontal right	0.995	0.791	0.88	1

mAP at IOU equals to 0.5 are widely accepted detection metric for many real-life detection applications [13,57,58,66]. YOLOv3 presented promising performance with the highest accuracy, indicating that YOLOv3 was a successful detector at detecting third-molar impacted teeth. It was superior to the Faster-RCNN and its use with ResNet50, AlexNet, and VGG16 in terms of mAP and classification accuracy.

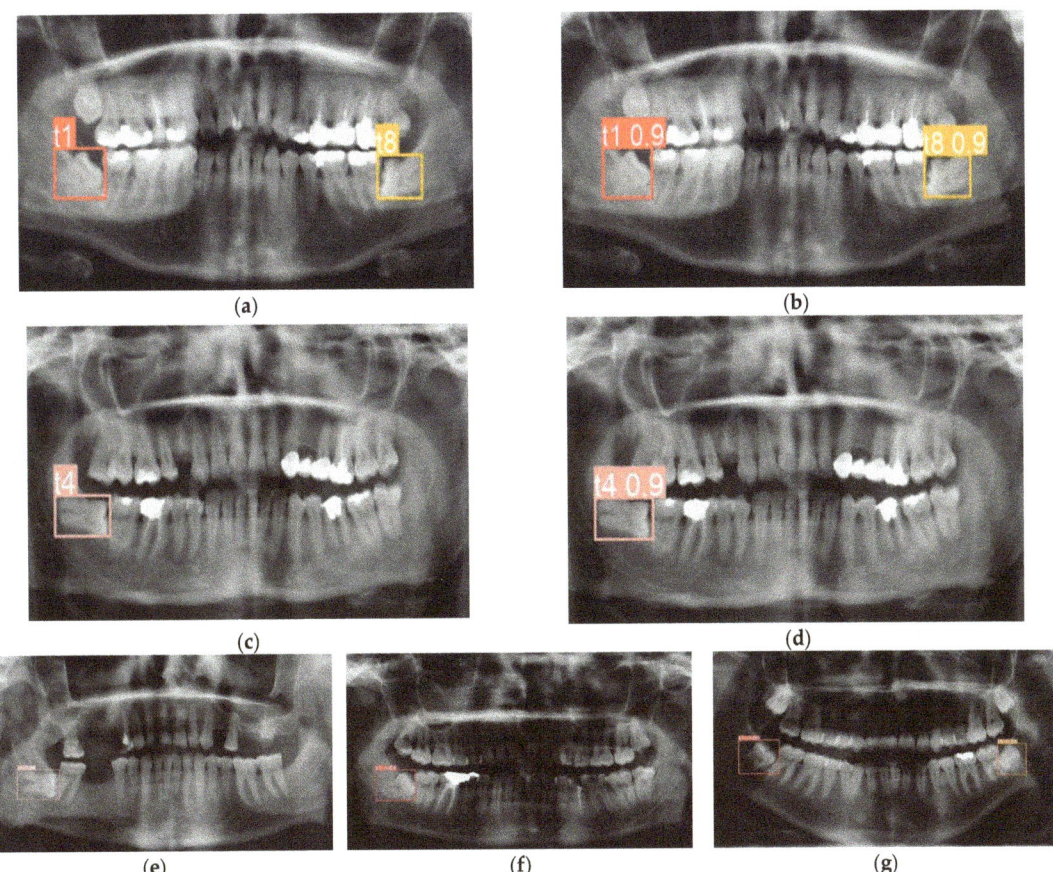

Figure 6. Detection result samples from YOLOv3 (**a**–**d**), ground truths (**a**–**c**), predictions (**b**–**d**) and Faster RCNN with ResNet (**e**), AlexNet (**f**) and VGG16 (**g**).

4. Discussion

A significant increase in the number of studies on artificial intelligence-based decision support systems has been seen in the field of dentistry as well as other fields of healthcare. In dentistry, an automated analysis and interpretation system in which radiographs are automatically analyzed to find defects is a fundamental goal. Previous studies used images from different imaging modalities like panoramic, periapical, and bitewing radiographs for detection, segmentation, and classification purposes. Common topics included studies on tooth detection, tooth numbering, and many other conditions like carries, lesions, anatomical structures, cysts, etc. [17–27,46–54,70]. Contrarily, it was observed that previous studies on mandibular third molar detection alone were rare and explored only one model architecture performance.

Lee et al. (2018) suggested a deep learning model to diagnose and predict periodontally compromised teeth. It consisted of 1740 periapical radiographic images, resulting in diagnostic accuracy of 76.7% for molar teeth. It was concluded that the CNN algorithm was helpful for diagnosing periodontally compromised teeth with different expectations of improved systems for better performance in time [71]. They compared the agreement between the expert observer and AI application. The proposed work presented a higher performance in accuracy for YOLOv3 and Faster RCNN ResNet50. Other metrics were not reported.

Faure et al. (2021) proposed a method to automatically diagnose impacted teeth using Faster-RCNN with ResNet101, identifying impacted teeth with performances between 51.7% and 88.9% [38]. Angulation was not investigated; only one class for impacted third molars was used. The proposed work provided a more elaborative analysis by using two detectors with three backbones and a higher number of classes.

Basaran et al. (2021) suggested a model for the diagnostic charting of ten dental conditions, including impacted teeth, in panoramic radiography. Their model was based on Faster R-CNN Inception v2, including 1084 graphs with 796 impacted teeth. It was reported that sensitivity and precision for impacted teeth were 0.96 and 0.77 [41]. When it was compared, this work presented higher precision, but mAP was not reported.

Tobel et al. (2017) used CNNs to develop an automated technique to monitor the development stages of the lower third molar on panoramic radiographs. They classified their growth into ten classes. They concluded that the performance was similar to staging by human observers but needed to be optimized for age estimation [72].

Vinayahalingam et al. (2019) implemented CNNs to detect and segment inferior alveolar nerve and lower third molars on panoramic radiographs. The mean dice-coefficient for the third molar was 0.947 ± 0.033 [26]. Contrary to traditional simple architectures, deep CNNs succeed in edge detection thanks to multiple convolutional and hidden layers featuring hierarchical feature presentation [73].

Kuwada et al. (2020) performed detection and classification for impacted supernumerary teeth in the anterior maxillary area [4]. This region was completely different from the region of third molars. Zhang et al. (2018) used 15 patient-related factors to predict postoperative facial swelling following impacted mandibular third molars extraction [39]. They used angulation of the third molar with respect to the second molar as a parameter but did not perform detection. Orhan et al. (2021) performed segmentation to detect third molar teeth with a precision value of 0.77 [40]. They used Cone-Beam Computed Tomography images and compared agreement between the human observer and AI application. The proposed work used panoramic images with higher precision in addition to evaluation metrics for detection.

Considering previous works, this work demonstrated an immediate and comprehensive solution for automated detection of mandibular third molar teeth using two types of detection techniques for the first time. This work also included two different third molar impaction classes. Previous works had only one class for all third molars, which limited the corresponding comparison. Moreover, many previous works performed classification and segmentation tasks for different purposes. This work focused only mandibular third molar detection problem. Although mAP was a standard evaluation metric for detection tasks in the computer vision field, it was not reported in previous works. Briefly, it was not always possible to directly compare each work because of incompatibilities between (i) type of radiography used, (ii) evaluation metrics used, and (iii) purposes.

Multi-label classification used in YOLOv3 performed better for datasets with overlapping labels than using softmax, which assumed each bounding box had only one class, which was not the case in real-life applications. Additional techniques such as advanced image pre-processing, data augmentation, and more data can improve the proposed solution's results and make it more robust.

This work has two limitations. First, the amount of data is limited. More panoramic radiographs will be collected and annotated to perform deep learning for more robust, reliable results. Second, mandibular third molars were used in this work due to their wider prevalence. Later, maxillary third molars will be analyzed as more data are collected.

5. Conclusions

The proposed solution aims to help dentists in their decision-making process. It is shown that four different models are successful in detecting third molars. The use of machine learning in dentistry has significant potential in diagnosis with high accuracy and precision. Diagnostic tools based on state-of-the-art deep learning models are reliable and robust auxiliary techniques for clinical decision-making, resulting in more efficient treatment planning for patients and clinician health management. In time, AI-based devices can be used as a standard tool in clinical practice and play a crucial role in providing diagnostic recommendations.

Funding: This research received no external funding.

Institutional Review Board Statement: The study was conducted in accordance with the Declaration of Helsinki and approved by the Institutional Review Board (or Ethics Committee) of Ankara Yildirim Beyazit University (protocol code 2021-69 and date of approval 16 February 2021).

Informed Consent Statement: Not applicable.

Data Availability Statement: The data supporting this study's findings are not available and accessible due to ethical issues, patients' and institutions' data protection policies.

Conflicts of Interest: The author declares no conflict of interest.

References

1. Zadrożny, Ł.; Regulski, P.; Brus-Sawczuk, K.; Czajkowska, M.; Parkanyi, L.; Ganz, S.; Mijiritsky, E. Artificial Intelligence Application in Assessment of Panoramic Radiographs. *Diagnostics* **2020**, *12*, 224. [CrossRef] [PubMed]
2. Prados-Privado, M.; Villalón, J.G.; Martínez-Martínez, C.H.; Ivorra, C. Dental Images Recognition Technology and Applications: A Literature Review. *Appl. Sci.* **2020**, *10*, 2856. [CrossRef]
3. Perschbacher, S. Interpretation of panoramic radiographs. *Aust. Dent. J.* **2012**, *57*, 40–45. [CrossRef] [PubMed]
4. Kuwada, C.; Ariji, Y.; Fukuda, M.; Kise, Y.; Fujita, H.; Katsumata, A.; Ariji, E. Deep learning systems for detecting and classifying the presence of impacted supernumerary teeth in the maxillary incisor region on panoramic radiographs. *Oral Surg. Oral Med. Oral Pathol. Oral Radiol.* **2020**, *130*, 464–469. [CrossRef]
5. Panetta, K.; Rajendran, R.; Ramesh, A.; Rao, S.P.; Agaian, S. Tufts Dental Database: A Multimodal Panoramic X-ray Dataset for Benchmarking Diagnostic Systems. *IEEE J. Biomed. Health Inform.* **2021**. [CrossRef]
6. Hassoun, M.H. *Fundamentals of Artificial Neural Networks*; MIT Press: London, UK, 1995.
7. Yegnanarayana, B. *Artificial Neural Networks*; PHI Learning Pvt. Ltd.: Delhi, India, 2009.
8. Krogh, A. What are artificial neural networks? *Nat. Biotechnol.* **2008**, *26*, 195–197. [CrossRef]
9. Bishop, C.M.; Nasrabadi, N.M. *Pattern Recognition and Machine Learning*; Springer: New York, NY, USA, 2006; Volume 4, p. 768.
10. Jordan, M.I.; Mitchell, T.M. Machine learning: Trends, perspectives, and prospects. *Science* **2015**, *349*, 255–260. [CrossRef]
11. Wang, S.; Summers, R.M. Machine learning and radiology. *Med. Image Anal.* **2012**, *16*, 933–951. [CrossRef]
12. Skansi, S. *Introduction to Deep Learning: From Logical Calculus to Artificial Intelligence*; Springer: Berlin/Heidelberg, Germany, 2018.
13. Goodfellow, I.; Bengio, Y.; Courville, A. *Deep Learning*; MIT Press: London, UK, 2016.
14. Shin, H.C.; Roth, H.R.; Gao, M.; Lu, L.; Xu, Z.; Nogues, I.; Summers, R.M. Deep convolutional neural networks for computer-aided detection: CNN architectures, dataset characteristics and transfer learning. *IEEE Trans. Med. Imag.* **2016**, *35*, 1285–1298. [CrossRef]
15. Liu, L.; Ouyang, W.; Wang, X.; Fieguth, P.; Chen, J.; Liu, X.; Pietikäinen, M. Deep learning for generic object detection: A survey. *Int. J. Computerv.* **2020**, *128*, 261–318. [CrossRef]
16. Khan, A.; Sohail, A.; Zahoora, U.; Qureshi, A.S. A survey of the recent architectures of deep convolutional neural networks. *Artif. Intell. Rev.* **2020**, *53*, 5455–5516. [CrossRef]
17. Schwendicke, F.; Golla, T.; Dreher, M.; Krois, J. Convolutional neural networks for dental image diagnostics: A scoping review. *J. Dent.* **2019**, *91*, 103226. [CrossRef] [PubMed]
18. Leite, A.F.; Gerven, A.V.; Willems, H.; Beznik, T.; Lahoud, P.; Gaêta-Araujo, H.; Vranckx, M.; Jacobs, R. Artificial intelligence driven novel tool for tooth detection and segmentation on panoramic radiographs. *Clin. Oral Investig.* **2021**, *25*, 2257–2267. [CrossRef] [PubMed]
19. Parvez, M.F.; Kota, M.; Syoji, K. Optimization technique combined with deep learning method for teeth recognition in dental panoramic radiographs. *Sci. Rep.* **2020**, *10*, 19261.
20. Tuzoff, D.V.; Tuzova, L.N.; Bornstein, M.M.; Krasnov, A.S.; Kharchenko, M.A.; Nikolenko, S.I.; Sveshnikov, M.M.; Bednenko, G.B. Tooth detection and numbering in panoramic radiographs using convolutional neural networks. *Dentomaxillofac. Radiol.* **2019**, *48*, 20180051. [CrossRef]
21. Chen, H.; Zhang, K.; Lyu, P.; Li, H.; Zhang, L.; Wu, J.; Lee, C.H. A deep learning approach to automatic teeth detection and numbering based on object detection in dental periapical films. *Sci. Rep.* **2019**, *9*, 1–11. [CrossRef]
22. Kim, C.; Kim, D.; Jeong, H.; Yoon, S.J.; Youm, S. Automatic tooth detection and numbering using a combination of a CNN and heuristic algorithm. *Appl. Sci.* **2020**, *10*, 5624. [CrossRef]
23. Kuwana, R.; Ariji, Y.; Fukuda, M.; Kise, Y.; Nozawa, M.; Kuwada, C.; Muramatsu, C.; Katsumata, A.; Fujita, H.; Ariji, E. Performance of deep learning object detection technology in the detection and diagnosis of maxillary sinus lesions on panoramic radiographs. *Dentomaxillofac. Radiol.* **2021**, *50*, 20200171. [CrossRef]

24. Chang, H.J.; Lee, S.J.; Yong, T.H.; Shin, N.Y.; Jang, B.G.; Kim, J.E.; Huh, K.H.; Lee, S.S.; Heo, M.S.; Choi, S.C.; et al. Deep learning hybrid method to automatically diagnose periodontal bone loss and stage periodontitis. *Sci. Rep.* **2020**, *10*, 7531. [CrossRef]
25. Zheng, Z.; Yan, H.; Setzer, F.C.; Shi, K.J.; Mupparapu, M.; Li, J. Anatomically constrained deep learning for automating dental CBCT segmentation and lesion detection. *IEEE Trans. Autom. Sci. Eng.* **2020**, *18*, 603–614. [CrossRef]
26. Vinayahalingam, S.; Xi, T.; Bergé, S.; Maal, T.; de Jong, G. Automated detection of third molars and mandibular nerve by deep learning. *Sci. Rep.* **2019**, *9*, 9007. [CrossRef] [PubMed]
27. Hiraiwa, T.; Ariji, Y.; Fukuda, M.; Kise, Y.; Nakata, K.; Katsumata, A.; Fujita, H.; Ariji, E. A deep-learning artificial intelligence system for assessment of root morphology of the mandibular first molar on panoramic radiography. *Dentomaxillofac. Radiol.* **2019**, *48*, 20180218. [CrossRef] [PubMed]
28. Carrillo-Perez, F.; Pecho, O.E.; Morales, J.C.; Paravina, R.D.; Della Bona, A.; Ghinea, R.; Herrera, L.J. Applications of artificial intelligence in dentistry: A comprehensive review. *J. Esthet. Restor. Dent.* **2022**, *34*, 259–280. [CrossRef] [PubMed]
29. World Health Organization. *International Statistical Classification of Diseases and Related Health Problems*; 10th Revision; WHO: Geneva, Italy, 2011; Volume 2.
30. Rantanen, A. The age of eruption of the third molar teeth. A clinical study based on Finnish university students. *Acta Odontol. Scand.* **1967**, *25*, 1–86.
31. Hugoson, A.; Kugelberg, C. The prevalence of third molars in a Swedish population. An epidemiological study. *Commun. Dent. Health* **1988**, *5*, 121–138.
32. Royal College of Surgeons Faculty of Dental Surgery. Parameters of Care for Patients Undergoing Mandibular Third Molar Surgery. 2020. Available online: https://www.rcseng.ac.uk/-/media/files/rcs/fds/guidelines/3rd-molar-guidelines--april-2021.pdf (accessed on 23 April 2021).
33. Doğan, N.; Orhan, K.; Günaydin, Y.; Köymen, R.; Ökçu, K.; Üçok, Ö. Unerupted mandibular third molars: Symptoms, associated pathologies, and indications for removal in a Turkish population. *Quintessence Int.* **2007**, *38*, e497–e505.
34. Gümrükçü, Z.; Balaban, E.; Karabağ, M. Is there a relationship between third-molar impaction types and the dimen-sional/angular measurement values of posterior mandible according to Pell and Gregory/Winter Classification? *Oral Radiol.* **2021**, *37*, 29–35. [CrossRef]
35. McGrath, C.; Comfort, M.B.; Lo, E.C.; Luo, Y. Can third molar surgery improve quality of life? A 6-month cohort study. *J. Oral. Maxillofac. Surg.* **2003**, *61*, 759–763. [CrossRef]
36. Savin, J.; Ogden, G. Third molar surgery—A preliminary report on aspects affecting quality of life in the early postoperative period. *Br. J. Oral Maxillofac. Surg.* **1997**, *35*, 246–253. [CrossRef]
37. McArdle, L.; Renton, T. The effects of NICE guidelines on the management of third molar teeth. *Br. Dent. J.* **2012**, *213*, E8. [CrossRef]
38. Faure, J.; Engelbrecht, A. Impacted Tooth Detection in Panoramic Radiographs. In *International Work-Conference on Artificial Neural Networks*; Springer: Cham, Switzerland, 2021; pp. 525–536.
39. Zhang, W.; Li, J.; Li, Z.B.; Li, Z. Predicting postoperative facial swelling following impacted mandibular third molars extraction by using artificial neural networks evaluation. *Sci. Rep.* **2018**, *8*, 12281. [CrossRef]
40. Orhan, K.; Bilgir, E.; Bayrakdar, I.S.; Ezhov, M.; Gusarev, M.; Shumilov, E. Evaluation of artificial intelligence for detecting impacted third molars on cone-beam computed tomography scans. *J. Stomatol. Oral Maxillofac. Surg.* **2021**, *122*, 333–337. [CrossRef]
41. Başaran, M.; Çelik, Ö.; Bayrakdar, I.S.; Bilgir, E.; Orhan, K.; Odabaş, A.; Jagtap, R. Diagnostic charting of panoramic radiography using deep-learning artificial intelligence system. *Oral Radiol.* **2021**, 1–7. [CrossRef] [PubMed]
42. Yasa, Y.; Çelik, Ö.; Bayrakdar, I.S.; Pekince, A.; Orhan, K.; Akarsu, S.; Atasoy, S.; Bilgir, E.; Odabaş, A.; Aslan, A.F. An artificial intelligence proposal to automatic teeth detection and numbering in dental bite-wing radiographs. *Acta Odontol. Scand.* **2020**, *11*, 275–281. [CrossRef] [PubMed]
43. Winter, G. *Impacted Mandibular Third Molars*; American Medical Book, Co.: St Louis, MO, USA, 1926.
44. Pell, G.J. Impacted mandibular third molars: Classification and modified techniques for removal. *Dent Digest.* **1933**, *39*, 330–338.
45. Tzutalin. LabelImg. Git Code. 2015. Available online: https://github.com/tzutalin/labelImg (accessed on 5 October 2015).
46. Carter, K.; Worthington, S. Predictors of third molar impaction: A systematic review and meta-analysis. *J. Dent. Res.* **2016**, *95*, 267–276. [CrossRef]
47. Jaroń, A.; Trybek, G. The pattern of mandibular third molar impaction and assessment of surgery difficulty: A Retrospective study of radiographs in east Baltic population. *Int. J. Environ. Res. Public Health* **2021**, *18*, 6016. [CrossRef]
48. Zaman, M.U.; Almutairi, N.S.; Abdulrahman Alnashwan, M.; Albogami, S.M.; Alkhammash, N.M.; Alam, M.K. Pattern of Mandibular Third Molar Impaction in Nonsyndromic 17760 Patients: A Retrospective Study among Saudi Population in Central Region, Saudi Arabia. *BioMed Res. Int.* **2021**, *2021*, 1880750. [CrossRef]
49. Demirel, O.; Akbulut, A. Evaluation of the relationship between gonial angle and impacted mandibular third molar teeth. *Anat. Sci. Int.* **2020**, *95*, 134–142. [CrossRef]
50. Hashemipour, M.A.; Tahmasbi-Arashlow, M.; Fahimi-Hanzaei, F. Incidence of impacted mandibular and maxillary third molars: A radiographic study in a Southeast Iran population. *Med. Oral Patol. Oral Cir. Bucal.* **2013**, *18*, e140. [CrossRef]
51. Eshghpour, M.; Nezadi, A.; Moradi, A.; Shamsabadi, R.M.; Rezaer, N.M.; Nejat, A. Pattern of mandibular third molar impaction: A cross-sectional study in northeast of Iran. *Niger. J. Clin. Pract.* **2014**, *17*, 673–677. [PubMed]

52. Goyal, S.; Verma, P.; Raj, S.S. Radiographic evaluation of the status of third molars in Sriganganagar population—A digital panoramic study. *Malays. J. Med. Sci.* **2016**, *23*, 103. [CrossRef] [PubMed]
53. Enabulele, J.E.; Obuekwe, O.N. Prevalence of caries and cervical resorption on adjacent second molar associated with impacted third molar. *J. Oral Maxillofac. Surg. Med. Pathol.* **2017**, *29*, 301–305. [CrossRef]
54. Passi, D.; Singh, G.; Dutta, S.; Srivastava, D.; Chandra, L.; Mishra, S.; Dubey, M. Study of pattern and prevalence of mandibular impacted third molar among Delhi-National Capital Region population with newer proposed classification of mandibular impacted third molar: A retrospective study. *Nat. J. Maxillofac. Surg.* **2019**, *10*, 59.
55. Jiao, L.; Zhang, F.; Liu, F.; Yang, S.; Li, L.; Feng, Z.; Qu, R. A survey of deep learning-based object detection. *IEEE Access* **2019**, *7*, 128837–128868. [CrossRef]
56. He, X.; Zhao, K.; Chu, X. AutoML: A survey of the state-of-the-art. *Knowl. Based Syst.* **2021**, *212*, 106622. [CrossRef]
57. Ren, S.; He, K.; Girshick, R.; Sun, J. Faster r-cnn: Towards real-time object detection with region proposal networks. *Adv. Neural Inf. Process. Syst.* **2015**, *28*, 91–99. [CrossRef]
58. Redmon, J.; Farhadi, A. YOLOv3: An incremental improvement. *arXiv* **2018**, arXiv:1804.02767.
59. Liu, W.; Anguelov, D.; Erhan, D.; Szegedy, C.; Reed, S.; Fu, C.Y.; Berg, A.C. SSD: Single Shot MultiBox Detector. In *Computer Vision–ECCV 2016, ECCV 2016 Lecture Notes in Computer Science*; Leibe, B., Matas, J., Sebe, N., Welling, M., Eds.; Springer: Cham, Switzerland, 2016; Volume 9905. [CrossRef]
60. Lin, T.Y.; Goyal, P.; Girshick, R.; He, K.; Dollár, P. Focal loss for dense object detection. In Proceedings of the IEEE International Conference on Computer Vision, Venice, Italy, 22–29 October 2017; pp. 2980–2988.
61. Krizhevsky, A.; Sutskever, I.; Hinton, G.E. Imagenet classification with deep convolutional neural networks. In Proceedings of the 25th International Conference on Neural Information Processing Systems-Volume 1 (NIPS'12), Red Hook, NY, USA, 3–6 December 2012; p. 25.
62. Simonyan, K.; Zisserman, A. Very deep convolutional networks for large-scale image recognition. *arXiv* **2014**, arXiv:1409.1556.
63. He, K.; Zhang, X.; Ren, S.; Sun, J. Deep residual learning for image recognition. In Proceedings of the IEEE Conference on Computer Vision and Pattern Recognition, Las Vegas, NV, USA, 27–30 June 2016; pp. 770–778.
64. Mao, Q.C.; Sun, H.M.; Liu, Y.B.; Jia, R.S. Mini-YOLOv3: Real-time object detector for embedded applications. *IEEE Access* **2019**, *7*, 133529–133538. [CrossRef]
65. Girshick, R.; Donahue, J.; Darrell, T.; Malik, J. Rich feature hierarchies for accurate object detection and semantic segmentation. In Proceedings of the IEEE Conference on Computer Vision and Pattern Recognition (CVPR), Columbus, OH, USA, 24–27 June 2014; pp. 580–587.
66. Everingham, M.; Van Gool, L.; Williams, C.K.I.; Winn, J.; Zisserman, A. The Pascal visual object classes (VOC) challenge. *Int. J. Comput. Vis.* **2009**, *88*, 303–338. [CrossRef]
67. Bell, S.; Zitnick, C.L.; Bala, K.; Girshick, R. Inside-outside net: Detecting objects in context with skip pooling and recurrent neural networks. In Proceedings of the IEEE Conference on Computer Vision and Pattern Recognition, Las Vegas, NV, USA, 27–30 June 2016; pp. 2874–2883.
68. Huang, J.; Rathod, V.; Sun, C.; Zhu, M.; Korattikara, A.; Fathi, A.; Murphy, K. Speed/accuracy trade-offs for modern convolutional object detectors. In Proceedings of the IEEE Conference on Computer Vision and Pattern Recognition, Honolulu, HI, USA, 21–26 July 2017; pp. 7310–7311.
69. Van Etten, A. Satellite imagery multiscale rapid detection with windowed networks. In Proceedings of the IEEE Winter Conference on Applications of Computer Vision (WACV), Waikoloa Village, HI, USA, 7–11 January 2019; pp. 735–743.
70. Ekert, T.; Krois, J.; Meinhold, L.; Elhennawy, K.; Emara, R.; Golla, T.; Schwendicke, F. Deep learning for the radiographic detection of apical lesions. *J. Endod.* **2019**, *45*, 917–922. [CrossRef] [PubMed]
71. Lee, J.H.; Kim, D.H.; Jeong, S.N.; Choi, S.H. Diagnosis and prediction of periodontally compromised teeth using a deep learning-based convolutional neural network algorithm. *J. Periodontal Implant. Sci.* **2018**, *48*, 114–123. [CrossRef] [PubMed]
72. De Tobel, J.; Radesh, P.; Vandermeulen, D.; Thevissen, P.W. An automated technique to stage lower third molar development on panoramic radiographs for age estimation: A pilot study. *J. Forensic Odontol. Stomatol.* **2017**, *35*, 42.
73. Wang, R. Edge detection using convolutional neural network. In *Advances in Neural Networks–ISNN 2016, Proceedings of the 13th International Symposium on Neural Networks, ISNN 2016, St. Petersburg, Russia, 6–8 July 2016*; Springer International Publishing: Cham, Switzerland, 2016; pp. 12–20.

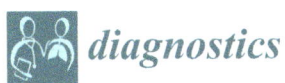

Article

Comparison of Tongue Characteristics Classified According to Ultrasonographic Features Using a K-Means Clustering Algorithm

Ariya Chantaramanee [1], Kazuharu Nakagawa [2,*], Kanako Yoshimi [2], Ayako Nakane [2], Kohei Yamaguchi [2] and Haruka Tohara [2]

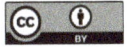

Citation: Chantaramanee, A.; Nakagawa, K.; Yoshimi, K.; Nakane, A.; Yamaguchi, K.; Tohara, H. Comparison of Tongue Characteristics Classified According to Ultrasonographic Features Using a K-Means Clustering Algorithm. *Diagnostics* 2022, 12, 264. https://doi.org/10.3390/diagnostics12020264

Academic Editors: Daniel Fried and Jae-Hong Lee

Received: 24 November 2021
Accepted: 19 January 2022
Published: 21 January 2022

Publisher's Note: MDPI stays neutral with regard to jurisdictional claims in published maps and institutional affiliations.

Copyright: © 2022 by the authors. Licensee MDPI, Basel, Switzerland. This article is an open access article distributed under the terms and conditions of the Creative Commons Attribution (CC BY) license (https://creativecommons.org/licenses/by/4.0/).

[1] Department of Preventive Dentistry, Naresuan University, Phitsanulok 65000, Thailand; tam_jantra@hotmail.com
[2] Department of Dysphagia Rehabilitation, Graduate School of Medical and Dental Sciences, Tokyo Medical and Dental University (TMDU), Tokyo 113-8510, Japan; k.yoshimi.gerd@tmd.ac.jp (K.Y.); a.nakane.swal@tmd.ac.jp (A.N.); yanma627@yahoo.co.jp (K.Y.); harukatohara@hotmail.com (H.T.)
* Correspondence: nakagerd@tmd.ac.jp; Tel.: +81-03-5803-4560

Abstract: The precise correlations among tongue function and characteristics remain unknown, and no previous studies have attempted machine learning-based classification of tongue ultrasonography findings. This cross-sectional observational study aimed to investigate relationships among tongue characteristics and function by classifying ultrasound images of the tongue using a K-means clustering algorithm. During 2017–2018, 236 healthy older participants (mean age 70.8 ± 5.4 years) were enrolled. The optimal number of clusters determined by the elbow method was 3. After analysis of tongue thickness and echo intensity plots, tongues were classified into three groups. One-way ANOVA was used to compare tongue function, tongue pressure, and oral diadochokinesis for /ta/ and /ka/ in each group. There were significant differences in all tongue functions among the three groups. The worst function was observed in patients with the lowest values for tongue thickness and echo intensity (tongue pressure [P = 0.023], /ta/ [P = 0.007], and /ka/ [P = 0.038]). Our results indicate that ultrasonographic classification of tongue characteristics using K-means clustering may aid clinicians in selecting the appropriate treatment strategy. Indeed, ultrasonography is advantageous in that it provides real-time imaging that is non-invasive, which can improve patient follow-up both in the clinic and at home.

Keywords: artificial intelligence; ultrasonography; tongue; algorithm; dysphagia

1. Introduction

Several recent studies have investigated the use of ultrasonography for evaluating the muscles of the head and neck, as it enables assessment of both muscle quality and quantity [1]. The tongue is the major organ involved in normal oropharyngeal swallowing [2], consisting of four intrinsic muscles (superior longitudinal, inferior longitudinal, transversus, and verticalis) and four extrinsic muscles (palatoglossus, genioglossus, hyoglossus, and styloglossus) [3], which serve to move and alter the shape of the tongue, respectively [4]. Given that the tongue consists of eight unique muscles, ultrasonography represents an effective strategy for investigating its characteristics in detail.

In addition to qualitative characteristics such as tongue thickness (TT) and cross-sectional area, ultrasonography can be used to assess qualitative characteristics of the tongue, such as the presence of intramuscular adipose tissue and muscle density. These qualitative parameters are represented in terms of echo intensity (EI) on grayscale ultrasonography images [5,6]. One recent study reported that lower EI values are associated with decreased tongue function and increased TT [7], while another identified decreased tongue EI as an independent risk factor for sarcopenic dysphagia in older adults [8]. However, despite a few relevant studies, the precise correlations among EI, TT, and tongue function remain unknown. We hypothesized that ultrasonography images of the tongue would provide insight into these relationships.

However, tongue classification based on ultrasonography is challenging due to the complicated structure of the tongue [9]. As such, researchers have investigated various strategies to aid in classification, including the use of linear classifiers (logistic regression), decision trees (random-forest analysis), support vector machines, and clustering algorithms [10]. Among these, clustering is widely utilized given its simplicity and efficiency [11]. Recent studies have reported that clustering algorithms are highly accurate in distinguishing malignant and benign brain tumors with 95% confidence [12]. For example, Ding et al. reported an accuracy of 91.07% and area under the curve of 0.96 when a clustering algorithm was used to classify breast tumors on ultrasonography [13] ($p < 0.05$). Übeyli and Doğdu also reported that a clustering algorithm could be used to classify erythemato-squamous disease into five categories with an accuracy of 94.22% [14].

In the present study, we aimed to investigate the relationships between tongue characteristics and tongue function, including tongue pressure (TP) and diadochokinesis (OD), by classifying ultrasound images of the tongue. Among the various clustering methods available (e.g., K-means clustering, hierarchical clustering, Gaussian mixture models, and density-based clustering [10,15]), we selected K-means clustering because we used two parameters (EI and TT) to describe the characteristics of the tongue, making this method simple and efficient [11].

2. Materials and Methods

2.1. Sample Size

The sample size was calculated using G*Power 3.1 (Kiel University, Kiel, Germany). The alpha value (α, probability of a type I error) and power (1-β, probability of not making a type II error) were set to 0.05 and 0.90, respectively. For this study, we selected a medium effect size of 0.25 [16,17]. The calculation indicated a required sample size of 207 participants across the three groups.

2.2. Participation

The participants included 236 healthy older individuals (71 men, 165 women; mean age: 70.8 ± 5.4 years) from Oyama City (Tochigi, Japan) recruited during 2017–2018. All participants self-reported normal swallowing function and understanding following an explanation of the study. Individuals with a history of neurologic disease, cognitive dysfunction, head and neck cancer or surgery, or any problems related to swallowing function were excluded. Demographic data such as age, sex, weight, height, and body mass index were recorded for each patient.

All study participants provided written informed consent. The study protocols conformed to the guidelines outlined in the Declaration of Helsinki and were approved by the ethics committee of the Faculty of Dentistry at Tokyo Medical and Dental University (D2014-047).

2.3. Assessment of Tongue Characteristics

Tongue ultrasonography was performed in Brightness mode using a portable ultrasound machine (M-Turbo; Fujifilm SonoSite, Tokyo, Japan) equipped with a convex transducer (5–10 MHz). All ultrasound examinations were performed by one well-trained examiner, with the participant in a relaxed, seated position. For measurement, the probe was placed underneath the chin, and the angle of the probe was positioned perpendicular to the Frankfurt horizontal plane at the first premolar area (Figure 1A,B) [7–9] using passive pressure. Echo gain was maintained at the same level for all measurements, which were obtained with the tongue in the resting position after swallowing saliva. This process was repeated thrice, and the mean of the three values was recorded for each measurement.

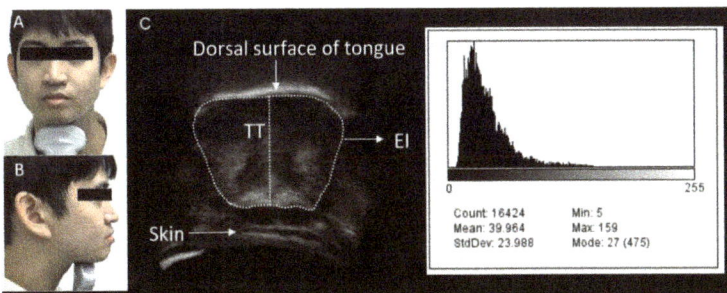

Figure 1. Points of measurement. (**A**) Position of the ultrasonography probe (anterior view). (**B**) Position of the ultrasonography probe (lateral view). (**C**) Ultrasonographic image and grayscale histogram of the tongue.

TT and EI measurements were analyzed using ImageJ (version 1.37, National Institutes of Health, Rockville, MD, USA). TT was measured from the dorsal surface of the tongue to the upper border of the geniohyoid muscle. A region of interest that included as much tongue muscle tissue as possible while avoiding the surrounding fascia was selected to determine EI (Figure 1C) [7]. The mean EI was measured via a histogram-based grayscale analysis, with values ranging from 0 (black) to 255 (white).

2.4. Assessment of Tongue Function

Tongue function was described in terms of tongue strength and tongue skill. Tongue strength was measured as the maximum TP using a JMS TP manometer (JMS Co. Ltd., Tokyo, Japan). An air-filled balloon probe was placed on the dorsal aspect of the tongue. The participant was then instructed to raise the tongue and compress the balloon toward the palate as forcefully as possible [7,18]. Three measurements were obtained, and the average value was recorded as the maximum TP.

Tongue skill was measured based on OD using an oral cavity function testing device. The device, which had a built-in microphone, was placed in front of the mouth, following which the participant was instructed to repeat each of two syllables (/ta/ or /ka/) as quickly as possible for 5 s. This requires using the middle portion and the base of the tongue, respectively [7,19]. The device automatically counted the total number of appropriately pronounced syllables. Repetition speed was calculated as repetitions per second.

2.5. Statistical Analysis

Data were analyzed using RStudio version 1.1423 (Rstudio Inc., Boston, MA, USA) and are presented as the mean ± standard deviation. The Kolmogorov–Smirnov test was used to verify that the data followed a normal distribution. Mean values for tongue function (including TP, /ta/, and /ka/) were compared between groups using one-way analysis of variance. Multiple comparisons were performed using Tukey's test. The level of significance was defined as $p < 0.05$.

Intraclass correlation coefficients (ICC) were used to assess the reliability of the TT and EI measurements. The ICCs were 0.755 and 0.765 for TT and EI, respectively. All intraclass correlation coefficient values were >0.75, indicating good reliability, with values ≥ 0.9 indicating excellent reliability.

2.6. Classification Using K-Means Clustering Algorithms

K-means clustering is performed using machine learning algorithms, which learn from input data and use statistical analyses to predict outcomes or perform specific tasks, without requiring explicit instructions [10].

The K-means clustering algorithms are unsupervised clustering algorithms that classify input data-points into classes based on their inherent distance from each other (i.e., centroid-based clustering). When the number of clusters is fixed to K clusters or groups (Figure 2A), initial k centroids (center of the group) are randomly created and placed onto the data plot (Figure 2B), following which the Euclidean distance from each data-point to the centroids is calculated (Equation (1)) (Figure 2C,D) [10,20].

$$d_{euc}(x, y) = \sqrt{\sum_{i=1}^{n}(x_i - y_i)^2} \quad (1)$$

where x and y are the two vectors of length n.

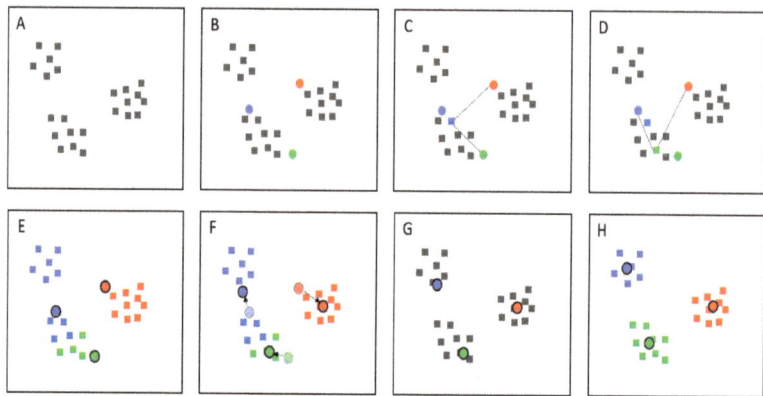

Figure 2. Demonstration of the K-means clustering algorithm, $k = 3$. (**A**) Data plot. (**B**) Three centroids are randomly created, and (**C**) the distance from each data-point to the centroids is calculated using Euclidean distance. (**D**) The step is repeated for all data-points, (**E**) each of which is classified into a group according to its closest centroid. (**F**) The centroid is updated to the new location based on the mean value of all data-points in the group. (**G**) The distance between each data-point and the new centroids is calculated again. (**H**) These steps are repeated until the mean value of all data-points stops changing.

In this study, each data-point was classified into a group according to its closest centroid, based on the Euclidean distance between the data-point and the centroid (Figure 2E). After the first classification, the centroid was updated to the new location (i.e., the actual center of the group) based on the mean value of all data-points in the group (Figure 2F), following which the distance between each data-point and the new centroid was calculated (Figure 2G). These steps were repeated until the mean value of all data-points stopped changing (i.e., the new centroids remained in the same location) (Figure 2H) [10,15].

The most popular methods for determining the optimal number of clusters are the silhouette method and the elbow method—the latter of which was used in this study [21]. This method aims to minimize the sum of the square of the Euclidean distances between each point and its corresponding centroid (total intra-cluster variation, also known as total within-cluster sum of squares (*tot.withinss*; Equation (2)). A smaller value for *tot.withinss* indicates that the data-points are close to the centroid; therefore, it measures the compactness of the clustering and should ideally be as small as possible [10,20].

$$tot.withinss = \sum_{i=1}^{k}\sum_{x_i \in C_k}(x_i - \mu_i)^2 \quad (2)$$

where k is the number of clusters, C is the cluster ($C = C2, C3, \ldots, Ck$), x_i is a data-point belonging to cluster C_k, and μ is the mean value of the data-points assigned to cluster C_k.

For the optimal cluster calculation, the data were first assessed using K-means clustering algorithms in which k varied from 1 to 10. Then, *tot.withinss* was calculated for each

k and plotted according to the number of clusters, k (Figure 3). The location of a bend in the plot is generally considered to indicate the appropriate number of clusters because it indicates that adding another cluster does not markedly improve *tot.withinss* [15,22,23]. Figure 3 shows that the bend occurred at three clusters ($k = 3$).

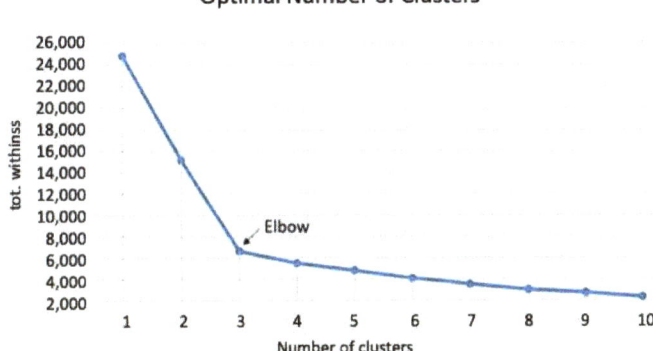

Figure 3. Linear plot between *tot.withinss* and the number of clusters (varying from 1 to 10). The bending point is located at $k = 3$, which represents the optimal number of clusters.

In this study, we plotted EI on the x axis and TT on the y axis (Figure 4). The "kmeans" (d, centers) function in R software was used to calculate the Euclidean distance, locate the centroid, and repeat all steps of the calculation. In this context, "d" refers to the numeric matrix of data (EI, TT), while "centers" refers to the number of clusters (i.e., 3).

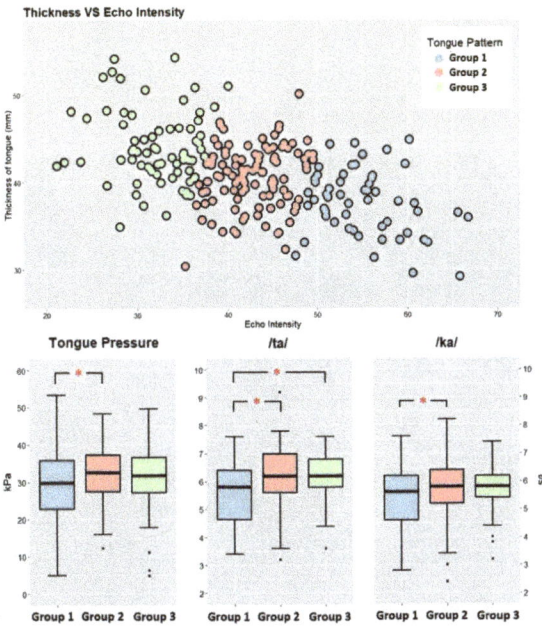

Figure 4. Scatter plot of echo intensity and tongue thickness using the K-means for the three groups. Box plot comparison of tongue function (tongue pressure, /ta/, and /ka/) among the groups based on tongue characteristics. Tongue pressure: Group 1 vs. Group 2, P = 0.023 (* p value < 0.05). /ta/: Group 1 vs. Group 3, P = 0.001 (* p value < 0.05); Group 1 vs. Group 2, P = 0.007 (* p value < 0.05). /ka/: Group 1 vs. Group 2, P = 0.038 (* p value < 0.05).

3. Results

3.1. Determining Optimal Clusters

The plot exhibited a sharp bend at three clusters ($k = 3$), indicating the optimal number of clusters for the dataset (Figure 3). Therefore, tongue characteristics were classified into three groups (Group 1, Group 2, and Group 3).

3.2. Tongue Characteristics

EI and TT data were plotted and divided into three groups using K-means clustering algorithms (Figure 4). Average TT and EI were 37.6 ± 3.7 mm and 55.1 ± 4.7 in Group 1, 40.5 ± 3.5 mm and 42.8 ± 3.5 in Group 2, and 44.0 ± 4.2 mm and 32.2 ± 4.1 in Group 3, respectively (Table 1). These findings indicate that Group 1 exhibited decreased TT and increased brightness when compared with Groups 2 and 3. The tongues of participants in Group 3 were the thickest and darkest (Figure 5).

Table 1. Participant characteristics ($n = 236$).

Variables	Group 1 (Mean ± Standard Deviation)	Group 2 (Mean ± Standard Deviation)	Group 3 (Mean ± Standard Deviation)	Range	p-Value (ANOVA [†])
Physical data					
Number	54	109	73	-	-
Sex (female, %)	71.6	74.1	64.4	-	-
Age (years)	72.6 ± 5.0	69.8 ± 5.6	71.0 ± 5.2	65.0–86.0	0.007
BMI [‡] (kg/m^2)	23.4 ± 2.9	22.7 ± 2.9	22.4 ± 2.7	14.0–32.4	0.154
Ultrasonographic data					
Tongue thickness (mm)	37.6 ± 3.7	40.5 ± 3.5	44.0 ± 4.2	29.2–54.3	<0.001
Echo intensity	55.1 ± 4.7	42.8 ± 3.5	32.2 ± 4.1	21.1–66.8	<0.001
Tongue function data					
Tongue pressure (kPa)	28.7 ± 9.9	32.3 ± 7.1	31.4 ± 8.2	4.9–53.3	0.030
/ta/	5.6 ± 1.1	6.1 ± 1.2	6.2 ± 0.8	3.2–9.2	0.005
/ka/	5.4 ± 1.1	5.8 ± 1.1	5.7 ± 0.8	2.4–10.2	0.040

[†] ANOVA, analysis of variance; [‡] BMI, body mass index.

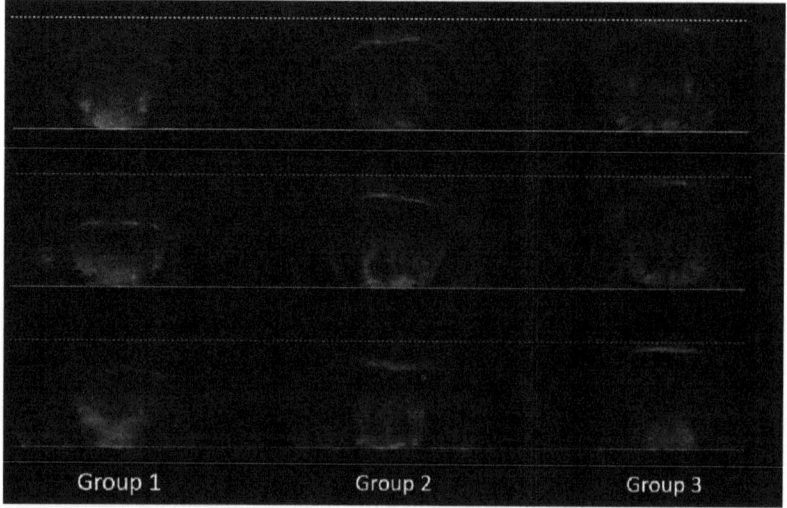

Figure 5. Comparison of illustrative ultrasound images in each group. The solid and dashed lines represent the lowest and the highest parts of the tongue (dorsal surface of the tongue) in Group 3, respectively.

3.3. Tongue Function

TP was highest in Group 2 (32.3 ± 7.1 kPa) and lowest in Group 1 (28.7 kPa), with a significant difference between the two groups ($p < 0.023$). However, there was no significant difference in TP between Groups 2 and 3 (Figure 4).

The average /ta/ and /ka/ values (6.1 and 5.8 time/sec, respectively) were highest in Group 2, and the differences between Groups 2 and 1 were significant ($p < 0.007$ and $p < 0.038$, respectively). The average /ta/ value was also greater in Group 3 than in Group 1 ($p < 0.012$), which had the lowest average /ta/ and /ka/ values (5.6 and 5.4 times/sec, respectively). However, the average /ta/ and /ka/ values did not significantly differ between Groups 2 and 3 (Figure 4).

Overall, the findings indicate that tongue function was poorest in Group 1, but that there was no significant difference in tongue function between Groups 2 and 3.

4. Discussion

In this study, we utilized K-means clustering to classify patterns of tongue characteristics based on ultrasound measurements. Our findings indicated that participants in Group 1 exhibited the poorest tongue function in terms of both TP and OD. Moreover, our analysis suggests that K-means clustering is useful for predicting tongue function based on ultrasonography findings.

4.1. Relationship between Tongue Group and TP

Group 1 exhibited the lowest values for TT and TP and the highest value for EI. TP is an important indicator of tongue muscle strength and swallowing during the oral phase [24,25]. Previous studies have demonstrated a correlation between TT and TP, which is plausible given that muscle mass is commonly associated with muscle strength [26,27]. EI reflects intramuscular adipose tissue content: Higher EI indicates greater adiposity, which may affect tongue function, as indicated by the findings in Group 1 [7,28–30]. Thus, when the tongue appears thinner and brighter on ultrasonography, as noted in Group 1, tongue strength is likely to be lower.

However, another study suggested that EI itself may not be related to TP [7]. This discrepancy may be explained by differences in study design. The authors of the previous study used regression analysis to identify factors that could predict EI, which identified TT and OD as the only significant factors. However, the present study classified ultrasonographic tongue characteristics into three groups, following which TP was compared among the groups.

4.2. Relationship between Tongue Groups and OD

OD refers to the rate of articulation, reflecting the speed of tongue movement [31]. Group 1 exhibited the lowest TP and OD values. Both TP and OD are commonly used to determine the efficacy of speech production. Previous research has highlighted the relationship between strength and speed during speech production. Hence, TP and OD should be related, as observed in the present study [2,31,32]. Although muscle mass is clearly associated with muscle strength, no previous studies have reported a direct relationship between TT and OD. However, one study noted a relationship between EI and /ta/ or /ka/ [7].

Based on the above, patients in Group 1 should exhibit the poorest tongue function, followed by those in Group 2, while patients in Group 3 should exhibit the best tongue function. However, in our study, patients in Group 2 exhibited the strongest tongue function, except for /ta/ (Table 1). Furthermore, there were no statistically significant differences between Groups 2 and 3. This finding suggests that muscle quantity and quality may be sufficient for maintaining tongue function in Groups 2 and 3, but not in Group 1. Further studies are required to fully elucidate the relationships between tongue characteristics and tongue function.

4.3. Categorizing Tongue Characteristics Using K-Means Clustering Algorithms

Previous studies have investigated various methods for applying medical image segmentation [12–14,33]. Generally, segmentation methods are used to detect diseases such as brain cancer based on magnetic resonance images [12,33], breast cancer based on ultrasonographic images [13], or skin diseases based on clinical features [14]. While these studies have highlighted the accuracy of K-means clustering, the final diagnosis of all medical images was known, and the clustering method was mainly used to detect disease based on imaging, following which the findings were compared with the true diagnosis to establish the accuracy of the method. However, as we did not know the diagnosis in each case, we were unable to determine the accuracy of the current classification method.

Several studies have investigated whether EI can be used for tongue classification. The EI of the tongue increases with age [34]. Research has also indicated that the EI of the tongue is significantly higher in patients with amyotrophic lateral sclerosis (ALS) than in healthy participants [35], suggesting that EI can be used to distinguish between healthy and diseased tongue muscle. However, no previous studies have examined these associations using detailed classifications based on ultrasonography or significant differences in tongue function to define each group. Our findings indicate that K-means clustering may be an effective approach for classification of the tongue. Future studies should aim to collect data for various patient groups based on age, sex, and disease status, as this may help to determine whether our method can be used to improve diagnosis.

4.4. Clinical Implications

Several studies have indicated that older individuals are more likely to experience dysphagia due to age-related decreases in muscle mass [26,36–38]. Thus, assessments of muscle mass and the strength/function of the perioral muscles are necessary for maintaining oral function in older adults. Our analysis indicated that patients in Group 1 exhibited the thinnest, brightest, and most easily detectable tongues on ultrasonography (Figure 5). Establishing standard diagnostic criteria based on ultrasonography patterns may represent a more useful and non-invasive strategy for assessing and preventing oral hypofunction. Furthermore, identifying the risks associated with each ultrasonography pattern may aid in determining the appropriate treatments and exercises for community-dwelling older adults. Indeed, one recent study demonstrated that training the tongue by pushing it against a hard palate, (i.e., tongue-pressure resistance training) can improve both tongue (TP and OD) and suprahyoid muscle function [37]. Another study suggested that 3 months of oral training can improve swallowing function and OD in older adults who are at high risk of deterioration in oral health [39].

Furthermore, aging leads to atrophy of the tongue papillae, and several studies have reported an association between tongue function and the characteristics of the tongue surface [40,41]. Appropriate diagnostic assessment of tongue function can aid clinicians in selecting the proper treatment strategy, which may in turn aid older adults in maintaining oral hygiene, feeding ability, and swallowing function. Given that these strategies can help to prevent sarcopenic dysphagia, our classification method has important implications regarding quality of life in older individuals.

4.5. Limitations

Our study had some limitations. First, the dataset used for training the classification model was based on only 236 participants, which may have been insufficient for determining the outcome without error. Thus, a larger sample size required to verify our model. Second, all study participants were healthy; none of them had compromised tongue function or neurological status. As such, we were unable to investigate the effects of aging and disease such as neuromuscular diseases on tongue characteristics. In addition, muscle fibrosis and adiposity are major characteristics of sarcopenia, and in general, age-related fibrosis of muscle tissue is also associated with increased EI [42]. In our method, we categorized the participants' tongue using EI and TT. Therefore, the influence of aging on EI could not be eliminated. Furthermore, it is difficult to distinguish diseases such as neuromuscular disorders using our classification. Longitudinal studies that include participants with poor tongue function, systemic sarcopenia, and various diseases may aid in determining the usefulness of our classification method.

5. Conclusions

We used K-mean clustering algorithms on ultrasonographic images to categorize tongue characteristics based on muscle luminance and TT of healthy older individuals. In this study, the elbow method was used to calculate *tot.withinss* for each k and plotted it according to the number of clusters. The optimal number of clusters determined by this method was three. EI was plotted on the x-axis and TT on the y-axis for analysis, and the subjects were classified into three groups.

The results showed that Group 1, which had the highest EI, had the lowest TT and TP and significantly lower OD. The classification of tongue images using K-mean clustering algorithms could be applied for predicting tongue function and for diagnosis. If used by clinicians as a tool to prevent the decline of oral and swallowing functions, it may help to provide functional training and follow-up for older adults. For accurate classification, more sample analysis is needed in the future to establish an algorithm.

Ultrasonography is not only easy to use for real-time imaging but is also radiation-free, painless, portable, and can be used not only in hospitals but also in home-visits. However, it is difficult at present to distinguish the cause of changes in EI from the images. EI is affected by aging and diseases, as well as sarcopenia. The limitation of this study is that the effect of aging cannot be excluded. Therefore, it is necessary to analyze the imaging characteristics of the tongue and related factors for various ages and diseases in the future.

Author Contributions: A.C.: involved in study conception and design, involved in analysis and interpretation of data, drafting of the manuscript; K.N.: involved in drafting of the manuscript, critical revision of the manuscript for important intellectual content; K.Y. (Kanako Yoshimi): involved in acquisition of data, drafting of the manuscript; A.N.: involved in acquisition of data; K.Y. (Kohei Yamaguchi): involved in acquisition of data; H.T.: involved in study conception and design. All authors have read and agreed to the published version of the manuscript.

Funding: This research received no external funding.

Institutional Review Board Statement: The study protocols were approved by the ethics committee of the Faculty of Dentistry, Tokyo Medical and Dental University (D2014-047). The study conformed to the guidelines of Declaration of Helsinki.

Informed Consent Statement: All study participants provided written informed consent. Written informed consent was obtained from the patients for publication of this paper.

Conflicts of Interest: The authors declare no conflict of interest.

References

1. Watanabe, Y.; Yamada, Y.; Fukumoto, Y.; Ishihara, T.; Yokoyama, K.; Yoshida, T.; Miyake, M.; Yamagata, E.; Kimura, M. Echo Intensity Obtained from Ultrasonography Images Reflecting Muscle Strength in Elderly Men. *Clin. Interv. Aging* **2013**, *8*, 993–998. [CrossRef]
2. Robbins, J.; Humpal, N.S.; Banaszynski, K.; Hind, J.; Rogus-Pulia, N. Age-Related Differences in Pressures Generated During Isometric Presses and Swallows by Healthy Adults. *Dysphagia* **2016**, *31*, 90–96. [CrossRef] [PubMed]
3. Sanders, I.; Mu, L. A Three-Dimensional Atlas of Human Tongue Muscles. *Anat. Rec.* **2013**, *296*, 1102–1114. [CrossRef]
4. Sakamoto, Y. Structural Arrangement of the Intrinsic Muscles of the Tongue and Their Relationships with the Extrinsic Muscles. *Surg. Radiol. Anat.* **2018**, *40*, 681–688. [CrossRef] [PubMed]
5. Fukumoto, Y.; Ikezoe, T.; Yamada, Y.; Tsukagoshi, R.; Nakamura, M.; Mori, N.; Kimura, M.; Ichihashi, N. Skeletal Muscle Quality Assessed from Echo Intensity Is Associated with Muscle Strength of Middle-Aged and Elderly Persons. *Eur. J. Appl. Physiol.* **2012**, *112*, 1519–1525. [CrossRef]
6. Fukumoto, Y.; Ikezoe, T.; Yamada, Y.; Tsukagoshi, R.; Nakamura, M.; Takagi, Y.; Kimura, M.; Ichihashi, N. Age-Related Ultrasound Changes in Muscle Quantity and Quality in Women. *Ultrasound Med. Biol.* **2015**, *41*, 3013–3017. [CrossRef]

7. Chantaramanee, A.; Tohara, H.; Nakagawa, K.; Hara, K.; Nakane, A.; Yamaguchi, K.; Yoshimi, K.; Junichi, F.; Minakuchi, S. Association Between Echo Intensity of the Tongue and Its Thickness and Function in Elderly Subjects. *J. Oral Rehabil.* **2019**, *46*, 634–639. [CrossRef] [PubMed]
8. Ogawa, N.; Mori, T.; Fujishima, I.; Wakabayashi, H.; Itoda, M.; Kunieda, K.; Shigematsu, T.; Nishioka, S.; Tohara, H.; Yamada, M.; et al. Ultrasonography to Measure Swallowing Muscle Mass and Quality in Older Patients with Sarcopenic Dysphagia. *J. Am. Med. Dir. Assoc.* **2018**, *19*, 516–522. [CrossRef]
9. Tamura, F.; Kikutani, T.; Tohara, T.; Yoshida, M.; Yaegaki, K. Tongue Thickness Relates to Nutritional Status in the Elderly. *Dysphagia* **2012**, *27*, 556–561. [CrossRef]
10. Shalev-Shwartz, S.; Ben-David, S. *Understanding Machine Learning: From Theory to Algorithms*; Cambridge University Press: Cambridge, UK, 2014.
11. Kambatla, K.; Kollias, G.; Kumar, V.; Grama, A. Trends in Big Data Analytics. *J. Parallel Distrib. Comput.* **2014**, *74*, 2561–2573. [CrossRef]
12. Al-Naami, B.; Bashir, A.; Amasha, H.; Al-Nabulsi, J.; Almalty, A.M. Statistical Approach for Brain Cancer Classification Using a Region Growing Threshold. *J. Med. Syst.* **2011**, *35*, 463–471. [CrossRef]
13. Ding, J.; Cheng, H.D.; Huang, J.; Liu, J.; Zhang, Y. Breast Ultrasound Image Classification Based on Multiple-Instance Learning. *J. Digit. Imaging* **2012**, *25*, 620–627. [CrossRef] [PubMed]
14. Übeyli, E.D.; Doğdu, E. Automatic Detection of Erythemato-Squamous Diseases Using k-Means Clustering. *J. Med. Syst.* **2010**, *34*, 179–184. [CrossRef] [PubMed]
15. Estivill-Castro, V. Why So Many Clustering Algorithms: A Position Paper. *SIGKDD Explor. Newsl.* **2002**, *4*, 65–75. [CrossRef]
16. Cohen, J. *Statistical Power Analysis for the Behavioral Science*, 2nd ed.; Routledge: New York, NY, USA, 1988.
17. Dupont, W.D.; Plummer, W.D. Power and Sample Size Calculations for Studies Involving Linear Regression. *Control. Clin. Trials* **1998**, *19*, 589–601. [CrossRef]
18. Utanohara, Y.; Hayashi, R.; Yoshikawa, M.; Yoshida, M.; Tsuga, K.; Akagawa, Y. Standard Values of Maximum Tongue Pressure Taken Using Newly Developed Disposable Tongue Pressure Measurement Device. *Dysphagia* **2008**, *23*, 286–290. [CrossRef]
19. Sarukawa, S.; Noguchi, T.; Miyazaki, K.; Itoh, H.; Nishino, H.; Kusama, M.; Sugawara, Y.; Kawada, K. Development of a Tool for Speech Intelligibility Evaluation After Glossectomy: The TKR Speech Test. *Jpn. J. Head Neck Cancer* **2013**, *39*, 374–378.
20. Alpaydin, E. *Introduction to Machine Learning, 3rd ed*; MIT Press: Cambridge, MA, USA, 2014.
21. Thinsungnoena, T.; Kaoungkub, N.; Durongdumronchaib, P.; Kerdprasopb, K.; Kerdprasop, N. (Eds.) The Clustering Validity with Silhouette and Sum of Squared Errors. In Proceedings of the 3rd International Conference on Industrial Application Engineering (ICIAE2015), Tokyo, Japan, 14–16 March 2015.
22. Bholowalia, P.; Kumar, A. EBK-Means: A Clustering Technique Based on Elbow Method and k-Means in WSN. *Int. J. Comput. Appl.* **2014**, *105*, 17–24.
23. Charrad, M.; Ghazzali, N.; Boiteau, V.; Niknafs, A. NbClust: An R Package for Determining the Relevant Number of Clusters in a Data Set. *J. Stat. Soft.* **2014**, *61*, 1–36. [CrossRef]
24. Hamahata, A.; Beppu, T.; Shirakura, S.; Hatanaka, A.; Yamaki, T.; Saitou, T.; Sakurai, H. Tongue Pressure in Patients with Tongue Cancer Resection and Reconstruction. *Auris Nasus Larynx* **2014**, *41*, 563–567. [CrossRef]
25. Shaker, R.; Cook, I.J.; Dodds, W.J.; Hogan, W.J. Pressure-Flow Dynamics of the Oral Phase of Swallowing. *Dysphagia* **1988**, *3*, 79–84. [CrossRef]
26. Larsson, L.; Degens, H.; Li, M.; Salviati, L.; Lee, Y.I.; Thompson, W.; Kirkland, J.L.; Sandri, M. Sarcopenia: Aging-Related Loss of Muscle Mass and Function. *Physiol. Rev.* **2019**, *99*, 427–511. [CrossRef] [PubMed]
27. Umemoto, G.; Furuya, H.; Arahata, H.; Sugahara, M.; Sakai, M.; Tsuboi, Y. Relationship Between Tongue Thickness and Tongue Pressure in Neuromuscular Disorders. *Neurol. Clin. Neurosci.* **2016**, *4*, 142–145. [CrossRef]
28. Akima, H.; Yoshiko, A.; Hioki, M.; Kanehira, N.; Shimaoka, K.; Koike, T.; Sakakibara, H.; Oshida, Y. Skeletal Muscle Size Is a Major Predictor of Intramuscular Fat Content Regardless of Age. *Eur. J. Appl. Physiol.* **2015**, *115*, 1627–1635. [CrossRef] [PubMed]
29. Akima, H.; Yoshiko, A.; Tomita, A.; Ando, R.; Saito, A.; Ogawa, M.; Kondo, S.; Tanaka, N.I. Relationship Between Quadriceps Echo Intensity and Functional and Morphological Characteristics in Older Men and Women. *Arch. Gerontol. Geriatr.* **2017**, *70*, 105–111. [CrossRef]
30. Strasser, E.M.; Draskovits, T.; Praschak, M.; Quittan, M.; Graf, A. Association Between Ultrasound Measurements of Muscle Thickness, Pennation Angle, Echogenicity and Skeletal Muscle Strength in the Elderly. *Age* **2013**, *35*, 2377–2388. [CrossRef]
31. Neel, A.T.; Palmer, P.M. Is Tongue Strength an Important Influence on Rate of Articulation in Diadochokinetic and Reading Tasks? *J. Speech Lang. Hear. Res.* **2012**, *55*, 235–246. [CrossRef]
32. Hiramatsu, T.; Kataoka, H.; Osaki, M.; Hagino, H. Effect of Aging on Oral and Swallowing Function After Meal Consumption. *Clin. Interv. Aging* **2015**, *10*, 229–235. [PubMed]
33. Zhang, J.; Jiang, W.; Wang, R.; Wang, L. Brain MR Image Segmentation with Spatial Constrained k-Mean Algorithm and Dual-Tree Complex Wavelet Transform. *J. Med. Syst.* **2014**, *38*, 93. [CrossRef]
34. Yamaguchi, K.; Nakagawa, K.; Yoshimi, K.; Chantaramanee, A.; Nakane, A.; Furuya, J.; Tohara, H. Age-related changes in swallowing muscle intramuscular adipose tissue deposition and related factors. *Exp. Gerontol.* **2021**, *1*, 111505. [CrossRef]

35. McIlduff, C.E.; Martucci, M.G.; Shin, C.; Qi, K.; Pacheck, A.K.; Gutierrez, H.; Mortreux, M.; Rutkove, S.B. Quantitative ultrasound of the tongue: Echo intensity is a potential biomarker of bulbar dysfunction in amyotrophic lateral sclerosis. *Clin. Neurophysiol.* **2020**, *131*, 2423–2428. [CrossRef]
36. Clegg, A.; Young, J.; Iliffe, S.; Rikkert, M.O.; Rockwood, K. Frailty in Elderly People. *Lancet* **2013**, *381*, 752–762. [CrossRef]
37. Namiki, C.; Hara, K.; Tohara, H.; Kobayashi, K.; Chantaramanee, A.; Nakagawa, K.; Saitou, T.; Yamaguchi, K.; Yoshimi, K.; Nakane, A.; et al. Tongue-Pressure Resistance Training Improves Tongue and Suprahyoid Muscle Functions Simultaneously. *Clin. Interv. Aging* **2019**, *14*, 601–608. [CrossRef]
38. Yamaguchi, K.; Tohara, H.; Hara, K.; Nakane, A.; Kajisa, E.; Yoshimi, K.; Minakuchi, S. Relationship of Aging, Skeletal Muscle Mass, and Tooth Loss with Masseter Muscle Thickness. *BMC Geriatr.* **2018**, *18*, 67. [CrossRef] [PubMed]
39. Sakayori, T.; Maki, Y.; Hirata, S.; Okada, M.; Ishii, T. Evaluation of a Japanese "Prevention of Long-Term Care" Project for the Improvement in Oral Function in the High-Risk Elderly. *Geriatr. Gerontol. Int.* **2013**, *13*, 451–457. [CrossRef] [PubMed]
40. Umemori, N.; Kakinoki, Y.; Karaki, J.; Kakigawa, H. New method for determining surface roughness of tongue. *Gerodontology.* **2012**, *29*, 90–95. [CrossRef]
41. Kikutani, T.; Tamura, F.; Nishiwaki, K.; Suda, M.; Kayanaka, H.; Machida, R.; Yoshida, M.; Akagawa, Y. The degree of tongue-coating reflects lingual motor function in the elderly. *Gerodontology* **2009**, *26*, 291–296. [CrossRef] [PubMed]
42. Pillen, S.; Arts, I.M.P.; Zwarts, M.J. Muscle ultrasound in neuromuscular disorders. *Muscle Nerve.* **2008**, *37*, 679–693. [CrossRef] [PubMed]

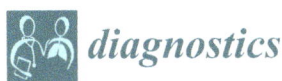

Article

Artificial Intelligence Application in Assessment of Panoramic Radiographs

Łukasz Zadrożny [1,*], Piotr Regulski [2], Katarzyna Brus-Sawczuk [3], Marta Czajkowska [4,*], Laszlo Parkanyi [5], Scott Ganz [6,7] and Eitan Mijiritsky [8,9]

1. Department of Dental Propaedeutics and Prophylaxis, Faculty of Dental Medicine, Medical University of Warsaw, 02-006 Warsaw, Poland
2. Department of Dental and Maxillofacial Radiology, Faculty of Dental Medicine, Medical University of Warsaw, 02-091 Warsaw, Poland; piotr.regulski@wum.edu.pl
3. Department of Comprehensive Dental Care, Faculty of Dental Medicine, Medical University of Warsaw, 02-091 Warsaw, Poland; kbrus@wum.edu.pl
4. Department of Laryngology, Medical University of Silesia, 40-027 Katowice, Poland
5. Department of Periodontology, Faculty of Dentistry, University of Szeged, 6720 Szeged, Hungary; parkanyilaci@gmail.com
6. Department of Restorative Dentistry Rutgers, The State University of New Jersey, Newark, NJ 07103, USA; drganz@drganz.com
7. Independent Researcher, Fort Lee, NJ 07024, USA
8. Tel-Aviv Sourasky Medical Center, Department of Otolaryngology, Head and Neck and Maxillofacial Surgery, Sackler Faculty of Medicine, Tel Aviv 6139001, Israel; mijiritsky@bezeqint.net
9. The Maurice and Gabriela Goldschleger School of Dental Medicine, Tel Aviv University, Tel Aviv 6997801, Israel

* Correspondence: lzadrozny@wum.edu.pl (Ł.Z.); mrtczajkowska@gmail.com (M.C.)

Citation: Zadrożny, Ł.; Regulski, P.; Brus-Sawczuk, K.; Czajkowska, M.; Parkanyi, L.; Ganz, S.; Mijiritsky, E. Artificial Intelligence Application in Assessment of Panoramic Radiographs. *Diagnostics* 2022, 12, 224. https://doi.org/10.3390/diagnostics12010224

Academic Editor: Jae-Hong Lee

Received: 29 December 2021
Accepted: 14 January 2022
Published: 17 January 2022

Publisher's Note: MDPI stays neutral with regard to jurisdictional claims in published maps and institutional affiliations.

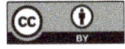

Copyright: © 2022 by the authors. Licensee MDPI, Basel, Switzerland. This article is an open access article distributed under the terms and conditions of the Creative Commons Attribution (CC BY) license (https://creativecommons.org/licenses/by/4.0/).

Abstract: The aim of this study was to assess the reliability of the artificial intelligence (AI) automatic evaluation of panoramic radiographs (PRs). Thirty PRs, covering at least six teeth with the possibility of assessing the marginal and apical periodontium, were uploaded to the Diagnocat (LLC Diagnocat, Moscow, Russia) account, and the radiologic report of each was generated as the basis of automatic evaluation. The same PRs were manually evaluated by three independent evaluators with 12, 15, and 28 years of experience in dentistry, respectively. The data were collected in such a way as to allow statistical analysis with SPSS Statistics software (IBM, Armonk, NY, USA). A total of 90 reports were created for 30 PRs. The AI protocol showed very high specificity (above 0.9) in all assessments compared to ground truth except from periodontal bone loss. Statistical analysis showed a high interclass correlation coefficient (ICC > 0.75) for all interevaluator assessments, proving the good credibility of the ground truth and the reproducibility of the reports. Unacceptable reliability was obtained for caries assessment (ICC = 0.681) and periapical lesions assessment (ICC = 0.619). The tested AI system can be helpful as an initial evaluation of screening PRs, giving appropriate credibility reports and suggesting additional diagnostic methods for more accurate evaluation if needed.

Keywords: AI; panoramic radiograph; screening; diagnosis; dentistry

1. Introduction

Radiological examination is an essential part of patient management in modern dentistry. The panoramic radiograph (PR) is a common extraoral radiograph used to identify the hard tissues of the oral cavity and surrounding skeletal structures. Although resolution is not as detailed as intra-oral radiographs for examination of the teeth, many changes in calcification of the dental structures and in ossification of the surrounding bone can aid in the identification of dental diseases, such as caries (decay), periodontal bone loss, and bone lesions [1]. As far as cone-beam computed tomography (CBCT) systems are developed and becoming more and more popular for imaging comprehensive 3D volumetric information concerning oral soft tissues, bones, and teeth, PRs remain a very common initial X-ray and screening tool in the diagnostic process in dentistry [1–12]. However, although CBCT provides more data, the analysis is laborious and time-consuming [3,7,13]. PR analysis is faster than CBCT, but the accurate evaluation of all PR aspects still requires time and specialized knowledge. Thus, computer-aided systems have been developed to assist in medical and dental imaging diagnosis [14–17] and processing of the treatment [1,13,18,19]. One of the artificial intelligence (AI)-based systems based on the convolutional neural networks (CNN) is Diagnocat (LLC Diagnocat, Moscow, Russia). This is an online platform where different X-rays can be uploaded and analyzed by the algorithm. PR evaluation takes up to 2 min and the software generates a report (Figure 1). Such a report may focus the attention of the clinician on a specific problem or may be used as a communication aid with the patient to explain a required treatment. Moreover, the report contains suggestions for additional diagnoses, e.g., with use of CBCT or suggested consultations regarding specific sites with appropriate specialists. The aim of this study was to assess the reliability of Diagnocat software in the automatic evaluation of panoramic radiological images.

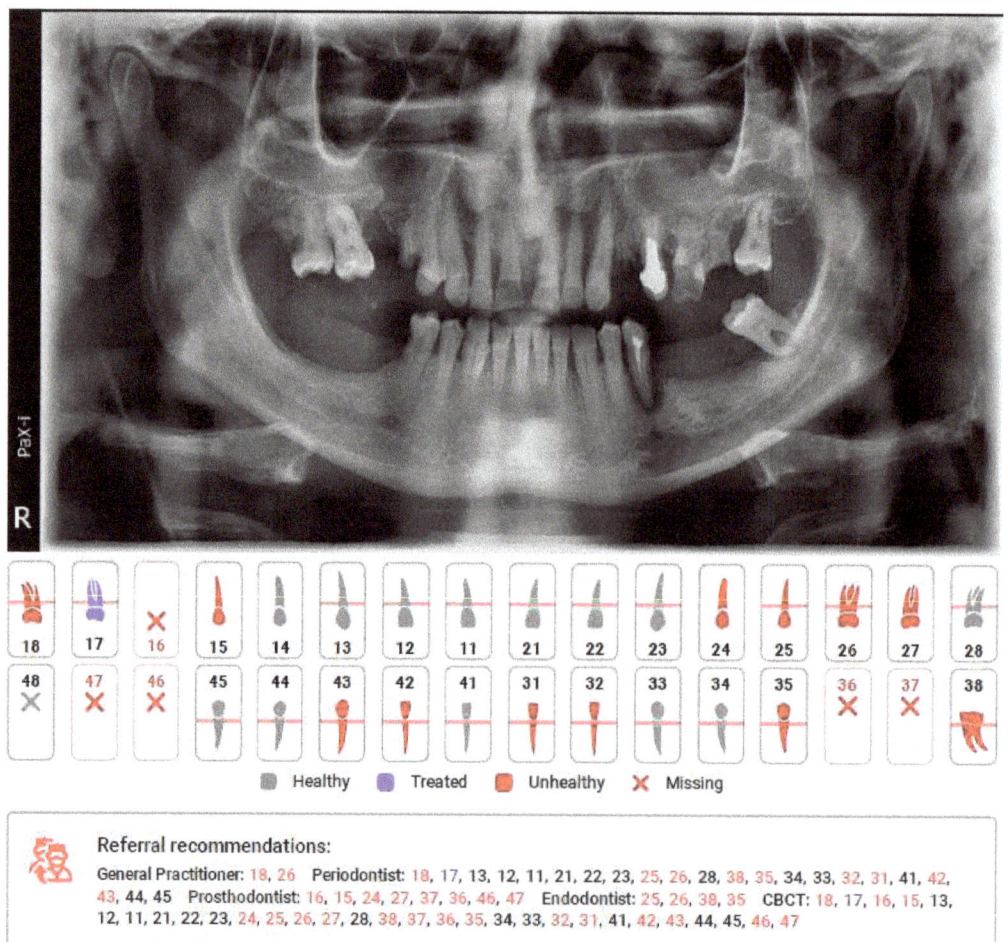

(A)

Figure 1. Cont.

Tooth 18 Periodontal bone loss [88%], Dental calculus [79%], Signs of caries [99%].

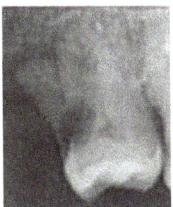

Tooth 17 Periodontal bone loss [95%], Filling [83%].

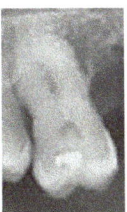

Tooth 16 Missing [100%].

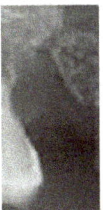

Tooth 15 Root fragment [99%].

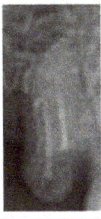

Tooth 14

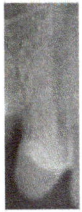

(B)

Figure 1. (**A**). First page of the DC report including simple diagram of teeth with a legend of findings and referral recommendations pointing specific specialists for specific teeth. (**B**). One of the following pages of the DC report including specific teeth captions and description with percent of accuracy.

2. Materials and Methods

This retrospective research was performed following the principles of the Declaration of Helsinki and was approved by the Ethical Comity by the Medical University of Warsaw, Poland (Approval code: AKBE 221/2021). Thirty panoramic radiographs (PR) of 16 women and 14 men collected from the Dental and Maxillofacial Radiology Department, Medical University of Warsaw, Poland, taken from November 2019 to May 2021 were included in the study. Diagnostically acceptable or excellent quality radiographs, covering at least six teeth with the possibility of assessing the marginal and apical periodontium, were included. The exclusion criteria were: radiographs with unacceptable quality, containing severe artifacts, such as motion artifacts, shadow of the spine, or air projected on the region under assessment, radiographs containing developmental disorders. All PRs were listed and numbered. Then, all PRs were uploaded to the Diagnocat software (DC, Diagnocat LCC, Moscow, Russia) account, and the radiologic report of each was generated as the basis of automatic evaluation. The same PRs were manually evaluated by three independent dentists (evaluators) with 12, 15, and 28 years of experience in dentistry, respectively. One of the dentists (P.R) is experienced in dentomaxillofacial radiology. The missing teeth, presence of carries, dental fillings, prosthetic restorations (crowns or posts), endodontically treated teeth (with underfilled, overfilled or with inhomogeneous filling in the root canals), residual roots, periapical lesion (osteolytic, osteosclerotic or mixed), and periodontal bone loss were assessed. A special form was created to completed by each evaluator for each radiograph. Each evaluator assessed each radiograph independently and separately (without knowing the Diagnocat software evaluation). The reports were transferred to spreadsheets according to each pathology (category), tooth number, and evaluator. For each tooth, two possible values (presence of pathology or absence of pathology) were acceptable.

In order to assess the reliability of Diagnocat reports, they were compared with ground truth, obtained on the basis of analysis of three evaluators. If two or three evaluators agreed on the assessment, the diagnosis was considered as ground truth. Statistical analysis was done with SPSS Statistics software (IBM, Armonk, NY, USA). The sensitivity and specificity assessment was performed. Statistical analysis was performed for each pathology. Interclass correlation coefficient (ICC) analysis with a two-way mixed model was performed. It was assumed that ICC values greater than 0.75 would guarantee good reliability. In order to assess the interevaluator consistency, the ICC was also calculated.

The average time of evaluation was estimated for the creation of reports by different evaluators and AI software.

3. Results

In total, 90 reports were created for 30 PRs. Overall numbers of evaluated pathologies are listed in the Table 1. The average time to prepare a single report was up to 2.0 min for DC and 8.5 min for evaluators.

The AI protocol showed very high specificity (above 0.9) in all assessments compared to ground truth except from periodontal bone loss. Sensitivity was very high (above 0.9) for the assessment of missing teeth and prosthetic restorations, and high (above 0.8) for dental fillings, endodontically treated teeth, residual roots, and periodontal bone loss. Low sensitivity was obtained for caries, periapical lesion, as well as over and underfilled canals assessment (see Table 1).

Statistical analysis showed high ICC (ICC > 0.75) for all interevaluator assessments, proving the good credibility of the ground truth and the reproducibility of the reports. The detailed results are shown in Table 2.

Table 1. Sensitivity and specificity assessment of Diagnocat software.

Categories	Correctly Diagnosed (True Positive)	Mis-Diagnosed (False Negative)	Over-Diagnosed (False Positive)	Total Assessments	Sensitivity	Specificity
missing tooth	149	6	15	960	0.961	0.981
caries	89	111	11	805	0.445	0.982
filling	223	45	7	805	0.832	0.987
prosthetic restoration (crown or post)	44	2	4	805	0.957	0.995
endodontically treated tooth	95	14	4	805	0.872	0.994
underfilled canal	28	18	0	109	0.609	1.000
overfilled canal	5	6	0	109	0.455	1.000
inhomogeneous filling in canal	4	1	6	109	0.800	0.942
residual root	32	7	1	805	0.821	0.999
periapical lesion (osteolytic, osteosclerotic or mixed)	23	36	14	805	0.390	0.981
periodontal bone loss	189	47	87	805	0.801	0.847

Table 2. ICC for all interevaluator assessments (ICC >075).

Categories	ICC Interevaluator
missing tooth	0.977
caries	0.829
filling	0.928
prosthetic restoration (crown, post)	0.984
endodontically treated tooth	0.989
underfilled canal	0.924
overfilled canal	0.886
inhomogeneous filling in canal	0.834
residual root	0.969
periapical lesion (osteolytic, osteosclerotic or mixed)	0.903
periodontal bone loss	0.842

The statistical assessment between ground truth and Diagnocat software results showed acceptable reliability (ICC > 0.75) for missing teeth, fillings assessment, prosthetic restoration, endodontically treated teeth (including under and overfilled canals), residual roots, and periodontal bone loss. Unacceptable reliability was obtained for caries assessment (ICC = 0.681) and periapical lesions assessment (ICC = 0.619) (see Table 3).

Table 3. ICC over ground truth for different evaluated objects.

Groups	ICC Diagnocat/Ground Truth
missing tooth	0.959
carries	0.681
filling	0.920
prosthetic restoration (crown, post)	0.968
endodontically treated tooth	0.948
underfilled canal	0.784
overfilled canal	0.752
inhomogeneous filling in canal	0.671
residual root	0.938
periapical lesion (osteolytic, osteosclerotic or mixed)	0.619
periodontal bone loss	0.764

4. Discussion

The application of AI in medicine and dentistry has increased in recent years, which may be seen in the number of published studies [1,18–27]. The CNN based automatic protocol for X-ray evaluation used within this study presented high or very high sensitivity for dental fillings, endodontically treated teeth, residual roots, periodontal bone loss, missing teeth, and prosthetic restorations. Low sensitivity was obtained for periapical lesions, caries, as well as over and underfilled canals. Diagnocat did not detect any of the three periapical cysts, nor either of the two intramaxillary cysts or two broken endodontic instruments. However, the protocol did not name these specific pathologies. All teeth connected to these pathologies were marked as unhealthy and suggested for additional diagnostics using CBCT or referral for additional evaluation by a general practitioner (GP), endodontist (ED), or periodontist (PD) depending on the problem (see Figure 1 tooth 26, Figure 2 tooth 44, Figure 3 tooth 16). Our study shows the lowest reliability for apical periodontitis, which can be detected radiographically as periapical translucencies (a widened periodontal ligament or clearly detectable lesions). The detection and interpretation of a radiolucency in the periapical region is considered an important sign of periapical pathology. Although PRs represent the first, basic radiological overview X-rays, the detection of apical lesions on panoramic radiographs comes with limited sensitivity [28]. Nardi et al. in a retrospective study evaluated the diagnostic accuracy of panoramic radiographs in the detection of clinically/surgically confirmed asymptomatic apical lesions using CBCT imaging as the reference standard. Sensitivity, specificity, diagnostic accuracy, positive predictive value, and negative predictive value for panoramic radiographs with respect to CBCT imaging were analysed. Panoramic pictures showed good diagnostic accuracy, high specificity, and low sensitivity for the detection of endodontically treated apical periodontitis. The accuracy of detection also depends on the localisation and quality of the X-ray. The best identified apical lesions were located in the lower canine/premolar and molar areas, whereas the worst identified apical lesions were located in the upper/lower incisor area and upper molar area (anatomical conditions). These authors also found that the radiographic detection of apical lesions is subject to the large variation between examiners in terms of their experience. In our study, three experienced evaluators separately evaluated all the radiographic data from panoramic radiographs. In the inclusion criteria, we included the OPG quality criterion to limit the issue of localisation mentioned above. Among 805 assessments to reveal the presence or absence of the periapical lesions, obtained values of sensitivity and specificity were 0.390 and 0.981, respectively.

The application of CNNs to assist in the detection of apical lesions could improve the ability to detect the apical lesions. The AI and deep learning protocol described by Ekert at al. [29] revealed that a moderately deep CNN trained on a limited amount of image data showed satisfying discriminatory ability to detect apical lesions on panoramic radiographs. The reference test was the majority vote of six independent examiners who detected apical lesions on an ordinal scale (0, no apical lesion; 1, uncertain apical lesion; 2, clearly detectable apical lesion, certain apical lesion) in comparison with the CNN protocol. The CNN based protocol revealed sensitivity and specificity values of 0.65 and 0.87, respectively. In molars, sensitivity was significantly higher than in other tooth types, whereas specificity was lower. The authors cautioned that the sensitivity of their system should be improved before clinical use. In our research, among 805 measurements, Diagnocat revealed unacceptable reliability with ICC = 0.619. The program failed to assess major osteolytic inflammatory lesions (e.g., cysts) in the periapical area. In a systematic review (search field 1862 titles, 50 studies included), the artificial intelligence models exhibited wide clinical applications in dentomaxillofacial radiology to identify maxillofacial pathologies including periodontitis/periapical disease. However, it is still necessary to further verify the reliability and applicability of the artificial intelligence models prior to transferring these models into clinical practice [14]. Regarding the diagnosis of periapical disease, Mol et al., as the pioneers of computer aided systems, concluded that interpretation could play an important role in the diagnosis of periapical bone lesions. Its objectivity and reproducibility can make it a valuable instrument for standardizing the diagnostic process [30]. It seems promising to use a more accurate radiologic tool as CBCT in artificial intelligence protocols. Orhan et al. used the same artificial intelligence system as we tested in our study, to detect periapical pathologies but on CBCT images. The images of 153 periapical lesions obtained from 109 patients were included in the study. The reliability of the artificial intelligence system in correctly detecting a periapical lesion was 92.8%. On the other hand, when analysing CBCT pictures by CNN: volumetric measurements of the lesions were similar to those with manual segmentation. There was no significant difference between the two measurement methods ($p > 0.05$). The authors concluded that artificial intelligence systems support the clinical diagnosis and can be useful for detecting apical lesions on CBCT. Under the conditions of these studies volume measurements performed by humans and by artificial intelligence systems were comparable to each other [31]. According to the literature, CBCT, as the modern radiologic tool, significantly increases the detection of periapical pathology compared to conventional periapical and panoramic radiographs [32,33]. Jae-Lee et al. evaluated the detection and diagnosis of three types of odontogenic cystic lesions, namely odontogenic keratocysts, dentigerous cysts, and periapical cysts, using dental panoramic radiography and CBCT based on a deep CNN. The pretrained model using CBCT images showed good diagnostic performance (sensitivity 96.1%, specificity 77.1%), which was significantly greater than that achieved by other models using panoramic images (sensitivity 88.2%, specificity 77.0%) ($p = 0.014$). The authors concluded that the CNN system trained with CBCT images obtained higher diagnostic performance than that trained with panoramic images [34]. Radiographic imaging for the diagnosis of caries lesions has been a part of clinical examinations for approximately a century. The value of radiography compared with a merely visual examination is especially emphasized in the diagnosis of caries lesions in clinically inaccessible surfaces, e.g., approximal. Detecting caries lesions on the radiographs can be questionable in some cases, depending on the experience of the person assessing the radiograph, localisation of the caries lesion, and type of radiograph (periapical, panoramic, bitewing, CBCT). Automated interpretation of the image with the aim to standardise diagnosis and optimise accuracy has been a research object in dentistry. Lee et al. evaluated the efficacy of CNN algorithms for detection of dental caries in periapical radiographs with rather high accuracy [35]. CNN systems were explored in the detection of caries lesions in bitewings. The research by Cantu et al. showed an accuracy of the system of 80%, while dentists' mean accuracy was lower (71%). The AI system was significantly more sensitive than dentists, while its specificity was not significantly lower [36]. The neural networks used in detecting and diagnosing dental caries were also assessed by Prados-Privado et al. in a systematic review. The way in which each of the studies analysed caries (definition, type, tooth), as well as the parameters of each neural network (type of network, characteristics of the database, and results), were studied. Unfortunately, under the conditions of these studies and variable parameters assessed, the authors could not reach conclusive findings. Not all studies have detailed how detected caries are defined and not all of them specify the type of caries. Each study included in this review used a different neural network. All these variabilities complicated the conclusions about the subject, the reliability, or absence of a neural network in the detection and diagnosis of caries. Then, a comparison between the neural networking and clinical dental results are obligatory [37].

There are limitations in this study. The evaluated group of 30 PR is relatively small, although it provides data for appropriate statistical analysis. The second limitation is setting the ground truth as the basis of three evaluators' reports. Furthers studies are needed in this field and authors of this research suggest involving a wider group of evaluators and performing analyses using larger samples.

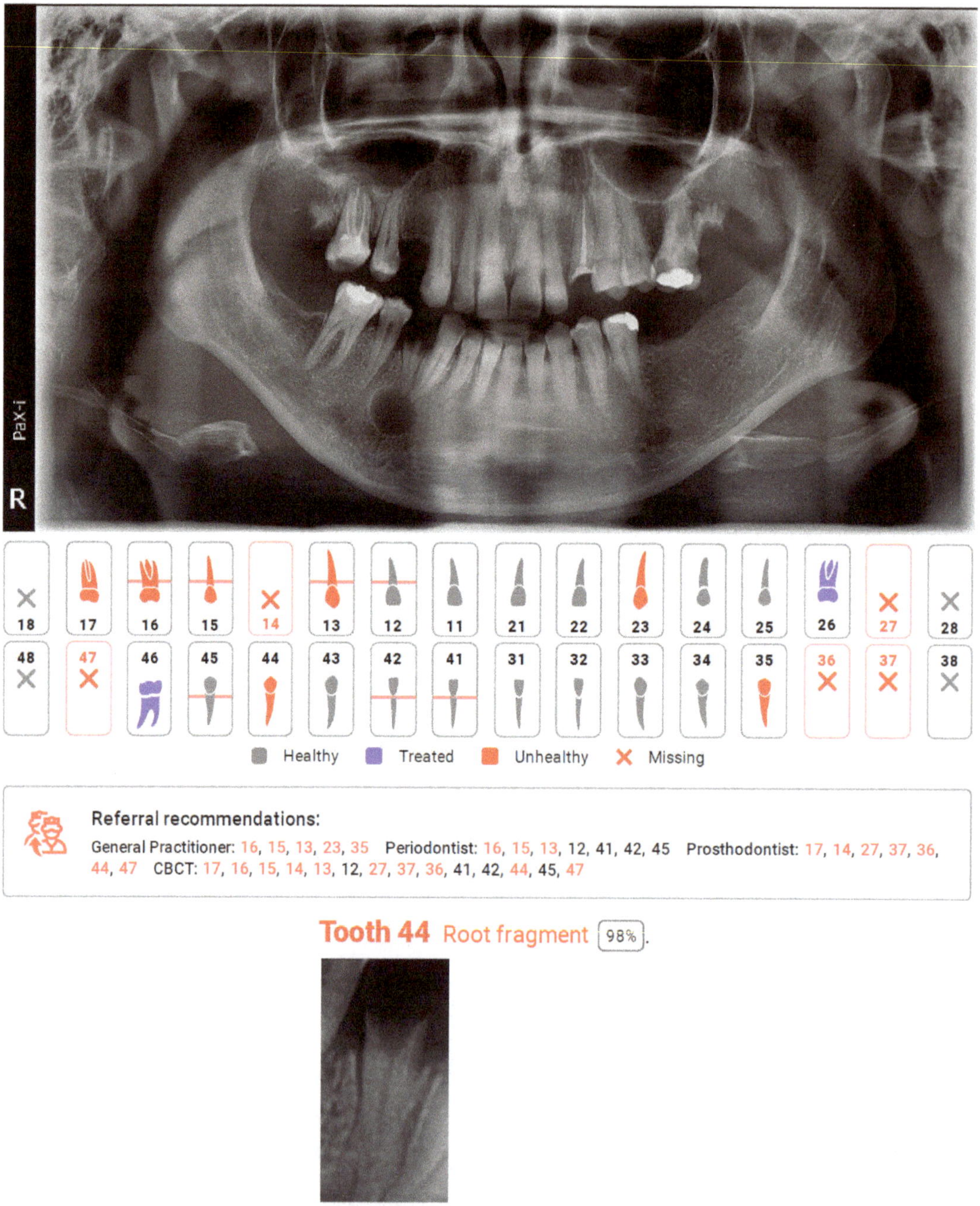

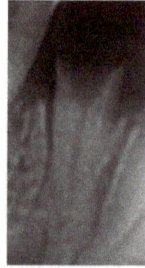

Figure 2. Diagnocat report, with missing detection of cyst connected with tooth 44, and automating caption of tooth recognized as a root fragment.

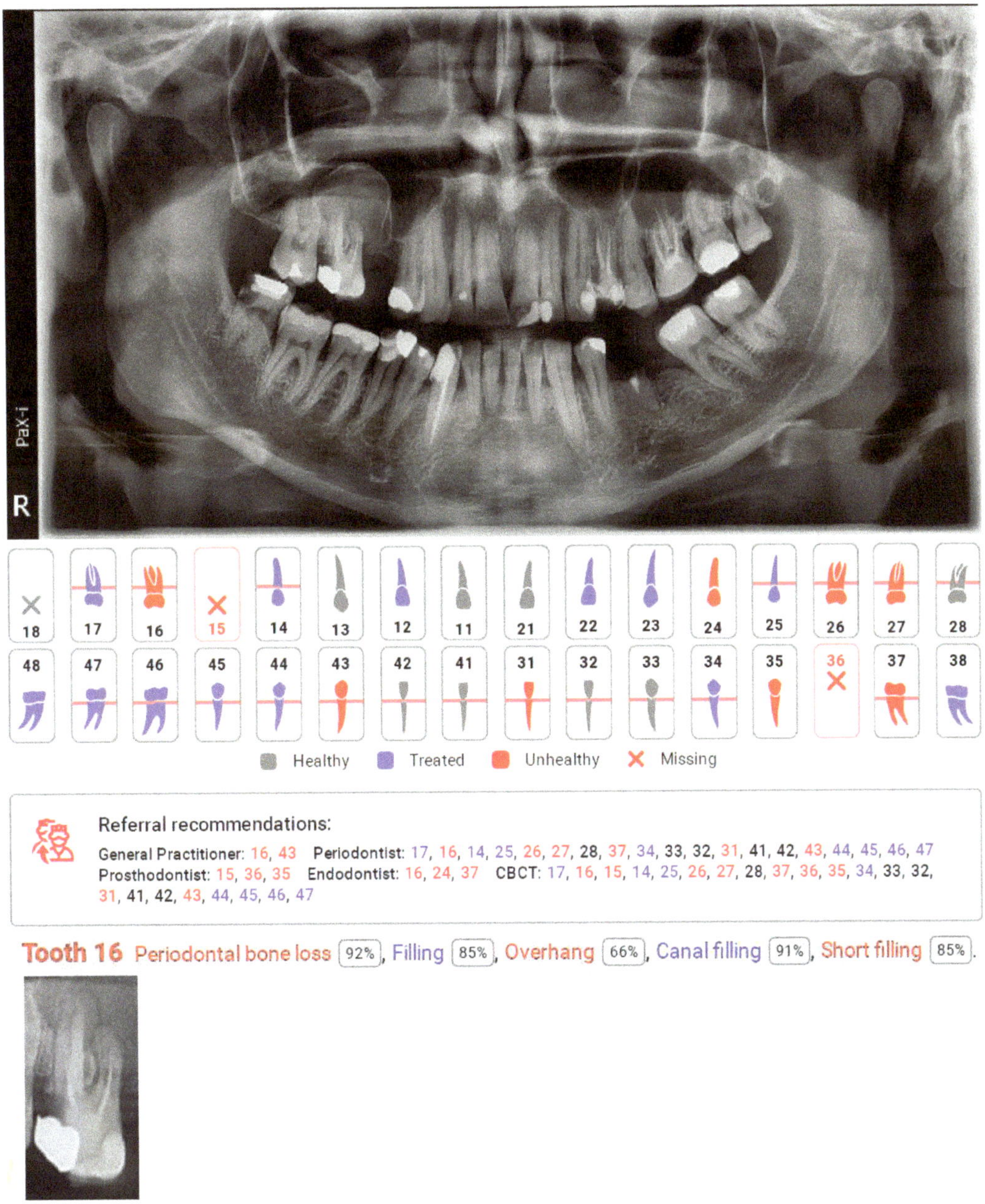

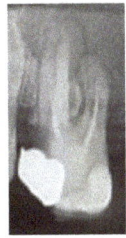

Figure 3. Diagnocat report, with missing detection of cyst in the right maxillary sinus in the region of tooth 16 and automating caption of tooth with detected other pathologies. Referral recommendations suggest additional CBCT diagnosis for this tooth as well as consultation with an endodontist.

5. Conclusions

Within the limitations of this retrospective study, we can draw the conclusion that the tested CNN based AI system can be helpful for an initial evaluation of screening PR for dental applications. Moreover, the report generated by the system refers to some potential pathologies to be evaluated by specific specialists or analysed with more accurate methods such as CBCT.

Author Contributions: Conceptualization, Ł.Z. and E.M.; methodology, Ł.Z., P.R. and E.M.; software, P.R. and L.P.; validation, Ł.Z. and E.M.; formal analysis, P.R.; investigation, Ł.Z., P.R. and K.B.-S.; resources, Ł.Z., E.M., P.R. and K.B.-S.; data curation, P.R.; writing—original draft preparation, Ł.Z. and K.B.-S. and E.M; writing—review and editing, Ł.Z., P.R., K.B.-S., M.C. and S.G.; visualization, Ł.Z. and L.P.; supervision, E.M. and S.G.; project administration, M.C.; funding acquisition, E.M. All authors have read and agreed to the published version of the manuscript.

Funding: This research received no external funding.

Institutional Review Board Statement: The study follows principles of the Declaration of Helsinki and was approved by the Ethical Comity by the Medical University of Warsaw, Poland. Approval code: AKBE 221/2021.

Informed Consent Statement: Patient consent was waived due to lack of possibility to identify participating patients (Ethical Committee by the Medical University of Warsaw, Poland; Approval code: AKBE 221/2021; Approval date: 13 December 2021).

Data Availability Statement: The data presented in this study are available on request from the corresponding author. The data are not publicly available due to privacy restrictions.

Acknowledgments: Authors would like to appreciate help and support of Piotr Nagadowski (Natrodent, Poland) and Evgeniy Shumilov (LCC Diagnocat, Russia) who instructed and introduced the application of Diagnocat software for research purposes.

Conflicts of Interest: The authors declare no conflict of interest.

References

1. Cosson, J. Interpreting an orthopantomogram. *Aust. J. Gen. Pract.* **2020**, *49*, 550–555. [CrossRef]
2. Vinayahalingam, S.; Goey, R.S.; Kempers, S.; Schoep, J.; Cherici, T.; Moin, D.A.; Hanisch, M. Automated chart filing on panoramic radiographs using deep learning. *J. Dent.* **2021**, *115*, 103864. [CrossRef]
3. Chan, M.; Dadul, T.; Langlais, R.; Russell, D.; Ahmad, M. Accuracy of extraoral bite-wing radiography in detecting proximal caries and crestal bone loss. *J. Am. Dent. Assoc.* **2018**, *149*, 51–58. [CrossRef]
4. Vandenberghe, B.; Jacobs, R.; Bosmans, H. Modern dental imaging: A review of the current technology and clinical applications in dental practice. *Eur. Radiol.* **2010**, *20*, 2637–2655. [CrossRef]
5. White, S.C.; Pharoah, M.J. *Oral Radiology-E-Book: Principles and Interpretation*; Elsevier Health Sciences: Amsterdam, The Netherlands, 2014.
6. Oz, U.; Orhan, K.; Abe, N. Comparison of linear and angular measurements using two-dimensional conventional methods and three-dimensional cone beam CT images reconstructed from a volumetric rendering program in vivo. *Dentomaxillofacial Radiol.* **2011**, *40*, 492–500. [CrossRef]
7. Farman, A.G.; Scarfe, W.C. Development of imaging selection criteria and procedures should precede cephalometric assessment with cone-beam computed tomography. *Am. J. Orthod. Dentofac. Orthop.* **2006**, *130*, 257–265. [CrossRef]
8. Scarfe, W.C.; Farman, A.G.; Sukovic, P. Clinical applications of cone-beam computed tomography in dental practice. *J. -Can. Dent. Assoc.* **2006**, *72*, 75.
9. Kobayashi, K.; Shimoda, S.; Nakagawa, Y.; Yamamoto, A. Accuracy in measurement of distance using limited cone-beam computerized tomography. *Int. J. Oral Maxillofac. Implant.* **2004**, *19*, 19.
10. Hatcher, D.C.; Dial, C.; Mayorga, C. Cone beam CT for pre-surgical assessment of implant sites. *CDA* **2003**, *31*, 825–834.
11. Miles, D.A. The future of dental and maxillofacial imaging. *Dent. Clin. North Am.* **2008**, *52*, 917–928. [CrossRef]
12. Kandelman, D.; Arpin, S.; Baez, R.J.; Baehni, P.C.; Petersen, P.E. Oral health care systems in developing and developed countries. *Periodontol 2000* **2012**, *60*, 98–109. [CrossRef]
13. Ralls, S.; Cohen, M.; Southard, T. Computer-assisted dental diagnosis. *Dent. Clin. North Am.* **1986**, *30*, 695–712.
14. Ezhov, M.; Gusarev, M.; Golitsyna, M.; Yates, J.M.; Kushnerev, E.; Tamimi, D.; Aksoy, S.; Shumilov, E.; Sanders, A.; Orhan, K. Clinically applicable artificial intelligence system for dental diagnosis with CBCT. *Sci. Rep.* **2021**, *11*, 15006. [CrossRef]
15. Hung, K.; Montalvao, C.; Tanaka, R.; Kawai, T.; Bornstein, M.M. The use and performance of artificial intelligence applications in dental and maxillofacial radiology: A systematic review. *Dentomaxillofacial Radiol.* **2020**, *49*, 20190107. [CrossRef]
16. Mahoor, M.H.; Abdel-Mottaleb, M. Classification and numbering of teeth in dental bitewing images. *Pattern Recognit.* **2005**, *38*, 577–586. [CrossRef]
17. Hosny, A.; Parmar, C.; Quackenbush, J.; Schwartz, L.H.; Aerts, H. Artificial intelligence in radiology. *Nat. Rev. Cancer* **2018**, *18*, 500–510. [CrossRef]

18. Chen, H.; Zhang, K.; Lyu, P.; Li, H.; Zhang, L.; Wu, J.; Lee, C.H. A deep learning approach to automatic teeth detection and numbering based on object detection in dental periapical films. *Sci. Rep.* **2019**, *9*, 3840. [CrossRef]
19. Estai, M.; Tennant, M.; Gebauer, D.; Brostek, A.; Vignarajan, J.; Mehdizadeh, M.; Saha, S. Deep learning for automated detection and numbering of permanent teeth on panoramic images. *Dentomaxillofac Radiol.* **2021**, *50*, 20210296. [CrossRef]
20. Ranschaert, E.; Topff, L.; Pianykh, O. Optimization of Radiology Workflow with Artificial Intelligence. *Radiol. Clin. N. Am.* **2021**, *59*, 955–966. [CrossRef]
21. Chen, Y.W.; Stanley, K.; Att, W. Artificial intelligence in dentistry: Current applications and future perspectives. *Quintessence Int.* **2020**, *51*, 248–257. [CrossRef]
22. Grischke, J.; Johannsmeier, L.; Eich, L.; Griga, L.; Haddadin, S. Dentronics: Towards robotics and artificial intelligence in dentistry. *Dent. Mater.* **2020**, *36*, 765–778. [CrossRef]
23. Kulkarni, S.; Seneviratne, N.; Baig, M.S.; Khan, A.H.A. Artificial Intelligence in Medicine: Where Are We Now? *Acad. Radiol* **2020**, *27*, 62–70. [CrossRef]
24. Loehfelm, T.W. Artificial Intelligence for Quality Improvement in Radiology. *Radiol. Clin. North Am.* **2021**, *59*, 1053–1062. [CrossRef]
25. Schwendicke, F.; Samek, W.; Krois, J. Artificial Intelligence in Dentistry: Chances and Challenges. *J. Dent. Res.* **2020**, *99*, 769–774. [CrossRef]
26. Shan, T.; Tay, F.R.; Gu, L. Application of Artificial Intelligence in Dentistry. *J. Dent. Res.* **2021**, *100*, 232–244. [CrossRef]
27. Steinkamp, J.; Cook, T.S. Basic Artificial Intelligence Techniques: Natural Language Processing of Radiology Reports. *Radiol. Clin. North Am.* **2021**, *59*, 919–931. [CrossRef]
28. Nardi, C.; Calistri, L.; Grazzini, G.; Desideri, I.; Lorini, C.; Occhipinti, M.; Mungai, F.; Colagrande, S. Is panoramic radiography an accurate imaging technique for the detection of endodontically treated asymptomatic apical periodontitis? *J. Endod.* **2018**, *44*, 1500–1508. [CrossRef]
29. Ekert, T.; Krois, J.; Meinhold, L.; Elhennawy, K.; Emara, R.; Golla, T.; Schwendicke, F. Deep learning for the radiographic detection of apical lesions. *J. Endod.* **2019**, *45*, 917–922.e915. [CrossRef]
30. Mol, A.; Van Der Stelt, P. Application of computer-aided image interpretation to the diagnosis of periapical bone lesions. *Dentomaxillofacial Radiol.* **1992**, *21*, 190–194. [CrossRef]
31. Orhan, K.; Bayrakdar, I.; Ezhov, M.; Kravtsov, A.; Özyürek, T. Evaluation of artificial intelligence for detecting periapical pathosis on cone-beam computed tomography scans. *Int. Endod. J.* **2020**, *53*, 680–689. [CrossRef]
32. Patel, S.; Wilson, R.; Dawood, A.; Foschi, F.; Mannocci, F. The detection of periapical pathosis using digital periapical radiography and cone beam computed tomography-part 2: A 1-year post-treatment follow-up. *Int. Endod. J.* **2012**, *45*, 711–723. [CrossRef]
33. Davies, A.; Mannocci, F.; Mitchell, P.; Andiappan, M.; Patel, S. The detection of periapical pathoses in root filled teeth using single and parallax periapical radiographs versus cone beam computed tomography—A clinical study. *Int. Endod. J.* **2015**, *48*, 582–592. [CrossRef]
34. Lee, J.H.; Kim, D.H.; Jeong, S.N. Diagnosis of cystic lesions using panoramic and cone beam computed tomographic images based on deep learning neural network. *Oral. Dis.* **2020**, *26*, 152–158. [CrossRef]
35. Lee, J.-H.; Kim, D.-H.; Jeong, S.-N.; Choi, S.-H. Detection and diagnosis of dental caries using a deep learning-based convolutional neural network algorithm. *J. Dent.* **2018**, *77*, 106–111. [CrossRef]
36. Cantu, A.G.; Gehrung, S.; Krois, J.; Chaurasia, A.; Rossi, J.G.; Gaudin, R.; Elhennawy, K.; Schwendicke, F. Detecting caries lesions of different radiographic extension on bitewings using deep learning. *J. Dent.* **2020**, *100*, 103425. [CrossRef]
37. Prados-Privado, M.; García Villalón, J.; Martínez-Martínez, C.H.; Ivorra, C.; Prados-Frutos, J.C. Dental Caries Diagnosis and Detection Using Neural Networks: A Systematic Review. *J. Clin. Med.* **2020**, *9*, 3579. [CrossRef]

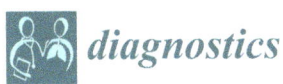

Article

Deep Learning-Based Microscopic Diagnosis of Odontogenic Keratocysts and Non-Keratocysts in Haematoxylin and Eosin-Stained Incisional Biopsies

Roopa S. Rao [1], Divya B. Shivanna [2], Kirti S. Mahadevpur [2], Sinchana G. Shivaramegowda [2], Spoorthi Prakash [2], Surendra Lakshminarayana [1] and Shankargouda Patil [3,*]

[1] Department of Oral Pathology and Microbiology, Faculty of Dental Sciences, Ramaiah University of Applied Sciences, Bengaluru 560054, India; drroopasrao1971@gmail.com (R.S.R.); drsuri29@gmail.com (S.L.)

[2] Department of Computer Science and Engineering, Faculty of Engineering and Technology, Ramaiah University of Applied Sciences, Bengaluru 560054, India; divyabies@gmail.com (D.B.S.); mkirtishankar@gmail.com (K.S.M.); sinchanagowda28@yahoo.com (S.G.S.); spoorthi.ambika@gmail.com (S.P.)

[3] Department of Maxillofacial Surgery and Diagnostic Science, Division of Oral Pathology, College of Dentistry, Jazan University, Jazan 45142, Saudi Arabia

* Correspondence: dr.ravipatil@gmail.com

Abstract: Background: The goal of the study was to create a histopathology image classification automation system that could identify odontogenic keratocysts in hematoxylin and eosin-stained jaw cyst sections. Methods: From 54 odontogenic keratocysts, 23 dentigerous cysts, and 20 radicular cysts, about 2657 microscopic pictures with 400× magnification were obtained. The images were annotated by a pathologist and categorized into epithelium, cystic lumen, and stroma of keratocysts and non-keratocysts. Preprocessing was performed in two steps; the first is data augmentation, as the Deep Learning techniques (DLT) improve their performance with increased data size. Secondly, the epithelial region was selected as the region of interest. Results: Four experiments were conducted using the DLT. In the first, a pre-trained VGG16 was employed to classify after-image augmentation. In the second, DenseNet-169 was implemented for image classification on the augmented images. In the third, DenseNet-169 was trained on the two-step preprocessed images. In the last experiment, two and three results were averaged to obtain an accuracy of 93% on OKC and non-OKC images. Conclusions: The proposed algorithm may fit into the automation system of OKC and non-OKC diagnosis. Utmost care was taken in the manual process of image acquisition (minimum 28–30 images/slide at 40× magnification covering the entire stretch of epithelium and stromal component). Further, there is scope to improve the accuracy rate and make it human bias free by using a whole slide imaging scanner for image acquisition from slides.

Keywords: dentigerous cysts; histopathology images; image classification; odontogenic keratocysts; radicular cysts; deep learning

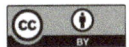

1. Introduction

Artificial Intelligence and machine learning has evoked interest and opportunities propagating research in health care. The newly developed automated tools that target varied aspects of medical/dental practice have provided a new dimension to translate the laboratory findings into clinical settings [1]. The automated tools act as an adjunct to a pathologist and meet the shortage of experts, which, furthermore, integrates experts of two disciplines, i.e., pathology and computer engineering. Although a pathologist provides a conclusive microscopic diagnosis to clinically challenging lesions, at times a pathologist may go for clinicopathological or radiographic correlation in case of inadequate biopsies [2].

However, if one focuses on the source and output, mere automation of images may not yield the desired results. Thereby, it is necessary to maintain the patient clinical details and follow-up data for a minimum of five years [1].

Pathology is the branch of medicine that deals with the microscopic examination of biopsied tissues for diagnostic purposes. The clinical diagnosis done by medical professionals mandates pathologist's consultations to tailor the treatment [3]. Thus, histopathology is traditionally considered a gold standard to confirm the clinical diagnosis.

A routine non-digitalized diagnostic pathology workflow involves procurement, preservation, processing, sectioning, and staining of the biopsied tissue to create glass slides followed by an interpretation [3]. The challenging cases are often consulted for multiple expert opinions. Other challenges encountered are ambiguity in diagnosis superimposed with inflammation, inter/intraobserver bias, etc. Although the diagnostic workflow is an exhaustive procedure, automation can ease out the pathologist's burden by providing a quick and reliable diagnosis [2].

The major Machine Learning challenges to analyze the histopathology images include (1) The requirement of a large dataset to analyze the histopathology images through machine learning algorithms. (2) Identification and assessment of biological structures such as nuclei, with varied shapes and sizes. (3) To detect, analyze, and segment tissue structures in the stroma, such as glands and tumor nests. (4) Lastly, to classify the entire slide image with stroma and epithelial cells [1,4,5].

Literature evidence shows that DL has been applied in analyzing images of major cancers such as breast, colon, and prostate affecting people globally, while rare diseases are seldom addressed by ML tools due to the paucity of data [2,6–8]. Furthermore, there are other wider applications of AI models in dentistry that are convolutional neural network (CNN) and artificial neural network (ANN) centric. These AI models have been used to detect and diagnose dental caries, vertical root fractures, apical lesions, salivary gland diseases, maxillary sinusitis, maxillofacial cysts, cervical lymph node metastasis, osteoporosis, alveolar bone loss, and for predicting orthodontic diagnosis and treatment [9,10], genomic studies of head and neck cancer [11], diagnosis and prediction of prognosis in oral cancer [9], and oncology [12,13], etc. Moreover, Majumdar B et al. (2018) highlighted the benefits of AI-based dental education as it can lower the cost of education and ease the strain on educators [14].

Odontogenic keratocysts (OKCs) are relatively rare jaw cysts that account for 3–11% of all jaw cysts[4]. It is found to be the third most common cyst in the Indian population. They are locally aggressive cystic lesions causing bony destruction of the jaws and root resorption of teeth [15–17].

A clinical feature that warrants its recognition as a distinct entity is an increased recurrence rate ranging from 2.55–62% and its malignant potential ranging between 0.13% and 2%. The high recurrence is a noted feature of OKCs in patients with nevoid basal cell carcinoma syndrome (NBCCS) [16]. Odontogenic keratocyst (OKC) was studied as a tumor to establish an impact of the reclassification and redefinition on the incidence of odontogenic tumors (OT) [18]. OKC may raise at any age [19].

OKCs have a unique microscopic appearance with 5–8 layers of para or orthokeratinized epithelium and a basal layer with tall columnar/cuboidal cells depicting a typical "tombstone" appearance with polarized nuclei, while other common jaw cysts (non-keratocysts), such as radicular and dentigerous cysts, account for 50% and 20%. Differentiating keratocysts from non-keratocysts is quite challenging with an absence of a unique microscopic appearance. Inflammation further complicates the microscopic evaluation. Rather location, dental procedures opted, or inflammation defines them [2].

The extent of the OKC lesion in the jaw, its aggressive clinical behavior, and high recurrence rate puts the clinicians into a dilemma with respect to therapeutic doctrine. Jaw cysts are frequently observed at dental institutes and are less frequently encountered by pathologists at medical institutes. There are no quantitative criteria in place which can eliminate the subjectivity bias and bring in more objectivity in the microscopic diagnosis of jaw cysts [2].

The treatment of odontogenic keratocysts remains controversial, with surgeons opting for conservative or radical approaches. Orthokeratinised keratocysts are treated less aggressively when compared to parakeratinized keratocysts and the associated syndrome. Clinicians continue to rely on their personal experience to opt for the most appropriate treatment.

Thereby, to resolve these issues, the study aimed to design a histopathology image classification automation system to diagnose and differentiate jaw cysts based on routine hematoxylin and eosin-stained slide images of incisional biopsies. This would deploy ML algorithms. This approach minimizes trauma to the patients and aids the surgeons to plan treatment management.

Here this study considered a relatively large image dataset of 2657 and each class had more than a thousand images, which is the basic requirement of the deep learning algorithm. The images were diverse. Thus, the proposed framework can be integrated into the automatic jaw cysts diagnosis system.

2. Materials and Methods

2.1. Tissue Specimens

Formalin-fixed (10% buffered) paraffin-embedded biological specimens that correspond to 54 cases of OKCs, 23 cases of DC, and 20 cases of RCs were retrieved from the archives of the Faculty of Dental Sciences, Dept. of Oral pathology, Ramaiah University of Applied Sciences. Next, 4 microns thick sections were cut and stained with hematoxylin and eosin (H&E). The patient's identity was concealed, while high-resolution images of microscopically confirmed cases of OKCs, RC, and DC were utilized for the present study. This work was approved by the Ethics Committee of Ramaiah University of Applied Sciences (Registry Number EC-20211/F/058).

2.2. Image Dataset

The dataset was obtained using Olympus BX53 Research Microscope with a digital Jenoptik camera and Gryphax imaging software. The images of the tissue specimens were of the dimension 3840 × 2160 pixel (px) and are saved in the jpg format.

Manually the images of the H&E-stained section of OKC, DC, and RC were captured at 40× magnification. The consistency of 30 images/slides could not be maintained, because pathological specimens differ from case to case. Furthermore, other factors, such as size, length, epithelial convolutions, and presentation of the pathognomonic features, do matter. This mandate exploring the entire stretch of epithelium. Those specimens with inflammation further bring about certain changes in the epithelium.

The manually obtained images were annotated by an experienced pathologist. Firstly, the jaw cysts were segregated into keratocysts and non-keratocysts employing the standard diagnostic criteria, as the keratocysts present with a distinct histologic appearance, such as parakeratinised squamous lining epithelium comprising of 5–8 layers of cells, while the basal cells are cuboidal or columnar, have elliptical nuclei, and are consistently aligned, resulting in a palisading pattern [20], while the non-keratocysts lack definitive histologic features. Inflamed keratocysts lacking typical epithelium, inadequate biopsies etc. were further classified as challenging ones.

Approximately 1384 images were of OKC and 1273 were images of the non-OKC class (where 636 were images of dentigerous cysts and 637 of radicular cysts). The images covered both the epithelial and the sub-epithelial-stromal components. Only a few cysts were completely devoid of epithelial components, consisting only of the fibrous or inflammatory stroma. 70% of the dataset was used as a training set, 15% as validation, and the remaining 15% as a test set (Figure 1).

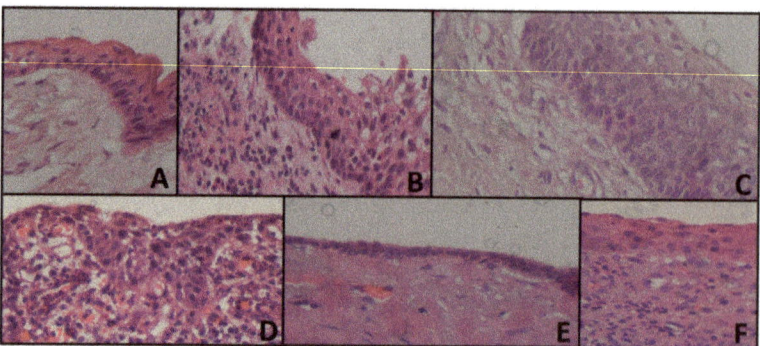

Figure 1. Representing histopathology images of the cyst (**A**) OKC with tombstone appearance of basal cells, corrugated epithelium without inflammation (**B**) Loss of classic appearance of OKC with underlying inflammation (**C**) Tombstone appearance, without corrugation with reversed polarity (**D**) Radicular cyst showing arcading pattern with inflammation (**E**) Dentigerous cyst, showing cystic lining without inflammation (**F**) Dentigerous cyst, showing inflammatory connective tissue.

2.3. Computational Framework

The computation mentioned in the algorithm was performed by using cloud computing environment Google Colab, GPU—Tesla K80, RAM 12 GB, personal computer (Intel$^{(R)}$ Core $^{(TM)}$ i3-4030U CPU @ 1.90 GHz) CNN was built with Keras.

Preprocessing

In the proposed framework preprocessing was one of the critical steps.

Step 1: Data-augmentation

In preprocessing, the dataset was augmented as the accuracy of DL algorithms increased with the increase in the number of images in the dataset. Data augmentation is a technique that assists machine learning programmers in significantly increasing the size of data available for training models.

Image Data Generator class was used for the dataset augmentation. The images size is set to (224, 224).

The data augmentation method is mainly used to get more images in the training dataset, so that we can improve the efficiency of the model and make it more generalized. This data augmentation will also help to overcome the overfitting problem posed by transfer learning. And this augmentation method only applied to the training set, and not on the validation, or test set (Table 1).

Table 1. Details of data augmentation Techniques.

Data Augmentation Technique	Value
Shear range	0.2
Rotation range	20
Horizontal flip	True
Vertical flip	False
Zoom range	0.5

The data augmentation methods used were as follows: Image shear is a bounding box transformation. Rotation of the image will be done by the rotation range. Image flipping is done by the horizontal flip and vertical flip. Zooming of the images is done by the zoom range.

The width-shift range and height-shift range arguments are provided to the data generator constructor to adjust the horizontal and vertical shift. For zooming of the images, the argument in the data generator class will take the float value. And the zoom-in operation will be performed when the given value to the argument is smaller than 1 and zoom-out will have performed when the value given is larger than 1. Table 1 shows the details of data augmentation.

Step 2: Region Selection

In the images two regions were majorly observed, the epithelial region and connective tissue region. The epithelial region of OKC had distinct features such as a palisading pattern of basal cells and parakeratinized surface which distinguishes from DC and RC, so here an attempt was made to retain only the epithelial region and remove the connective tissue region. The images were titled into nine patches, each patch of resolution 1280 × 720. The variance was calculated on each patch, the average was calculated over the variance values obtained, and the region with the variance less than the average was marked as connective tissue region. To confirm the connective tissue region, on the same patch, average intensity is calculated after converting into grayscale, then histogram was plotted for each patch. If the histogram had more values for the intensity above the average intensity, then this confirms the patch belongs to connective tissue. The confirmed patches pixel values were made zero. These tiles were concatenated again to get the original resolution (Figure 2).

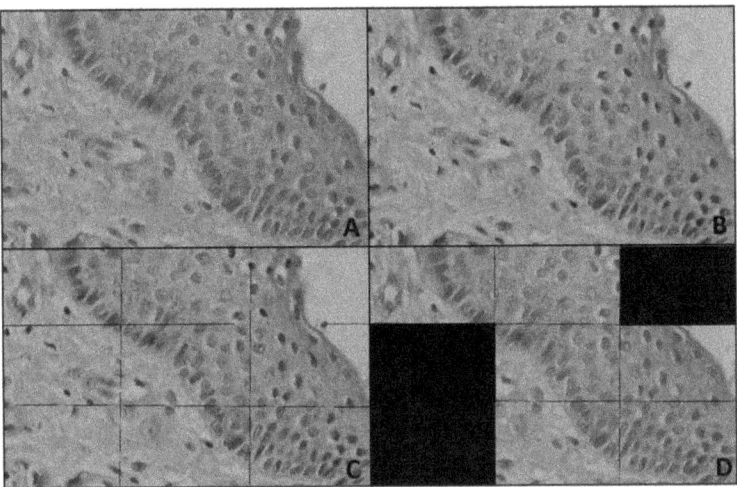

Figure 2. Representing preprocessing (**A**) Input image (**B**) Gray image (**C**) Titled gray image (**D**) Output of Preprocessing.

Region selection would have been achieved through an AI technique, such as semantic segmentation using Region CNN or UNet, where every pixel would be labeled to any of the classes, here, epithelial region and connective tissue region. These techniques needed massive, labeled data. Creating such labeled data, one should use a tool, such as the drawing pen tool of Photoshop or Adobe, to select the region of interest and label the pixels. This process would have been very time-consuming and tedious. Moreover, AI-based region selections, such as region-based convolutional neural networks or U-Net, were computationally expensive and need high-end machines. To make the developed technique usable for the public, these techniques had to be integrated with a desktop application, mobile application, or web application. In this case, the executable code may become too bulky to fit in the application and may take a longer time to execute and show the results. Therefore, in the present research, a very simple, computationally inexpensive, and very light image processing-based region selection technique was used.

2.4. Training of Convolutional Neural Networks

The experiment was conducted by training the comparatively simple CNN model VGG16 on the images with step 1 data augmentation and preprocessing.

The VGG model was developed by Simonyan with a very small convolutional in the network, as we know that it is a simple model, and it is a more widely applied model as compared to other models, because of its structure and the association between the convolutional layers. The VGG16 architecture has thirteen convolutional layers in the order Conv 1, Conv 2, Max pool 1, Conv 3, Cpnv 4, Max pool 2, Conv 5, Conv 6, Conv 7, Max pool 3, Conv 8, Conv 9, Conv 10, Max pool 4, Conv 11, Conv 12, Conv 13. This is followed by three fully connected layers with SoftMax as an activation function for the output layer. The Conv 1 and Conv 2 have sixty-four feature maps, which are resulted from sixty-four filters of size 3×3. Conv 3 and Conv 4 have a hundred and twenty-eight feature maps, resulting from a hundred and twenty-eight filters of size 3×3. Conv 5, Conv 6, and Conv 7 have two hundred and fifty-six feature maps, which are resulted from two hundred and fifty-six filters of size 3×3. Conv 8, Conv 9, and Conv 10 have five hundred and twelve feature maps, which are resulted from five hundred and twelve filters of size 3×3. Conv 11, Conv 12, and Conv 13 have, again, five hundred and twelve feature maps, which are resulted from five hundred and twelve filters of size 3×3. All the convolution layers were built with a one-pixel stride and one pixel of zero paddings. All the four max pooling's were done on a 2×2-pixel window and with stride 2.

Every convolutional layer will follow a ReLU layer and for sampling it has maximum pooling layers. For the classification, it has 3 layers that are fully linked for the classification, in which 2 serve as hidden layers and the last one will be the classification layer. The first layer had 25,088 perceptron's, the second had 4096, and the third had 2, as we were here performing binary classification of OKC and non-OKC.

Transfer learning is transferring the learned knowledge from a dataset by a network for solving similar kinds of problems on the dataset which has fewer instances in the dataset.

The belief in transfer learning is that the model trained on a huge and generic dataset may suit for classification of the dataset with a smaller number of images. One can use these learned feature maps, instead of training the model from scratch and in transfer learning, we have the privilege that we can consider only part of the model, or full model, as per our problem and we can take those considered part of the model weights to extract specific features from the dataset. Lower layers will be updated as per our classification problem.

In this work for the automation of OKC image classification, an already pre-trained VGG16 model was considered. VGG16 has 16 layers in total; the first thirteen layers are pre-trained on the data set ImageNet, which has nearly 1.2 million training images of 22,000 categories. The required image size for the transfer learning model is VGG16 ($224 \times 224 \times 3$). Only the last three layers were trained for the dataset in hand.

2.5. Experiment II

Experiment II was conducted by training the effective CNN model DenseNet169 on the preprocessed images with step 1 data augmentation.

Dense Net169 was trained on the given dataset. Dense Net is inspired by the study which showed that convolutional neural networks, which have short connections between the layers closer to the input layer than those which are closer to the output layer, are efficient to train and, at the same time, can grow deeper and have good accuracy. In Dense Net, each layer is connected to the other layer having the same feature-map size in a feed-forward manner. In the case of traditional networks, where the number of connections is equal to the number of layers, in Dense Net, the number of connections is calculated as $\frac{N(N+1)}{2}$ where N represents the number of layers.

This network architecture allows reusing the feature maps; it improves the information flow in the network through direct connections and reduces the number of parameters. The number of filters for each layer in Dense Net can be as small as 12. These densely connected links provide the effect of regularization which prevents overfitting in such cases where the training data are small.

Let y_0 represent an image, N is the number of layers in the network, Cn (.) is the composite function. The index of each layer is represented by n. Then, the input to the last layer is represented by Equation (1).

$$Y_n = C_n([y_0, y_1, y_2 \ldots, y_{n-1}]) \quad (1)$$

$[y_0, y_1, y_2, \ldots, y_{n-1}]$ is obtained by concatenating the feature maps from layers 0 to $n-1$. Cn is a composite function of three operations in the order: Batch normalization, ReLU, and 3×3 convolution.

The architecture of the Dense Net is divided into several blocks referred to as 'dense blocks. These blocks are separated by transition layers, which consist of convolution and pooling layers. This CNN captures the overall image features including the unique feature of OKC, separation between epithelium, and connective tissue region. This also helps in capturing the inflamed OKC, where the tombstone arrangement of basal cells was disturbed.

2.6. Experiment III

DenseNet169 was trained on the preprocessed dataset. This dataset was created by retaining the patches with epithelium layer in OKC and non-OKC (DC and RC) as explained in the preprocessing section. This CNN is trained to capture the regularity in basal cell arrangement (tombstone arrangement) and 5 to 8 layers of basal cell.

2.7. Experiment IV

The models trained in experiments II and III were integrated by averaging the resultant confidence scores to get the predicted output.

The overall architecture of experiment IV is as shown in Figure 3.

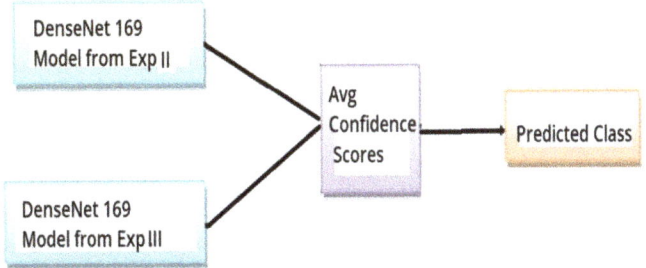

Figure 3. Overall architecture of experiment IV OKC classifier.

The optimizer used is the Adam optimizer, and binary cross entropy is the loss function.

3. Results

There were 1384 images of OKC and 1273 images of non-OKC; 15% of the images were used for testing the trained model. In total 207 images of OKC and 191 images of non-OKC were used for testing.

The loss function used in each classifier model discussed here is binary cross entropy. This is most used for binary classification problems. The formula for calculating the binary cross entropy loss or log loss is given by Equation (2).

$$\text{Loss} = -\frac{1}{N} \sum_{i=1}^{N} y_i \cdot \log(p(y_i)) + (1 - y_i) \cdot \log(1 - p(y_i)) \quad (2)$$

Accuracy is the fraction of several predictions done correctly by the model out of the total number of samples. The formula for calculating accuracy is given by Equation (3).

$$\text{Accuracy} = \frac{True\ positive + True\ negative}{True\ positive + True\ negative + False\ positive + False\ negative} \quad (3)$$

Precision is the fraction of several true positive cases out of the number of samples that are predicted positively by the model. The formula for calculating precision is given by Equation (4).

$$\text{Precision} = \frac{True\ positive}{true\ positive + False\ positive} \quad (4)$$

Recall is the fraction of many true positive cases out of the number of actual positive cases. The formula for calculating recall is given by Equation (5).

$$\text{Recall} = \frac{True\ positive}{true\ positive + False\ Negative} \quad (5)$$

The F1-score is the harmonic mean of precision and recall. The formula for calculating the F1-score is given by Equation (6).

$$F1 - score = 2 * \frac{Precision * Recall}{Precision + Recall} \quad (6)$$

ROC or Receiver Operator Characteristic curve is a graph that plots the true positive rate against the false-positive rates at different threshold values. This is particularly useful in binary classification problems.

A confusion matrix is a table that gives us a summary of the model's performance. The format of the confusion matrix for a binary classification problem is shown in (Table 2).

Table 2. Description of the confusion matrix.

	Actual Values	
Predicted Values	True positive True negative	False-positive False-negative

The macro-average gives the overall performance of the classifier. The macro average is the arithmetic mean of individual classes' precision, recall, and F1-score.

Weighted avg gives the function to compute precision, recall, and F1-score for each label and returns the average considering each label's proportion in the dataset.

3.1. The Training Phase

In the training phase the parameters given to the developed model were:

(a) 'Adam' optimizer

An optimization algorithm plays an important role in deep learning algorithms, as it is a strategy that is performed iteratively until an optimum solution is obtained. Adam optimizer is a hybrid of Adagrad and RMSProp algorithms to produce an optimum solution for a given problem.

(b) minimum batch size

Updating the internal model parameters would be tedious if done after every sample, so samples are grouped as batches and the model parameter is updated for these batches.

Batch size is a hyperparameter. Here, 11 histopathological images were grouped as batches.

(c) the number of training epochs

One epoch means the entire training dataset was used to update the internal model parameters once. The number of epochs is a hyperparameter.

(d) initial learning rate

The learning rate is also a hyperparameter. In the case of stochastic gradient descent optimization algorithm learning rate is the amount of the internal model parameter to change concerning the calculated error.

3.2. Results Experiment I

Hyperparameters such as the number of epochs and batch size are decided based on experimentation and comparing the results.

In experiment I the VGG16 model performed its best when trained for nine epochs with 12 as the batch size. At the end of nine epochs, the validation accuracy is 89.01% and test accuracy is 62% as shown in Figure 4.

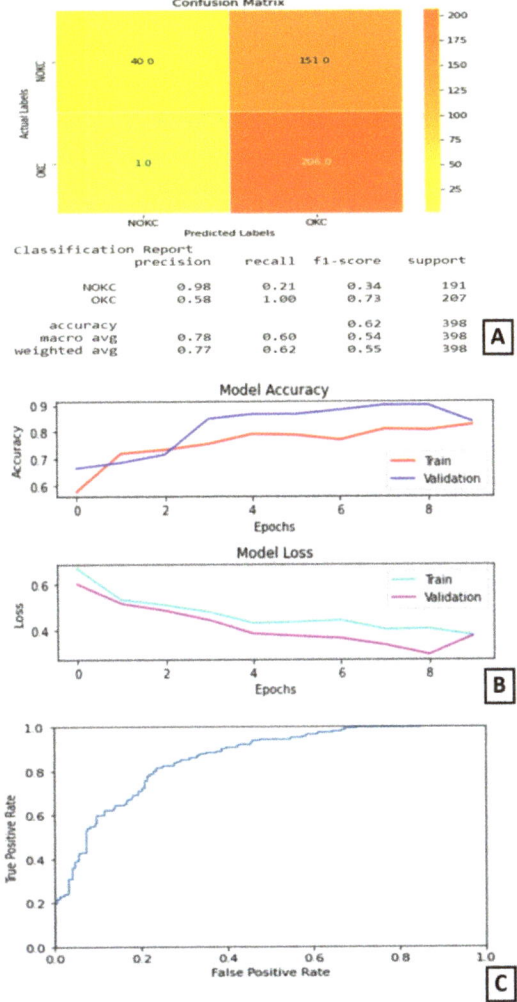

Figure 4. Results of Experiment I (**A**) Confusion matrix and performance metric (**B**) Training parameters (**C**) ROC curve.

3.3. Experiment II

In experiment II, only step 1 data augmentation was performed in preprocessing. That is, the CNN was trained only on the entire image.

In experiment II, the DenseNet169 model performed its best when trained for 15 epochs with 12 as the batch size. At the end of 15 epochs, the validation accuracy is 89.82% and test accuracy is 91%. The AUC for this model is 95.966%.

The plot of accuracy on training and validation data is as shown in Figure 5B. From this plot, we can find that the accuracy of the model for training and validation data converged and is stable at the end of 15 epochs, which indicates that the model is not overtrained and, also, did not overfit. The plot of loss on training and validation data is as shown in Figure 5B. From this plot, we can find that the loss of the model for training and validation data reduced as the training progressed. It converged after a few epochs and became stable later on. The confusion matrix and classification report are shown in Figure 5A. From the confusion matrix, we can understand that the number of true positives for this model is 181 out of 207 positive samples. The ROC curve is shown in Figure 5C.

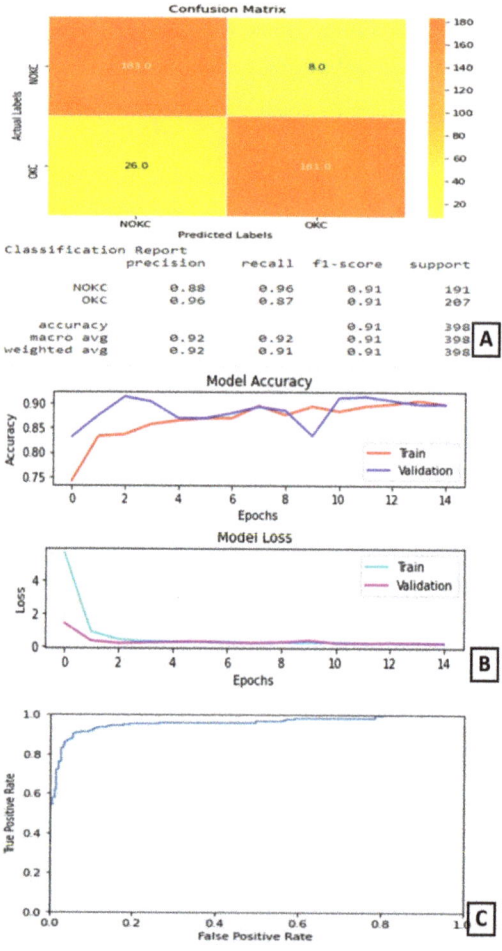

Figure 5. Results of Experiment II (**A**) Confusion matrix and performance metric (**B**) Training parameters (**C**) ROC curve.

3.4. Experiment III

In experiment III, both the steps were performed in preprocessing. That is, the CNN was trained only on the features of the epithelium.

On experimentation and comparison, Model-3 gave its best predictions when trained for 100 epochs with 16 as the batch size. At the end of 100 epochs, the test accuracy is noted as 91%. The AUC for this model is 96.375%.

The plot of accuracy on training and validation data is as shown in (Figure 6B). From this graph, we can observe that the validation accuracy is varying throughout the training, but, in the end, it stabilizes. The gap between the two lines shows some over-fitting on the validation data.

The plot of loss on training and validation data is as shown in (Figure 6B). From this graph, we can find that the training loss reduces in the first few epochs and then becomes completely stable. Similarly, the validation loss is almost stable with very little variation throughout the training (Figure 6B). The confusion matrix and classification report are shown in Figure 6A. On observing the confusion matrix, we can find that there are 191 correctly identified positive samples out of 207 positive samples. The ROC curve is as shown in Figure 6C.

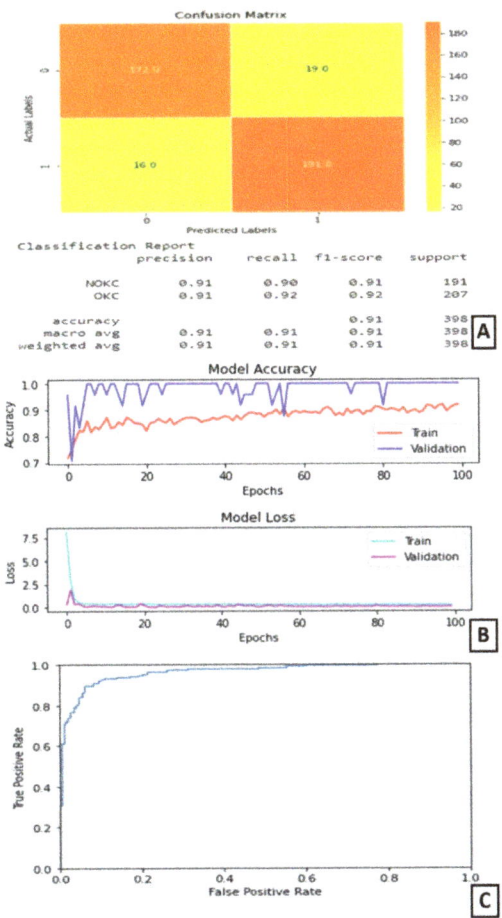

Figure 6. Results of Experiment III (**A**) Confusion matrix and performance metric (**B**) Training parameters (**C**) ROC curve.

3.5. Experiment IV

In experiment IV, the models trained in experiments II and III were integrated by averaging the resultant confidence scores to get the predicted output. The confusion matrix and classification report are shown in Figure 7A. The confusion matrix shows that this combined architecture has correctly identified 189 samples out of 207 samples belonging to the true class. The ROC curve is as shown in Figure 7B.

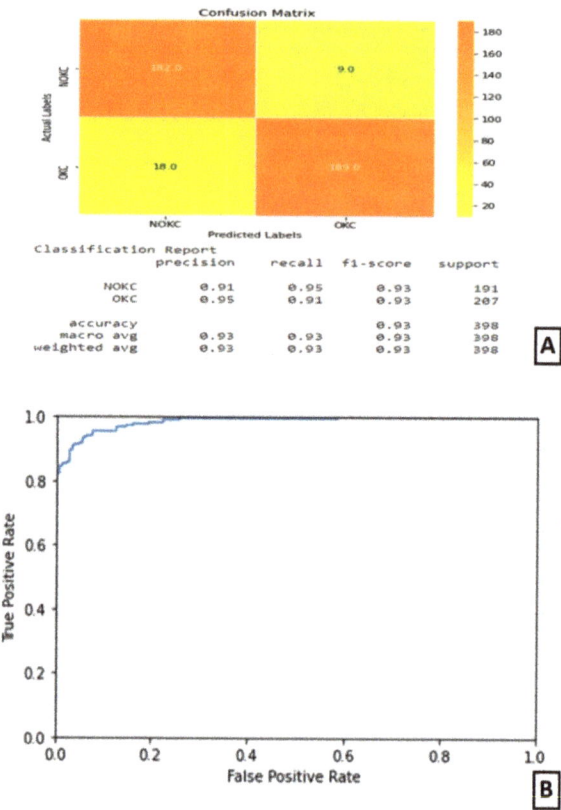

Figure 7. Results of Experiment IV (**A**) Confusion matrix and performance metric (**B**) ROC curve.

4. Discussion

The main features to look at in the OKC histopathology image pattern are thick epithelium, 5–6 layers of a regular arrangement of basal cells, also called tombstone arrangement, and the separation of epithelium and the connective tissue. On the other hand, DC has a thin epithelium layer with 2–3 layers of irregularly arranged basal cells and the epithelium layer is not properly distinguishable and has penetration into connective tissue in RC. The classification is more challenging when they undergo inflammation, the epithelium layer of DC becomes thick, which may be confused for OKC.

These images show large diversity within the class, posing a challenge for automation. Deep learning has shown promising results in the automation of digital histopathological image classification. Automation of digital histopathological image classification brings the standardization in the procedure, by eliminating the manual observation of the tissues under a microscope by the pathologists, which is completely subjective and suffers inter-laboratory variations.

In the proposed design, during preprocessing an attempt was made to select the epithelial region in the images. A Dense Net CNN was trained on these datasets to identify the features in the epithelium which distinguishes OKC from RC and DC. Another Dense Net was trained on the whole image to capture the separation of epithelium and the connective tissue feature. As the dataset had a limited number of images, transfer learning was adopted. The transfer learning approach results in better accuracy and reduced training time. Transfer learning is reusing a pre-built and pre-trained model on a new dataset. With transfer learning, we can reduce training time and get the best results even when many of data are unavailable. Both Dense Net CNNs obtained 91% accuracy over the dataset. An ensemble model of the Dense Net CNNs obtained an accuracy of 93%. Densenet169 was pre-trained on the ImageNet dataset only the last layer was trained for the given dataset. The problem of the OKC and non-OKC classification was addressed by using two CNN models. First, CNN was trained on the hand-crafted small patches of epithelium and the second on the whole image. They obtained a higher accuracy of 98% as they had a large dataset of 1704 OKC and 1635 non-OKC images [21].

The classification of periapical cysts (PCs), dentigerous cysts (DCs), ameloblastomas (ABs), odontogenic keratocysts (OKCs), and normal jaws with no diseases, considering the dataset for panoramic radiographs, were also attempted [22]. The classification performance of CNN for PCs, DCs, ABs, OKCs, and normal jaws for sensitivities, specificities, accuracies, and AUCs are: 82.8%, 99.2%, 96.2%, and 0.92 (PCs), 91.4%, 99.2%, 97.8%, and 0.96 (DCs), 71.7%, 100%, 94.3%, and 0.86 (ABs), 98.4%, 92.3%, 94.0%, and 0.97 (OKCs), and 100.0%, 95.1%, 96.0%, and 0.94 (normal jaws), respectively. The work process for assisting the dentist was analyzed, with emphasis on the automatic study of the cyst using texture analysis [23,24]. Keratocystic odontogenic tumor diagnosis automation is in the infancy stage [22]. A survey stated that feature retrieval for CNN accomplished fine-tuning in image classification [15]. The occurrence of several OKCs is one of the chief conditions for the analysis of nevoid basal cell carcinoma syndrome [25]. OKC lesions were commonly found more in females than males [26]. The recurrence of OKCs was in between five to seven years, but recurrence in the range of 12 to 102 months was also reported [27,28]. The management of OKCs did not accept any protocol [29]. An approach was proposed, known as the Bouligand–Minkowski descriptors (B–M), to evaluate the success rates based on the epithelial lining classification of these cysts using a histological image database [30].

The current investigation used H&E-stained sections on incisional biopsies, which are globally acknowledged, cost-effective, and time-tested. However, there are other ways to reduce the dataset by opting for immunohistochemical (IHC) staining specific to the nucleus. In the absence of a typical epithelium, in case of inadequate biopsy, the presence of non-keratinizing epithelium with basal palisading and an immunophenotype characteristic of OKC (basal bcl2, patchy or diffuse CK17, and upper layer CK10 positivity) may be consistent with the OKC diagnosis [31]. A basic nuclear staining approach like DAPI staining can be used to detect palisading patterns [2].

5. Conclusions

The hematoxylin and eosin-stained tissue specimens of OKC and NK were collected as a dataset. Two convolutional neural network models were trained on the region-selected dataset and the whole image dataset separately. These were ensemble by averaging their confidence scores, to give better accuracy. This architecture could be computationally expensive and may require a faster CPU to overcome. If IHC is opted for as a choice to reduce the dataset, utmost care must be taken on the economic viability while using IHC.

Author Contributions: Conceptualization, R.S.R. and D.B.S.; methodology, K.S.M.; software, S.L.; validation, S.G.S., R.S.R., and S.P. (Spoorthi Prakash); formal analysis, D.B.S.; investigation, S.L.; resources, K.S.M.; data curation, S.G.S. and S.P. (Spoorthi Prakash); writing—original draft preparation, R.S.R., S.L., D.B.S. and K.S.M.; writing—review and editing, S.G.S., S.P. (Spoorthi Prakash) and S.G.S.; visualization, D.B.S.; supervision, S.G.S. and S.P. (Spoorthi Prakash); project administration, S.P. (Shankargouda Patil). All authors have read and agreed to the published version of the manuscript.

Funding: This research received no external funding.

Institutional Review Board Statement: The study was conducted according to the guidelines of the Declaration of Helsinki, and approved by the Institutional Review Board (or Ethics Committee) of M S Ramaiah University of Applied Sciences (protocol code Registry Number EC-20211/F/058).

Informed Consent Statement: Informed consent was obtained from all subjects involved in the study.

Conflicts of Interest: The authors declare no conflict of interest.

References

1. Rashidi, H.H.; Tran, N.K.; Betts, E.V.; Howell, L.P.; Green, R. Artificial Intelligence and Machine Learning in Pathology: The Present Landscape of Supervised Methods. *Acad. Pathol.* **2019**, *6*. [CrossRef] [PubMed]
2. Sakamoto, K.; Morita, K.; Ikeda, T.; Kayamori, K. Deep-learning-based identification of odontogenic keratocysts in hematoxylin- and eosin-stained jaw cyst specimens. *arXiv* **2019**, arXiv:1901.03857.
3. Parwani, A.V. Next generation diagnostic pathology: Use of digital pathology and artificial intelligence tools to augment a pathological diagnosis. *Diagn. Pathol.* **2019**, *14*, 1–3. [CrossRef] [PubMed]
4. Chan, H.-P.; Samala, R.K.; Hadjiiski, L.M.; Zhou, C. Deep Learning in Medical Image Analysis. *Adv. Exp. Med. Biol.* **2020**, *1213*, 3–21. [CrossRef]
5. Hägele, M.; Seegerer, P.; Lapuschkin, S.; Bockmayr, M.; Samek, W.; Klauschen, F.; Müller, K.-R.; Binder, A. Resolving challenges in deep learning-based analyses of histopathological images using explanation methods. *Sci. Rep.* **2020**, *10*, 1–12. [CrossRef]
6. Schaefer, J.; Lehne, M.; Schepers, J.; Prasser, F.; Thun, S. The use of machine learning in rare diseases: A scoping review. *Orphanet J. Rare Dis.* **2020**, *15*, 1–10. [CrossRef]
7. Decherchi, S.; Pedrini, E.; Mordenti, M.; Cavalli, A.; Sangiorgi, L. Opportunities and Challenges for Machine Learning in Rare Diseases. *Front. Med.* **2021**, *8*. [CrossRef]
8. Brasil, S.; Pascoal, C.; Francisco, R.; Ferreira, V.D.R.; Videira, P.A.; Valadão, A.G. Artificial Intelligence (AI) in Rare Diseases: Is the Future Brighter? *Genes* **2019**, *10*, 978. [CrossRef]
9. Khanagar, S.B.; Al-Ehaideb, A.; Maganur, P.C.; Vishwanathaiah, S.; Patil, S.; Baeshen, H.A.; Sarode, S.C.; Bhandi, S. Developments, application, and performance of artificial intelligence in dentistry—A systematic review. *J. Dent. Sci.* **2021**, *16*, 508–522. [CrossRef]
10. Khanagar, S.B.; Al-Ehaideb, A.; Vishwanathaiah, S.; Maganur, P.C.; Patil, S.; Naik, S.; Baeshen, H.A.; Sarode, S.S. Scope and performance of artificial intelligence technology in orthodontic diagnosis, treatment planning, and clinical decision-making—A systematic review. *J. Dent. Sci.* **2021**, *16*, 482–492. [CrossRef]
11. Patil, S.; Awan, K.; Arakeri, G.; Seneviratne, C.J.; Muddur, N.; Malik, S.; Ferrari, M.; Rahimi, S.; Brennan, P.A. Machine learning and its potential applications to the genomic study of head and neck cancer—A systematic review. *J. Oral Pathol. Med.* **2019**, *48*, 773–779. [CrossRef]
12. Awan, K.H.; Kumar, S.S.; Sk, I.B.; Patil, S.; Raj, A.T. Potential Role of Machine Learning in Oncology. *J. Contemp. Dent. Pr.* **2019**, *20*, 529–530. [CrossRef]
13. Patil, S.; Moafa, I.H.; Alfaifi, M.M.; Abdu, A.M.; Jafer, M.A.; Raju, L.; Raj, A.T.; Sait, S.M. Reviewing the Role of Artificial Intelligence in Cancer. *Asian Pac. J. Cancer Biol.* **2020**, *5*, 189–199. [CrossRef]
14. Majumdar, B.; Sarode, S.; Sarode, G.; Patil, S. Technology: Artificial intelligence. *Br. Dent. J.* **2018**, *224*, 916. [CrossRef]
15. Latif, J.; Xiao, C.; Imran, A.; Tu, S. Medical Imaging using Machine Learning and Deep Learning Algorithms: A Review. In Proceedings of the 2019 2nd International Conference on Computing, Mathematics and Engineering Technologies (iCoMET), Sukkur, Pakistan, 30–31 January 2019. [CrossRef]
16. Augustine, D.; Rao, R.S.; Lakshminarayana, S.; Prasad, K.; Patil, S. Sub-epithelial hyalinization, incomplete cystic lining, and corrugated surface could be a predictor of recurrence in Odontogenic Keratocysts. *J. Oral Biol. Craniofacial Res.* **2021**, *11*, 423–429. [CrossRef]
17. Pinheiro, J.; De Carvalho, C.H.P.; Galvão, H.C.; Pinto, L.P.; De Souza, L.B.; Santos, P.P.D.A. Relationship between mast cells and E-cadherin in odontogenic keratocysts and radicular cysts. *Clin. Oral Investig.* **2019**, *24*, 181–191. [CrossRef]
18. Gaitán-Cepeda, L.; Quezada-Rivera, D.; Tenorio-Rocha, F.; Leyva-Huerta, E. Reclassification of odontogenic keratocyst as tumour. Impact on the odontogenic tumours prevalence. *Oral Dis.* **2010**, *16*, 185–187. [CrossRef]
19. Hadziabdic, N.; Dzinovic, E.; Udovicic-Gagula, D.; Sulejmanagic, N.; Osmanovic, A.; Halilovic, S.; Kurtovic-Kozaric, A. Nonsyndromic Examples of Odontogenic Keratocysts: Presentation of Interesting Cases with a Literature Review. *Case Rep. Dent.* **2019**, *2019*, 9498202. [CrossRef]
20. Shear, M. Developmental odontogenic cysts. An update1. *J. Oral Pathol. Med.* **1994**, *23*, 1–11. [CrossRef]
21. MacDonald-Jankowski, D.S. Keratocystic odontogenic tumour: Systematic review. *Dentomaxillofac. Radiol.* **2011**, *40*, 1–23. [CrossRef]
22. Kwon, O.; Yong, T.-H.; Kang, S.-R.; Kim, J.-E.; Huh, K.-H.; Heo, M.-S.; Lee, S.-S.; Choi, S.-C.; Yi, W.-J. Automatic diagnosis for cysts and tumors of both jaws on panoramic radiographs using a deep convolution neural network. *Dentomaxillofac. Radiol.* **2020**, *49*, 20200185. [CrossRef] [PubMed]

23. Vijayakumari, B.; Ulaganathan, G.; Banumathi, A.; Banu, A.F.S.; Kayalvizhi, M. Dental cyst diagnosis using texture analysis. In Proceedings of the 2012 International Conference on Machine Vision and Image Processing (MVIP), Coimbatore, India, 14–15 December 2012; pp. 117–120.
24. Banu, A.F.S.; Kayalvizhi, M.; Arumugam, B.; Gurunathan, U. Texture based classification of dental cysts. In Proceedings of the 2014 International Conference on Control, Instrumentation, Communication and Computational Tech-nologies (ICCICCT), Kanyakumari, India, 10–11 July 2014.
25. Borghesi, A.; Nardi, C.; Giannitto, C.; Tironi, A.; Maroldi, R.; Di Bartolomeo, F.; Preda, L. Odontogenic keratocyst: Imaging features of a benign lesion with an aggressive behaviour. *Insights Imaging* **2018**, *9*, 883–897. [CrossRef] [PubMed]
26. Chirapathomsakul, D.; Sastravaha, P.; Jansisyanont, P. A review of odontogenic keratocysts and the behavior of recurrences. *Oral Surg. Oral Med. Oral Pathol. Oral Radiol. Endodontol.* **2006**, *101*, 5–9. [CrossRef] [PubMed]
27. Zhao, Y.-F.; Wei, J.-X.; Wang, S.-P. Treatment of odontogenic keratocysts: A follow-up of 255 Chinese patients. *Oral Surg. Oral Med. Oral Pathol. Oral Radiol. Endodontol.* **2002**, *94*, 151–156. [CrossRef]
28. Ribeiro-Júnior, O.; Borba, A.M.; Alves, C.A.F.; de Gouveia, M.M.; Deboni, M.C.Z.; Naclério-Homem, M.D.G. Reclassification and treatment of odontogenic keratocysts: A cohort study. *Braz. Oral Res.* **2017**, *31*, e98. [CrossRef]
29. Titinchi, F. Protocol for management of odontogenic keratocysts considering recurrence according to treatment methods. *J. Korean Assoc. Oral Maxillofac. Surg.* **2020**, *46*, 358–360. [CrossRef]
30. Florindo, J.B.; Bruno, O.M.; Landini, G. Morphological classification of odontogenic keratocysts using Bouligand–Minkowski fractal descriptors. *Comput. Biol. Med.* **2016**, *81*, 1–10. [CrossRef]
31. Cserni, D.; Zombori, T.; Stájer, A.; Rimovszki, A.; Cserni, G.; Baráth, Z. Immunohistochemical Characterization of Reactive Epithelial Changes in Odontogenic Keratocysts. *Pathol. Oncol. Res.* **2019**, *26*, 1717–1724. [CrossRef]

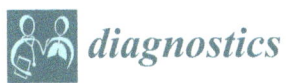

Article

Oral Cancer Discrimination and Novel Oral Epithelial Dysplasia Stratification Using FTIR Imaging and Machine Learning

Rong Wang [1], Aparna Naidu [1,2,†] and Yong Wang [1,*]

1 School of Dentistry, University of Missouri-Kansas City, Kansas City, MO 64108, USA; wangrong@umkc.edu
2 Oral Surgery and Pathology, Truman Medical Center, Kansas City, MO 64108, USA; aparna.naidu@tmcmed.org
* Correspondence: wangyo@umkc.edu
† Aparna Naidu was affiliated with University of Missouri during the time when the work was conducted, and she was affiliated with Truman Medical Center at the time when the manuscript was submitted.

Abstract: The Fourier transform infrared (FTIR) imaging technique was used in a transmission model for the evaluation of twelve oral hyperkeratosis (HK), eleven oral epithelial dysplasia (OED), and eleven oral squamous cell carcinoma (OSCC) biopsy samples in the fingerprint region of 1800–950 cm^{-1}. A series of 100 µm × 100 µm FTIR imaging areas were defined in each sample section in reference to the hematoxylin and eosin staining image of an adjacent section of the same sample. After outlier removal, signal preprocessing, and cluster analysis, a representative spectrum was generated for only the epithelial tissue in each area. Two representative spectra were selected from each sample to reflect intra-sample heterogeneity, which resulted in a total of 68 representative spectra from 34 samples for further analysis. Exploratory analyses using Principal component analysis and hierarchical cluster analysis showed good separation between the HK and OSCC spectra and overlaps of OED spectra with either HK or OSCC spectra. Three machine learning discriminant models based on partial least squares discriminant analysis (PLSDA), support vector machines discriminant analysis (SVMDA), and extreme gradient boosting discriminant analysis (XGBDA) were trained using 46 representative spectra from 12 HK and 11 OSCC samples. The PLSDA model achieved 100% sensitivity and 100% specificity, while both SVM and XGBDA models generated 95% sensitivity and 96% specificity, respectively. The PLSDA discriminant model was further used to classify the 11 OED samples into HK-grade (6), OSCC-grade (4), or borderline case (1) based on their FTIR spectral similarity to either HK or OSCC cases, providing a potential risk stratification strategy for the precancerous OED samples. The results of the current study support the application of the FTIR-machine learning technique in early oral cancer detection.

Citation: Wang, R.; Naidu, A.; Wang, Y. Oral Cancer Discrimination and Novel Oral Epithelial Dysplasia Stratification Using FTIR Imaging and Machine Learning. *Diagnostics* **2021**, *11*, 2133. https://doi.org/10.3390/diagnostics11112133

Academic Editor: Jae-Hong Lee

Received: 21 October 2021
Accepted: 15 November 2021
Published: 17 November 2021

Publisher's Note: MDPI stays neutral with regard to jurisdictional claims in published maps and institutional affiliations.

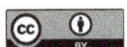

Copyright: © 2021 by the authors. Licensee MDPI, Basel, Switzerland. This article is an open access article distributed under the terms and conditions of the Creative Commons Attribution (CC BY) license (https://creativecommons.org/licenses/by/4.0/).

Keywords: Fourier transform infrared spectroscopy; FTIR imaging; spectral biomarker; multivariate analysis; machine learning; discriminant model; oral squamous cell carcinoma; oral epithelial dysplasia; oral potentially malignant disorder; risk stratification; early oral cancer detection

1. Introduction

Oral cancer refers to a subgroup of head and neck malignancies that affect the lips, tongue, salivary glands, gingiva, floor of the mouth, buccal surfaces, and other intra-oral locations. It is one of the most prevalent cancers worldwide, with especially high incidence in low- and middle-income countries. Despite easy access to the oral cavity and new management strategies, oral cancer is still characterized by high morbidity and low survival rates, which are partially due to late diagnosis [1]. More than 90% of oral cancers are oral squamous cell carcinoma (OSCC), which are a heterogeneous group of cancers arising from the mucosal lining of the oral cavity. Most oral cancer cases are associated with lifestyle habits including smoking, smokeless tobacco use, excessive alcohol consumption, and betel quid chewing. OSCC is 2–3 times more prevalent in men than it is in women, and its incidence is the highest in people who are older than 50 years of age. Genetic predisposition also plays an important role in the development of OSCC [2,3].

Oral carcinogenesis is a highly complex, multifactorial, and multistep process that can begin as hyperplasia/hyperkeratosis and can evolve to epithelial dysplasia, carcinoma in situ, and OSCC [4]. Most OSCC are preceded by asymptomatic clinical lesions that are referred to as oral potentially malignant disorders (OPMDs), which include leukoplakia, erythroplakia, reverse smoker's palate, erosive lichen planus, oral submucous fibrosis, lupus erythematosus, and actinic keratosis [5,6]. The clinical presentations of OPMDs can be further diagnosed as hyperplasia/ hyperkeratosis (HK), oral epithelial dysplasia (OED), or OSCC via histopathological evaluation. Epithelial HK are a benign overgrowth of cells in the oral epithelium. They may represent the initial stage of cancer development. OED is defined as a precancerous lesion in the oral epithelial region where cells exhibit atypia up to a certain level of the epithelium. The diagnosis and grading of OED are mainly based on the combination of architectural changes and the appearance of specific histological features [7]. An OED can be graded as mild, moderate, or severe based on the WHO's three-tier classification system. It has been estimated that 7–50% of severe, 3–30% of moderate, and <5% of mild OED lesions can transform into OSCC [8–10].

The gold standard WHO 2017 three-tier grading system for OED has some limitations, including subjectivity, inter- and intra-observer variations, and limited capability in predicting the malignant transformation risk of OED in individual cases [11]. Suggestions to overcome these limitations include the use of clinical determinants and molecular markers to supplement the grading system [12]. However, no single clinical-pathological predicting factor or molecular biomarker has achieved the clinical criteria for that purpose [13]. Accurate risk assessment and the effective management of OPMD and OED play critical roles for improving oral cancer survival rates and prognosis. Therefore, there is a need for new biomarkers or modern techniques that can provide objective and accurate OPMD/OED risk stratification for early oral cancer detection and prevention.

One promising technique is Fourier transform infrared (FTIR) spectroscopy. FTIR spectroscopy is based on the vibrational energy state changes of molecules after absorbing infrared radiation at certain frequencies. The unique absorption pattern of a sample produces characteristic bands in its FTIR spectrum. The FTIR spectrum for a biological sample provides a biochemical profile of proteins, nucleic acids, lipids, and carbohydrates in the sample, called "biomolecular fingerprinting" [14]. Not only can FTIR spectroscopy measure the relative quantity of a certain biomolecule, but it is also sensitive enough to probe subtle changes in molecular structure and microenvironment, such as the secondary structure of proteins, the mutation of nucleic acids, and the peroxidation of phospholipids [15–19]. It has been shown that FTIR spectroscopy can detect bimolecular changes that are associated with carcinogenesis much earlier than the appearance of morphological abnormalities, supporting its promising role in early cancer detection [20–22]. In FTIR imaging, each individual pixel comprises a full FTIR spectrum, and both the spectral and spatial information of the sample is integrated into a three-dimensional hyperspectral data cube [23]. Since the middle of the 20th century, FTIR spectroscopy and imaging techniques have been studied as label-free, non-invasive, highly sensitive, and specific analytical tools for the detection and characterization of malignancies in a wide variety of tissues, including skin, brain, breast, colon, cervix, lung, stomach, ovary, prostate, leukemia, lymphoma, and squamous epithelium [22,24,25].

In the field of oral disease research, FTIR spectroscopy and imaging techniques have been used to investigate oral cancer and precancer using a variety of biological samples, including oral tissues, exfoliated oral cells, biofluids (e.g., serum, plasma, saliva, sputum), and extracellular vesicles. Those studies provide early evidence for the usefulness of FTIR in oral cancer characterization and the differentiation of cancerous samples from noncancerous ones [26]. However, the number of published studies so far is still relatively small in this area, and more research is needed to better understand the promise of FTIR in oral cancer detection and the potential for clinical translation.

In the current study, we report an accurate discrimination of OSCC biopsy samples from HK samples using transmission FTIR imaging technique together with machine learning algorithms. Particularly, we introduce a novel classification strategy for OED samples based on their FTIR spectral similarities to either HK or OSCC samples for the first time. This novel classification strategy is easy to implement computationally and may provide a potential risk stratification solution to the malignant progression assessment of OED. The specific objectives of the current study were: 1. to develop an effective and practical method of generating representative epithelial FTIR spectra from formalin-fixed paraffin-embedded (FFPE) biopsy samples; 2. to characterize HK, OED, and OSCC samples based on their representative spectra; 3. to build machine learning models for discriminating OSCC from HK samples; and 4. to develop a novel strategy for classifying OED samples for potential risk stratification applications.

2. Materials and Methods

The overall flowchart of the experiment is illustrated in Figure 1.

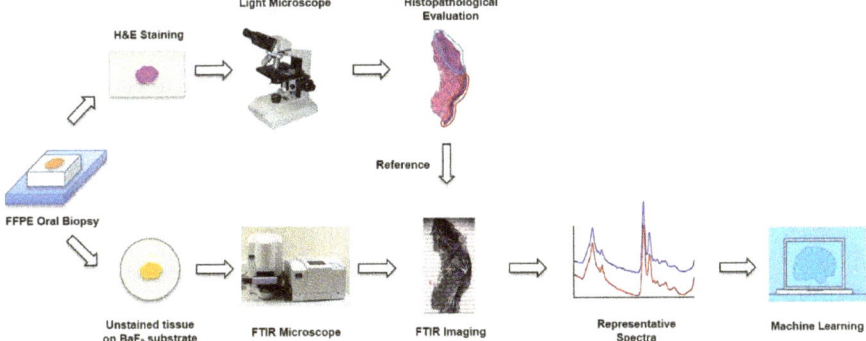

Figure 1. Flowchart of the experiment.

2.1. Sample Preparation

The current study received approval from the Institutional Review Board of University of Missouri at Kansas City (UMKC) for the use of archived human oral tissues. Specifically, 34 FFPE archived oral biopsy samples were obtained from the Pathology Department of the UMKC School of Dentistry, including 12 HK samples, 11 moderate-to-severe OED samples, and 11 OSCC samples. The samples were cut into 5-µm sections using a manual microtome (Leica RM2125, RTS, Leica Biosystems Inc., Buffalo Grove, IL, USA). One section was placed on positively charged glass slides for hematoxylin and eosin (H&E) staining and histological evaluation. The H&E-stained sections were imaged with a light microscope (Keyence BZ-X810, Keyence Corporation, Osaka, Japan), and the digital images were sent to a pathologist, who subsequently annotated areas of interest (AOI) based on histopathological evaluation. The annotated H&E images were then used as references for FTIR imaging. An adjacent tissue section was placed on a BaF$_2$ disc (REFLEX Analytical Corporation, Ridgewood, NJ, USA) for FTIR imaging. The tissue samples on the BaF$_2$ discs were deparaffinized through immersion in histological grade xylene (CAS number 1330-20-7, Sigma-Aldrich, St. Louis, MO, USA) for 5 min × 3 times at room temperature. The deparaffinized samples were air-dried and stored in a vacuum desiccator.

2.2. FTIR Imaging

FTIR images of tissue sections were acquired in transmission mode using a Perkin Elmer FTIR Spectrum Spotlight imaging system (Spectrum one, Spotlight 300, Perkin Elmer, Waltham, MA, USA). The Spotlight 300 imaging system features a dual-mode detector with a 1 ×16 narrow band mercury cadmium telluride (MCT) array and 100 μm medium band MCT single point detector operating at liquid nitrogen temperature. The following parameters were used for FTIR imaging: spectral resolution of 4 cm^{-1}, spectral range of 4000–950 cm^{-1}, pixel resolution of 6.25 μm, and co-adding spectra of 16 per pixel. Specifically, an overall survey image was first generated using the built-in light microscope in the FTIR Spotlight system for the sample section. Then, a series of 100 μm × 100 μm (16 × 16 pixels) imaging areas were defined in the survey image in reference to the diagnostic AOI in the corresponding digital H&E image. The diagnostic AOI was the sample region(s) that were used for pathological diagnosis. For example, if an OSCC sample consisted of hyperkeratotic region(s), dysplastic region(s), and OSCC region(s), only the OSCC region(s) were used as the diagnostic AOI. The imaging areas that were chosen were primarily in the epithelial regions for the HK and OED samples and in the invasive regions for the OSCC samples. Areas with poor tissue structural integrity were avoided to ensure high quality of spectra. The number of the imaging areas was mainly determined by the size and quality of each AOI. Right before the scan, a background spectrum was collected outside the sample area from the clean BaF$_2$ substrate to be subtracted from the single beam spectra for background correction. The imaging area size of 100 μm × 100 μm was chosen to ensure that there was enough tissue/cell content to obtain a local representative spectrum while limiting the acquisition time to ensure a valid background correction. FTIR image acquisition was performed using the Spectrum IMAGE software by Perkin Elmer. Figure 2 illustrates the FTIR imaging areas as described above.

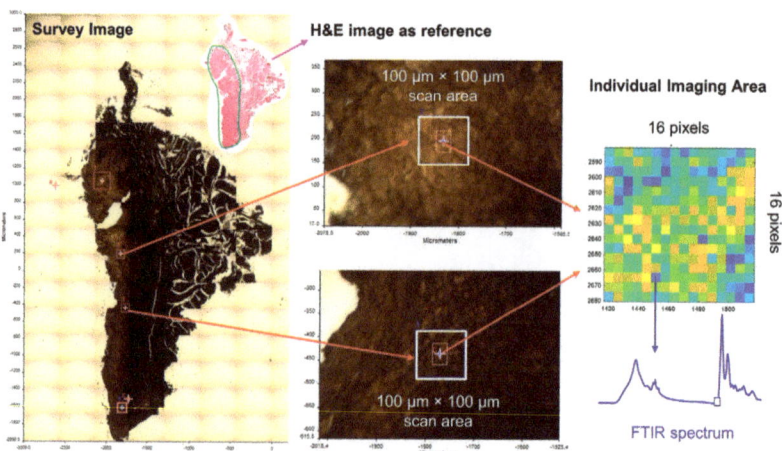

Figure 2. Illustration of FTIR imaging areas for a sample section.

2.3. Data Analysis

FTIR hyperspectral images are high-dimensional data containing thousands of variables (spatial coordinates and wavenumbers) for many objects (samples). An FTIR hyperspectral dataset holds an enormous amount of biochemical information and requires appropriate multivariate analyses to identify patterns and trends as well as to build classification models.

2.3.1. Spectral Preprocessing

All of the FTIR spectra were first preprocessed to remove or reduce biochemically irrelevant signal contributions from physical, macro-structural, and environmental factors. Spectral preprocessing can improve the accuracy of subsequent multivariate data analyses toward building better classification models. The data analysis was performed using the Eigenvector PLS_Toolbox software (Eigenvector research incorporated Inc., Manson, WA, USA) in MATLAB (R2020b, MathWorks, Inc., Natick, MA, USA). Specifically, the original hyperspectral image datasets were subject to the following general preprocessing: 1, transmission to absorbance conversion (A = log(1/T)); 2, selection of fingerprint region (1800–950 cm^{-1}); 3, Savitzky–Golay smoothing; 4, EMSC (extended multiplicative signal correction) for light-scattering; 5, automated weighted least squares (AWLS) baseline correction; and 6, vector normalization. The general preprocessing allowed the spectra to stay in their non-derivative form for easy observation and interpretation. Secondary derivative spectral differentiation (7-point window size) was used as an additional preprocessing step during model building.

2.3.2. Unsupervised Exploratory Analysis Using PCA and HCA

After signal preprocessing, unsupervised exploratory analyses were used to identify cluster patterns and data trends and to help understand the nature of the samples, including outliers and experimental errors. Principal component analysis (PCA) is the most widely used unsupervised multivariate exploratory analysis method for reducing the complexity of a spectral dataset by linearly transforming the original coordinate system into a new coordinate system defined by the principal components (PCs) that best explains the variance in the dataset. The PCs are orthogonal to each other and are generated in a decreasing order of explained variance. PCA decomposition uses the following form:

$$X = tp^T + E$$

where X represents the preprocessed spectra data, t represents the PCA scores, p represents the loadings, and E represents the residuals. All of the components are in matrix format, and p^T represents the transpose of the loading matrix p [27]. The PCA scores represent the variance in the samples and are used to detect clustering patterns related to biochemical similarities or dissimilarities among the samples. The PCA loadings represent the variance in the wavenumbers and are used to identify important spectral variables for the pattern observed in the score distribution [28]. The PCA loadings are often used for identifying spectral biomarkers that distinguish samples in different biological or pathological classes.

An observation of each individual image dataset revealed some outlier spectra, which were removed using PCA. Specifically, a reduced Hotelling's T^2 versus Q residuals scattering plot chart was generated by PCA. The x-axis (reduced Hotelling's T^2) is the sum of the normalized squares scores, which is the distance from the multivariate mean to the sample projection onto the PCA PCs space. The y-axis (reduced Q residuals) is the sum of squares of each sample in the PCA error matrix. The pixel spectra with high value in Hotelling's T^2 or Q residual or both were investigated and were subsequently removed from the dataset.

Some FTIR imaging areas contained both epithelial and nonepithelial (e.g., stroma) tissues. Unsupervised hierarchical cluster analysis (HCA) was used to separate epithelial spectra from other types of spectra. Due to the distinct spectral features of different tissue types, HCA was able to separate them at the highest or the next highest hierarchical levels. The pixel spectra corresponding to the epithelial tissue were selected and averaged to generate a representative epithelial FTIR spectrum for each imaging area (referred to as "representative spectra" later).

Multiple representative spectra were generated for each sample and were visually examined for quality check. Intra-sample variations of representative spectra were observed for some samples. To address this issue, two high-quality representative spectra from the diagnostic AOI of each sample were selected to reflect the intra-sample heterogeneity. As a result, a total of 68 representative spectra were selected from 34 samples and were consolidated into one combined dataset for further exploratory and discriminant analyses. Each representative spectrum in the combined dataset was labelled with a class ID according to its histopathological diagnosis (H for HK, D for dysplasia, and C for OSCC). The class average spectra for the three classes were compared for the visual identification of spectral differences. Additional exploratory analyses using unsupervised PCA and HCA were performed on all 68 representative spectra in the combined dataset to identify patterns and trends.

2.3.3. Supervised Discrimination between HK and OSCC Samples

Following exploratory analyses, discriminant machine learning models were built using three different supervised algorithms: partial least squares discriminant analysis (PLSDA), support vector machines discriminant analysis (SVMDA), and extreme gradient boosting discriminant analysis (XGBDA). PLSDA is a feature extraction and classification algorithm that is widely used for spectral data analysis. It is adapted from the partial least square regression (PLSR) technique, which aims to build a linear regression model using a latent variable (LV) approach to find the multidimensional direction in the X space that explains the maximum multidimensional variance direction in the Y space. The underlying mathematical model of PLSR is:

$$X = tp^T + E$$
$$Y = uq^T + F$$

in which X and Y are the observable variable matrix and predicted variable matrix, respectively; t and u represent projected scores of X and Y; p and q represent orthogonal loading matrices for the projected X and Y scores; and E and F are the error terms. When the predicted variables Y are categorical, such as in the current study (e.g., HK and OSCC classes), it becomes a discriminant technique called PLSDA. The PLSDA model is applied to X, reducing the original observable variables to a small number of LVs, which are linear combinations of the original variables that attempt to explain the maximum covariance between X and Y. Then, a linear discriminant classifier is used for classifying the samples [29]. PLSDA is an effective and powerful method for spectral data classification. It works well when high dimensionality and high collinearity are present in small-sample data, such as in the case in the current study. However, its performance may be subject to degradation under complex conditions such as nonlinearity, class imbalance, and multiclass [30]. An SVM is a binary linear classifier with a non-linear step called the kernel transformation [31]. A kernel function can transform the input spectral space into a feature space by applying a non-linear mathematical transformation. Then, a linear decision boundary is fit between the closest samples to the border of each class (called support vectors) and is used for determining the class memberships of new samples. In the current study, the radial basis function (RBF) kernel was used in SVM modeling. SVMDA is an effective algorithm for high dimensional spaces, especially when the number of dimensions is greater than the number of samples. With its kernel function, it can handle some non-linearity in the data. However, it is more time consuming and more susceptible to overfitting compared to PLSDA. The third algorithm XGBDA is an implementation of gradient boosted decision trees, that produces a prediction model in the form of an ensemble of weak prediction models, typically decision trees [32]. It is used in Kaggle competition and has shown superior efficiency and high prediction accuracy. The XGBDA algorithm is a class of lifting algorithm composes of a series of base classifiers. The original dataset is divided into multiple sub-datasets, and each sub-dataset is randomly assigned to the base classifier for classification/prediction. The results from the weak base classifiers are combined based on a certain weight, generating a final result for the XGBDA [33]. The advantages of XGBDA include its ability to handle non-linear parameters better than PLSDA and SVM and its robustness to outliers. On the other hand, XGBDA has a tendency for overfitting, and its performance for spectral data analysis has not been widely tested. It would be interesting to compare it with the commonly used PLSDA and SVMDA in the current study.

2.3.4. A novel Strategy for OED Classification

Based on the results from the exploratory analyses, a novel strategy was developed for discriminant analysis. Specifically, in the first phase, 46 representative spectra from 12 HK samples and 11 OSCC samples were used as training data to build the discriminant models. Due to the relatively small sample size, venetian blind (10-fold with 2 spectra from the same sample per blind) cross-validation was used for model performance optimization and evaluation. The model performance was evaluated using receiver operating characteristic curves (ROC curves), area under the curve (AUC), and sensitivity and specificity. A confusion matrix provides information for true positive (TP), false positive (FP), true negative (TN), and false negative (FN). Sensitivity is defined as the probability of achieving a positive test result in subjects with the disease and can be calculated by TP/(TP + FN). Specificity is defined as the probability of obtaining a negative test result in subjects without the disease and can be calculated by TN/(TN + FP) [34]. In the second phase, the performances of the three discriminant models were compared, and the best performing model was further used to classify the 22 representative spectra from the 11 OED samples.

3. Results

Figure 3 compares the class-average spectra for the HK, OED, and OSCC samples. Specifically, the class average spectra were calculated from 24 representative spectra of HK samples (green), 22 representative spectra of OED samples (blue), and 22 representative spectra of OSCC samples (red), respectively. Based on visual observation, the spectral differences are mainly located in four spectral regions: the region around 1650 cm^{-1}, the region of 1600–1500 cm^{-1}, the region of 1350–1180 cm^{-1}, and the region of 1160–950 cm^{-1}. The 1650 cm^{-1} band is the amide I band of protein, which is mainly associated with the C=O stretching vibration in the peptide backbone structure [35]. The results show a descending band intensity in the order of HK > OED > OSCC for the amide I band. The 1600–1500 cm^{-1} region is the amide II band of the protein, which is mainly associated with the bending vibration of the N-H bond and the stretching vibration of the C-N bond in the peptide backbone [35]. The results show a descending band intensity at 1548 cm^{-1} in the order of HK > OED > OSCC and a red shift toward lower wavenumbers on the right shoulder of the amide II band for the OSCC and OED spectra (more shift for OSCC than OED). The spectral region of 1350–1180 cm^{-1} can be attributed to the amide III band of protein (1350–1250 cm^{-1}), which is mainly from N-H bending and C-N stretching vibration, to the asymmetric vibration of $-PO_2^-$ (1240 cm^{-1}), and to the deformational modes of the CH_3/CH_2 groups in phospholipid and nuclei acids [36,37]. The results show a descending band intensity at 1310 cm^{-1} in the order of HK > OED > OSCC and at 1240 cm^{-1} in the order of OSCC > OED > HK. The spectral region of 1160–950 cm^{-1} can be attributed to the stretching vibrations of the C–O/C–C groups in the carbohydrate (e.g., glycogen) (1154 and 1030 cm^{-1}) and to the symmetric vibration of $-PO_2^-$ in the phospholipid and nucleic acids (1080 cm^{-1}) [14,38]. The results show a descending band intensity in this region in the order of OSCC > OED > HK.

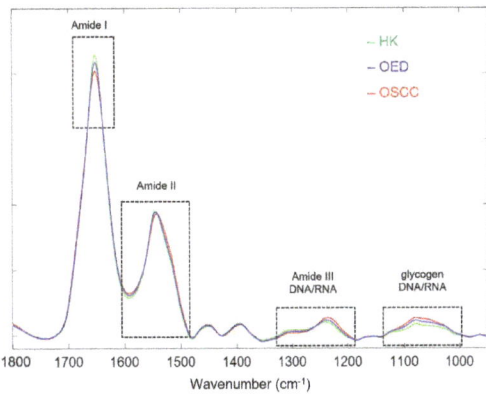

Figure 3. Three class-average spectra after general preprocessing for HK (green), OED (blue), and OSCC (red) samples, with visible spectral differences highlighted in dashed boxes.

Figure 4 shows the exploratory analysis results for all 68 representative spectra. (a-1) shows the reduced Hotelling T^2 versus Q residuals graph of PCA; (a-2) shows the score plot for PC1 and PC2; and (b) shows the HCA dendrogram graph. Both the PCA and HCA results showed good but not ideal separation between the HK and OSCC representative spectra. The OED representative spectra overlap with both the HK and OSCC representative spectra.

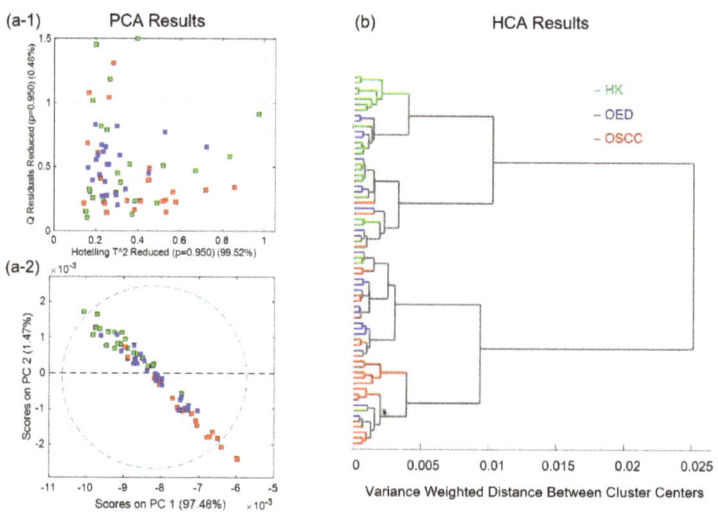

Figure 4. Unsupervised analysis results for all 68 representative spectra in the combined dataset: (**a-1**) Reduced Hotelling T^2 versus Q residuals graph of principle component analysis (PCA), and (**a-2**) score plot for principal components (PC1 and PC2) of PCA; (**b**) dendrogram graph of hierarchical cluster analysis (HCA).

Figure 5 summarizes the cross-validation performances of the three machine learning models built in the current study (PLSDA, SVMDA, and XGBDA) for discriminating the OSCC from HK samples. The PLSDA model showed a 100% sensitivity and 100% specificity, while both the SVMDA and the XGBDA models showed 95% sensitivities and 96% specificities.

	Model Cross-Validation Results							
	PLSDA Model			SVMDA Model			XGBDA Model		
Diagnostic Results		HK	OSCC		HK	OSCC		HK	OSCC
	HK	22	0	HK	23	1	HK	23	1
	OSCC	0	24	OSCC	1	21	OSCC	1	21
	Sensitivity = 100%			Sensitivity = 95%			Sensitivity = 95%		
	Specificity = 100%			Specificity = 96%			Specificity = 96%		

Figure 5. Cross-validation performances of three machine learning models for discriminating OSCC from HK samples. PLSDA—partial least square discriminant analysis, SVMDA—support vector machine discriminant analysis, and XGBDA—extreme gradient boosting discriminant analysis.

Figure 6a shows the average modeling errors on the y-axis versus the number of latent variables (LV) on the x-axis for the PLSDA model. Both the average classification errors for the calibration (orange curve) and cross-validation (blue curve) were displayed. The optimal number of latent variables was chosen to be four to minimize both errors. Figure 6b shows the loadings of the four chosen LVs for the PLSDA model. The loadings of LV1, LV2, LV3, and LV4 explain 94.50%, 4.48%, 0.38%, and 0.29% of the spectral variations between the HK and OSCC samples, respectively. Particularly, the loading of LV1 shows several prominent bands at 1670 (−), 1654 (+), 1548 (+),1516 (+), 1482 (−), 1238 (+), 1082 (+), 1026 (+), and 966 (+) cm^{-1}, and the loading of LV2 shows several prominent bands at 1704 (+), 1660 (−), 1640 (−), and 1482 (+), where "+" indicates positive bands and "−" indicates negative bands. Table 1 summarizes the 12 feature bands that were extracted from the top two loadings (LV1 and LV2) of the PLSDA model and their corresponding vibrational modes and biochemical assignment. Those bands are considered spectral biomarkers for discriminating OSCC from HK samples.

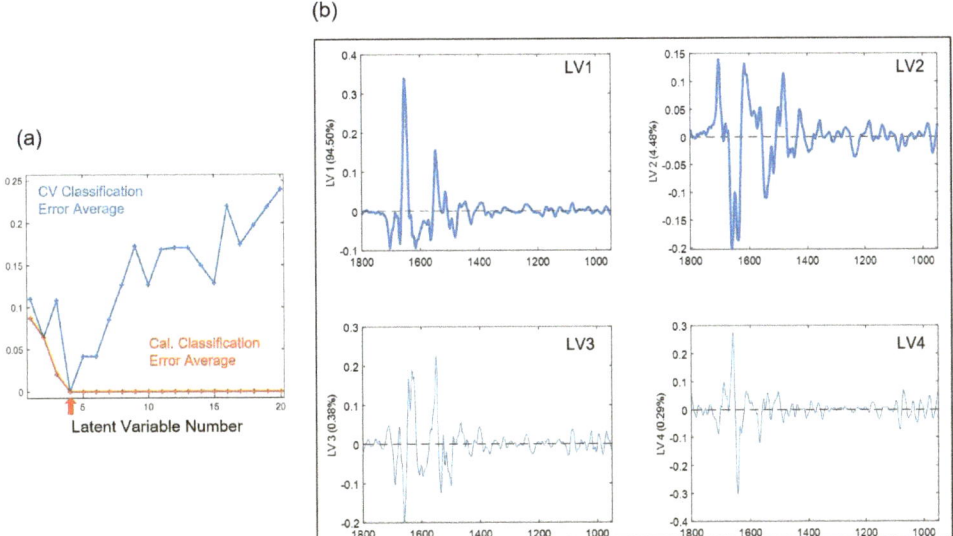

Figure 6. (a) Average calibration (Cal.) and cross-validation (CV) modeling errors versus the number of latent variables (LV) and (b) four chosen latent variable loadings (LV1–LV4) for the partial least square discriminant analysis (PLSDA) model.

Table 1. Spectral biomarkers identified using feature selection of the PLSDA model for discriminating OSCC from HK samples and their corresponding vibrational modes and biochemical assignments [14,39].

Wavenumber (cm^{-1})	Vibrational Modes and Biochemical Assignments
1704	Ester carbonyl C=O stretching, fatty acid esters, lipids
1670	Amide I, secondary structure of proteins
1660	Amide I, secondary structure of proteins
1654	C=O stretching of amide I, secondary structure of proteins,
1640	Amide I, secondary structure of proteins
1548	C-N and CN-H stretching of amide II, secondary structure of proteins
1516	Amide II, secondary structure of proteins
1482	deformation vibrations of –CH$_3$, lipid
1238	Asymmetric phosphodiester stretching ν_{as} (–PO$_2^-$), lipid, nuclei acid, amide III (C-N stretching, N-H bending) proteins
1082	Symmetric phosphodiester stretching ν_s (–PO$_2^-$), protein phosphorylation, phospholipids, collagen, DNA
1026	Vibrational frequency of -CH$_2$OH groups of carbohydrates (e.g., glucose, glycogen, etc.) C-O stretching, C-O stretching coupled with C-O bending of the C-OH groups of carbohydrates
966	C-O stretching of the phosphodiester, deoxyribose, C-C of DNA

Figure 7 shows (a) the ROC curves and AUC values, (b) the sensitivity and specificity curves, and (c) the confusion matrix for the PLSDA model. The AUC for calibration and cross-validation were both 1, and the sensitivity and specificity were both 100% at a threshold of 0.5 for the HK and OSCC samples. The results indicate a perfect discriminant model for the experimental HK and OSCC spectral data.

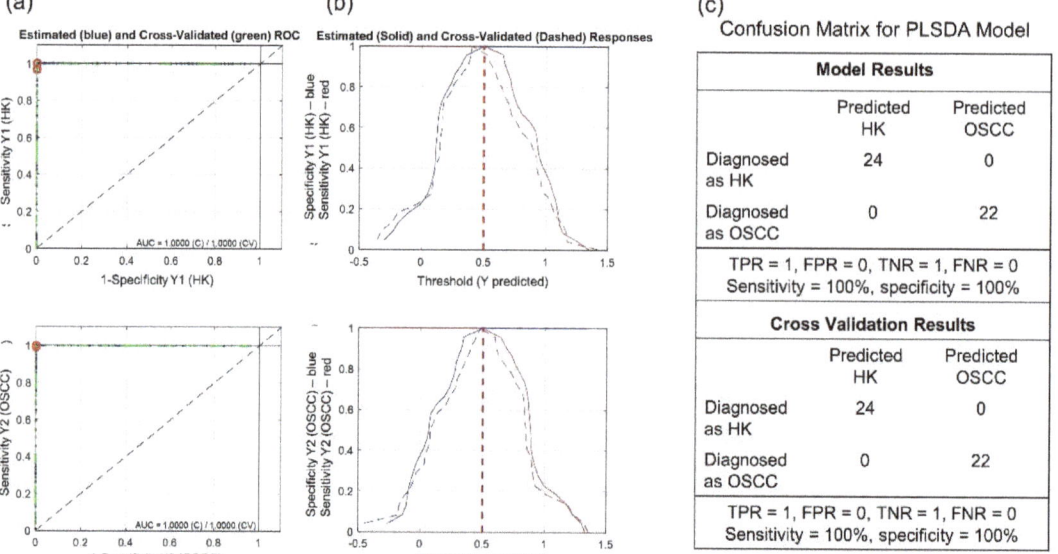

Figure 7. (a) Receiver operating characteristic (ROC) curves with area under the curve (AUC) values (AUC = 1); (b) sensitivity and specificity curves vs. threshold; and (c) confusion matrix for the partial least square discriminant analysis (PLSDA) model. TPR is true positive ratio, FPR is false positive ratio, TNR is true negative ratio, and FNR is false negative ratio.

Figure 8a shows the PLSDA model score plot for the top three latent variables (LV1–LV3) for all 68 representative spectra. Figure 8b visually summarizes the discrimination results for all 34 samples. The dashed purple line in the middle is the discrimination line of the PLSDA model. Two representative spectra connected with a solid line came from the same sample—a longer line suggests higher intra-sample spectral heterogeneity, while a shorter line suggests lower intra-sample spectral heterogeneity. The results show a complete discrimination between all of the HK samples and OSCC samples. For the OED samples, D-2, D-3, D-5, D-7, D-9, and D-11 were classified as "HK-grade", indicating more spectral similarities between the six OED samples and the HK samples; D-1, D-4, D-6, and D-8 were classified as "OSCC-grade", indicating more spectral similarities between the four OED samples and the OSCC samples. The two representative spectra of the sample D-10 were located in the vicinity of both sides of the discrimination line, indicating a borderline classification case.

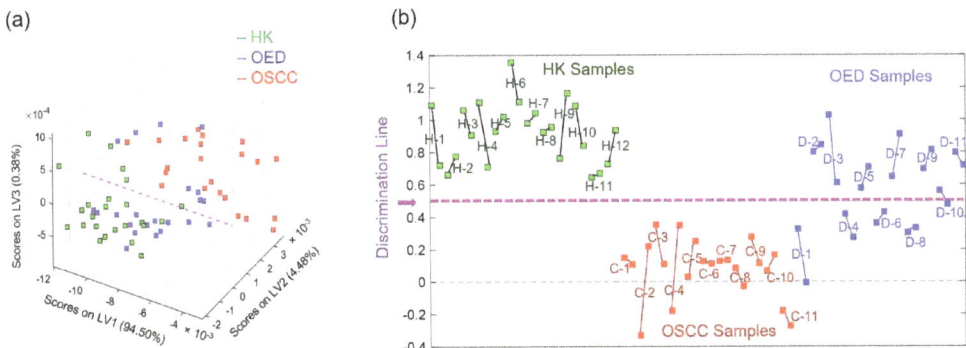

Figure 8. (a) Score plot for the top three latent variables (LV1–LV3) of the partial least square discriminant analysis (PLSDA) model; (b) visual illustration of the discrimination of all 34 samples by the PLSDA model (H for HK samples, C for OSCC samples, and D for OED samples).

4. Discussion

Despite cancer treatment advancements, oral cancer survival rates have not improved over the past several decades. The gold standard histopathological diagnosis of oral cancer and the grading of oral epithelial dysplasia have many limitations, including subjectivity, inconsistency, and inaccuracy. The lack of an effective screening program and the challenge of managing potentially malignant disorders and precancerous dysplasia lead to late diagnosis in >70% oral cancer patients, resulting in poor prognosis and survival rates. It has been shown that most oral cancer patients have pre-existing OPMDs, the majority of which are diagnosed as HK or OED [40]. OED is characterized by cytological and architectural alterations reflecting the loss of the normal maturation and stratification pattern of surface epithelium. Although these lesions have an increased statistical risk of progressing to malignancy, it is very difficult to predict the outcomes for individual patients with current histopathological diagnostic methods [12]. For example, even in the case of severe OED, the malignant transformation rate varies considerably from 3% to 50% [11]. According to Tilakaratne et al., a successful OED grading system should be (i) clinically relevant in terms of stratifying the cases for appropriate management plans, (ii) reproducible, minimizing intra- and inter-examiner variability, and (iii) biologically significant by identifying the lesions that are likely to undergo malignant transformation [41]. FTIR spectroscopy and imaging techniques show great promise to meet these criteria and to address the unmet medical needs for objective and accurate OED risk stratification.

A number of studies have applied FTIR techniques to investigate biochemical differences between normal and malignant oral tissues in the past two decades. Schultz et al. observed that poorly differentiated OSCC cells produced a relatively homogeneous and clearly abnormal cell biochemistry, whereas well-differentiated epithelial cells presented a very heterogeneous distribution of cellular components. The authors suggested that the FTIR analysis of cell components can be used to distinguish cancerous tissues from normal epithelial structures [42,43]. Fukuyama et al. observed FTIR spectral differences between normal oral mucosa and OSCC, including bands related to keratin, collagen, phosphate of nucleic acids, and membrane phospholipids [44]. A few studies on normal, pre-cancerous, and cancerous tissues of oral cavity have been conducted by one group from Università Politecnica delle Marche in Ancona, Italy, using reflectance FTIR mapping of thin tissue sections on a steel support. Distinct FTIR chemical maps of vibrational bands at 970 cm^{-1} (DNA), 1026 cm^{-1} (collagen), 1550 cm^{-1} (proteins), and 1735 cm^{-1} (lipids) were observed between normal and pathological oral tissues. The authors reported that the proliferating and regressive states of the tumors can be identified via the presence of a high content of DNA or collagen, respectively [45]. Pallua et al. investigated microarrays of

OSCC tissues using FTIR imaging with unsupervised methods including HCA and KMC (k-means cluster) and showed that intra-operative and surgical samples of the oral cavity can be characterized by FTIR microscopic imaging [46]. Bruni et al. reported increased DNA, lipid, and collagen levels in OSCC samples [45]. However, their attribution of the 1026 cm^{-1} band to collagen is debatable, as many other studies assigned the same band to glycogen instead [47–50]. Sabbatini et al. performed vibrational analyses of both epithelial and connective tissues of OSCC at various malignancy grades (G1–G3) and identified potential spectral markers for oral carcinogenesis, including the increase of free glycogen levels, structural alterations in nucleic acids, and a higher amount of RNA, which suggests an increase of the cellular transcriptional activity [51]. Banerjee et al. investigated FTIR-based spectral biomarkers towards the optimal differentiation of oral leukoplakia and cancer using a different sample preparation method. Specifically, deparaffinized FFPE tissue sections were treated as powder to prepare KBr pellets from which transmission spectra were acquired. The spectra represented a mixture of all of the components of the sample, including epithelial and connective tissues. They identified more than 20 spectral biomarkers using difference between mean spectra, forward feature selection, and Mann–Whitney U test techniques. The identified biomarkers were assigned to amide I, amide II, lipid, keratin, glycogen, DNA/RNA, etc. [48]. Naurecka et al. used the FTIR-ATR technique to study normal, leukoplakia, and cancerous oral tissues and reported spectral differences at amide I at 1650 cm^{-1}, amide II at 1535 cm^{-1}, nuclei acids at 1238 cm^{-1}, and glycogen at 1024–1030 cm^{-1} [49].

In the current study, the FTIR imaging technique combined with multivariate analyses were used to evaluate three classes of oral biopsy samples (HK, OED, and OSCC). Since whole sample FTIR imaging is very time consuming, a practical imaging method was developed to acquire representative spectra from the sample in a short time. Specifically, a series of 100 μm × 100 μm imaging areas (16 by 16 pixels) were defined in the AOI of the sample in reference to the corresponding H&E image. The area size of 100 μm × 100 μm was chosen so that each area contained enough tissue/cells to generate a local representative spectrum, while the acquisition time for each area was reasonably short (5–6 min) to ensure valid background correction. Representative spectra from multiple imaging areas in a sample were reviewed to understand the tissue heterogeneity of the specific sample. Different degrees of heterogeneity were observed for different samples. The consideration of intra-sample heterogeneity is particularly important for accurate model training when a relatively small number of training samples are used since a large number of training samples may contain high enough inter-sample heterogeneity to compensate for intra-sample heterogeneity. On the other hand, too many representative spectra from the same sample may cause a data redundancy problem, especially for samples with a low degree of intra-sample heterogeneity. As a result, a simple strategy was used to select the two representative spectra that best reflected the intra-sample heterogeneity of each sample for further analysis.

A series of spectral preprocessing was applied to the raw data to remove unwanted signal contributions, such as those from sample thickness variations and light scattering, and to prepare the data for optimal performance in later steps. The choice and quality of spectral preprocessing play an important role in the performance of multivariate analysis and classification. Even the order of the preprocessing steps can affect the analysis results. In the current study, different preprocessing steps and parameters were tried and the optimal procedure was decided as the following: the fingerprint region of 1800–950 cm^{-1} was selected due to its association with major biochemicals in tissues; second-order Savitzky–Golay smoothing was used to remove random noise (e.g., from instrument) while preserving useful biochemical spectral information; the EMSC algorithm was used to correct for resonant Mie scattering while maintaining the original spectral shape and scale; AWLS baseline correction was applied to remove background absorption interference, and vector normalization was then employed to correct for sample thickness variations. The above steps comprised the general preprocessing, which preserved the original shape of the spectra for easy visual comparison and interpretation. A comparison of the three class average spectra for the HK, OED, and OSCC samples (Figure 3) reveals an overall reduction in proteins and an increase in the nucleic acids as the oral tissues progress from HK to OED and further to OSCC. The amide II band exhibits a red shift for OED and OSCC samples, indicating some secondary structural changes in the collagen of the pathological tissues. Those findings are in good agreement with the literature that normal tissue spectra are characterized by higher protein contents, whereas more DNA and lipid signals are exhibited by malignant tissues [52]. In the current study, the typical lipid band between 1750–1700 cm^{-1} disappeared in all of the spectra, which is most likely due to the deparaffinization procedure which removed free lipids in the tissues as a side effect of removing the paraffin of the FFPE samples.

Exploratory analyses using PCA and HCA verified the overall quality and showed the trend of all 68 representative spectra. The reduced Hotelling T^2 versus Q residuals graph of PCA revealed no outliers among the data. The PCA and HCA results revealed a good but not ideal separation between the HK and OSCC spectra. The OED spectra were shown to overlap with both the HK and OSCC spectra. Exploratory analyses using unsupervised methods such as PCA and HCA serve well for quality inspection, patten observation, and trend discovery, but they usually cannot provide optimal classification for complicated pathological samples. Supervised methods are required for that purpose.

Based on the patterns revealed in the exploratory analyses, the OED spectra do not seem to separate well from either the HK spectra or the OSCC spectra. Instead, some OED spectra exhibit similarities to the HK spectra, while others exhibit similarities to the OSCC spectra. As a result, a novel strategy was developed to build an optimal discriminant model using the representative spectra of the HK and OSCC samples (first phase), which was subsequently used to classify the representative spectra of the OED samples (second phase).

Additional spectral preprocessing was applied to the representative spectra to optimize the discrimination model. First and second derivatives are commonly used preprocessing steps to highlight smaller spectral differences, which can be critical for finding the discriminative spectral features for complex biological samples. In the current study, the modeling results for non-derivative, first derivative, and second derivative representative spectra were compared. It was found that the second derivative preprocessing produced the best performance for the discrimination models. Therefore, it was used for final model building and validation.

In the first phase, three supervised discrimination models (PLSDA, SVMDA, and XGBDA) were trained and cross-validated using 24 HK spectra and 22 OSCC spectra. The results show better discrimination performance for the PLSDA model (100% sensitivity and 100% specificity) than the SVMDA and XGBDA models (95% sensitivity and 96% specificity). A total of 12 prominent bands were extracted from the top two latent variable loadings (LV1 and LV2) of the PLSDA model as discriminative spectral biomarkers in differentiating the OSCC from the HK samples (feature extraction/selection), as summarized in Table 1. The discriminative bands mainly came from proteins (amide I/II), nucleic acids ($-PO_2^-$), and carbohydrates (glucose and glycogen, etc.).

In the second phase, the optimal PLSDA model was used to classify the 22 representative spectra from 11 OED samples. The classification results show that 6 OED samples were classified as "HK-grade", indicating their spectral similarities to the HK samples, and 4 OED samples were classified as "OSCC-grade", indicating their spectral similarities to the OSCC samples. One OED sample was classified as "borderline case" because its two representative spectra were in proximity to and on both sides of the discrimination line. The 11 OED samples looked very similar in their morphological appearance and were all pathologically diagnosed as having a moderate-to-severe grade of dysplasia. However, The PLSDA model was able to classify them based on their FTIR spectral information as being biochemically similar either to the HK samples or to the OSCC samples. The results suggest that those morphologically similar tissue samples exhibit different biochemical profiles that can be detected using the FTIR-machine learning approach. The novel strategy developed in the current study provides a potential risk stratification method for OED.

A total of 68 representative FTIR spectra from 34 samples was used in the current pilot study. Future studies with a larger sample size are needed to further improve and validate the OSCC discrimination model. Moreover, archived OED cases with known OSCC transformation outcomes are needed to validate this novel strategy in its efficacy of predicting the malignant transformation risks of OED cases.

In the current study, a traditional Perkin Elmer FTIR spectrometer and imaging system (Spectrum one, Spotlight 300, Perkin Elmer, Waltham, MA, USA) with the spectral resolution of 4 cm^{-1} and spatial resolution of 6.25 μm was used. The current FTIR image acquisition and spectral preprocessing protocols generated good quality spectra in a reasonable time frame. Further improvements in spatial resolution and spectral quality can be achieved with added lenses, high-resolution infrared microscope optics, computational algorithms, and quantum cascade laser imaging systems, which offer advantages over traditional FTIR systems with respect to the speed of acquisition and field of view [53].

5. Conclusions

In summary, within the limitations of the study, our results show that an FTIR-machine learning approach can discriminant OSCC from HK oral biopsy samples with high accuracy. The novel OED classification strategy developed in the current study could potentially provide an objective risk stratification tool for OED or OPMDs and could therefore facilitate the early detection of oral cancer. Tissue sections from FFPE samples are routinely used for histopathological evaluation in cancer clinics. The use of the same tissue sections (unstained) for FTIR imaging can be easily integrated into existing diagnostic procedures. The integration of FTIR imaging techniques in existing histopathological diagnostic process provides valuable biochemical evaluation in addition to morphological evaluation and can assist pathologists in making a more accurate risk assessment for OPMDs/OED and for the earlier detection for OSCC.

Author Contributions: R.W. and Y.W. conceptualized the study; R.W. designed the study protocol and performed the sample preparation, data acquisition, data analyses, model building, and validation. Y.W. provided the hardware and software. A.N. provided the biopsy samples and sample pathological information. R.W. wrote the original manuscript draft and R.W., A.N. and Y.W. reviewed and edited the draft. All authors have read and agreed to the published version of the manuscript.

Funding: The study was partially supported by an internal award (#1901) from the Research Support Committee of UMKC school of dentistry.

Institutional Review Board Statement: The project was approved by UMKC Institutional Review Board on 27 June 2019 (IRB project number 2015501, IRB review number 249482). All procedures performed in studies involving human tissues were in accordance with the ethical standards of the institutional and/or national research committee and with the 1975 Helsinki declaration and its later amendments or comparable ethical standards.

Informed Consent Statement: Patient consent was waived because the current study was a secondary research involving only information collection and analysis.

Data Availability Statement: The data presented in this study are available on request.

Acknowledgments: The authors would like to thank Sarah Dallas's group in the School of Dentistry at UMKC for the use of their microtome, H&E staining station and microscope.

Conflicts of Interest: The authors declare no conflict of interest with respect to the authorship and publication of this article.

References

1. Siegel, R.L.; Miller, K.D.; Jemal, A. Cancer statistics, 2020. *CA: A Cancer J. Clin.* **2020**, *70*, 7–30. [CrossRef]
2. Ali, J.; Sabiha, B.; Jan, H.U.; Haider, S.A.; Khan, A.A.; Ali, S.S. Genetic etiology of oral cancer. *Oral Oncol.* **2017**, *70*, 23–28. [CrossRef]

3. Irani, S. New Insights into Oral Cancer-Risk Factors and Prevention: A Review of Literature. *Int. J. Prev. Med.* **2020**, *11*, 202. [CrossRef]
4. Shah, F.D.; Begum, R.; Vajaria, B.N.; Patel, K.R.; Patel, J.B.; Shukla, S.N.; Patel, P.S. A Review on Salivary Genomics and Proteomics Biomarkers in Oral Cancer. *Indian J. Clin. Biochem.* **2011**, *26*, 326–334. [CrossRef]
5. Van der Waal, I. Potentially malignant disorders of the oral and oropharyngeal mucosa; terminology, classification and present concepts of management. *Oral Oncol.* **2009**, *45*, 317–323. [CrossRef]
6. Warnakulasuriya, S. Oral potentially malignant disorders: A comprehensive review on clinical aspects and management. *Oral Oncol.* **2020**, *102*, 104550. [CrossRef] [PubMed]
7. Wenig, B.M. Squamous cell carcinoma of the upper aerodigestive tract: Precursors and problematic variants. *Mod. Pathol. Off. J. United States Can. Acad. Pathol. Inc.* **2002**, *15*, 229–254. [CrossRef]
8. Shirani, S.; Kargahi, N.; Razavi, S.M.; Homayoni, S. Epithelial dysplasia in oral cavity. *Iran. J. Med. Sci.* **2014**, *39*, 406–417. [PubMed]
9. Warnakulasuriya, S.; Reibel, J.; Bouquot, J.; Dabelsteen, E. Oral epithelial dysplasia classification systems: Predictive value, utility, weaknesses and scope for improvement. *J. Oral Pathol. Med.* **2008**, *37*, 127–133. [CrossRef] [PubMed]
10. Van der Waal, I. Oral potentially malignant disorders: Is malignant transformation predictable and preventable? *Med. Oral Patol. Oral Y Cir. Bucal* **2014**, *19*, e386–e390. [CrossRef]
11. Reibel, J. Prognosis of Oral Pre-malignant Lesions: Significance of Clinical, Histopathological, and Molecular Biological Characteristics. *Crit. Rev. Oral Biol. Med.* **2003**, *14*, 47–62. [CrossRef]
12. Ranganathan, K.; Kavitha, L. Oral epithelial dysplasia: Classifications and clinical relevance in risk assessment of oral potentially malignant disorders. *J. Oral Maxillofac. Pathol.* **2019**, *23*, 19–27. [PubMed]
13. Celentano, A.; Glurich, I.; Borgnakke, W.S.; Farah, C.S. World Workshop on Oral Medicine VII: Prognostic biomarkers in oral leukoplakia and proliferative verrucous leukoplakia—A systematic review of retrospective studies. *Oral Dis.* **2020**, *27*, 848–880. [CrossRef]
14. Talari, A.C.S.; Martinez, M.A.G.; Movasaghi, Z.; Rehman, S.; Rehman, I.U. Advances in Fourier transform infrared (FTIR) spectroscopy of biological tissues. *Appl. Spectrosc. Rev.* **2017**, *52*, 456–506. [CrossRef]
15. Fabian, H.; Naumann, D. Methods to study protein folding by stopped-flow FT-IR. *Methods* **2004**, *34*, 28–40. [CrossRef]
16. Ghimire, H.; Garlapati, C.; Janssen, E.A.M.; Krishnamurti, U.; Qin, G.; Aneja, R.; Perera, A.G.U. Protein conformational changes in breast cancer sera using infrared spectroscopic analysis. *Cancers* **2020**, *12*, 1708. [CrossRef]
17. Kelly, J.G.; Martin-Hirsch, P.L.; Martin, F.L. Discrimination of base differences in oligonucleotides using mid-infrared spectroscopy and multivariate analysis. *Anal. Chem.* **2009**, *81*, 5314–5319. [CrossRef]
18. Petibois, C.; Déléris, G. Evidence that erythrocytes are highly susceptible to exercise oxidative stress: FT-IR spectrometric studies at the molecular level. *Cell Biol. Int.* **2005**, *29*, 709–716. [CrossRef] [PubMed]
19. Benseny-Cases, N.; Klementieva, O.; Cotte, M.; Ferrer, I.; Cladera, J. Microspectroscopy (µFTIR) reveals co-localization of lipid oxidation and amyloid plaques in human Alzheimer disease brains. *Anal. Chem.* **2014**, *86*, 12047–12054. [CrossRef] [PubMed]
20. Bogomolny, E.; Huleihel, M.; Suproun, Y.; Sahu, R.K.; Mordechai, S. Early spectral changes of cellular malignant transformation using Fourier transform infrared microspectroscopy. *J. Biomed. Opt.* **2007**, *12*, 024003. [CrossRef] [PubMed]
21. Papamarkakis, K.; Bird, B.; Schubert, J.M.; Miljković, M.; Wein, R.; Bedrossian, K.; Laver, N.; Diem, M. Cytopathology by optical methods: Spectral cytopathology of the oral mucosa. *Lab. Investig.* **2010**, *90*, 589–598. [CrossRef] [PubMed]
22. Kumar, S.; Srinivasan, A.; Nikolajeff, F. Role of Infrared Spectroscopy and Imaging in Cancer Diagnosis. *Curr. Med. Chem.* **2018**, *25*, 1055–1072. [CrossRef]
23. Beć, K.; Grabska, J.; Huck, C. Biomolecular and bioanalytical applications of infrared spectroscopy—A review. *Anal. Chim. Acta* **2020**, *1133*, 150–177. [CrossRef]
24. Pallua, J.D.; Brunner, A.; Zelger, B.; Stalder, R.; Unterberger, S.H.; Schirmer, M.; Tappert, M. Clinical infrared microscopic imaging: An overview. *Pathol. Res. Pract.* **2018**, *214*, 1532–1538. [CrossRef]
25. Bel'skaya, L. Use of IR Spectroscopy in Cancer Diagnosis. A Review. *J. Appl. Spectrosc.* **2019**, *86*, 187–205. [CrossRef]
26. Wang, R.; Wang, Y. Fourier Transform Infrared Spectroscopy in Oral Cancer Diagnosis. *Int. J. Mol. Sci.* **2021**, *22*, 1206. [CrossRef]
27. Bro, R.; Smilde, A.K. Principal component analysis. *Anal. Methods* **2014**, *6*, 2812–2831. [CrossRef]
28. Morais, C.L.M.; Lima, K.M.G.; Singh, M.; Martin, F.L. Tutorial: Multivariate classification for vibrational spectroscopy in biological samples. *Nat. Protoc.* **2020**, *15*, 2143–2162. [CrossRef] [PubMed]
29. Ruiz-Perez, D.; Guan, H.; Madhivanan, P.; Mathee, K.; Narasimhan, G. So you think you can PLS-DA? *BMC Bioinform.* **2020**, *21*, 2. [CrossRef]
30. Song, W.; Wang, H.; Maguire, P.; Nibouche, O. Collaborative representation based classifier with partial least squares regression for the classification of spectral data. *Chemom. Intell. Lab. Syst.* **2018**, *182*, 79–86. [CrossRef]
31. Cortes, C.; Vapnik, V. Support-vector networks. *Mach. Learn.* **1995**, *20*, 273–297. [CrossRef]
32. Piryonesi, S.M.; El-Diraby, T.E. Data Analytics in Asset Management: Cost-Effective Prediction of the Pavement Condition Index. *J. Infrastruct. Syst.* **2020**, *26*, 04019036. [CrossRef]
33. Guang, P.; Huang, W.; Guo, L.; Yang, X.; Huang, F.; Yang, M.; Wen, W.; Li, L. Blood-based FTIR-ATR spectroscopy coupled with extreme gradient boosting for the diagnosis of type 2 diabetes: A STARD compliant diagnosis research. *Medicine* **2020**, *99*, e19657. [CrossRef]

34. Šimundić, A.-M. Measures of Diagnostic Accuracy: Basic Definitions. *EJIFCC* **2009**, *19*, 203–211.
35. Barth, A. Infrared spectroscopy of proteins. *Biochim. Et Biophys. Acta* **2007**, *1767*, 1073–1101. [CrossRef]
36. Casal, H.L.; Mantsch, H.H. Polymorphic phase behaviour of phospholipid membranes studied by infrared spectroscopy. *Biochim. Et Biophys. Acta (BBA)—Rev. Biomembr.* **1984**, *779*, 381–401. [CrossRef]
37. Baker, M.J.; Trevisan, J.; Bassan, P.; Bhargava, R.; Butler, H.J.; Dorling, K.M.; Fielden, P.R.; Fogarty, S.W.; Fullwood, N.J.; Heys, K.A.; et al. Using Fourier transform IR spectroscopy to analyze biological materials. *Nat. Protoc.* **2014**, *9*, 1771–1791. [CrossRef] [PubMed]
38. Wiercigroch, E.; Szafraniec, E.; Czamara, K.; Pacia, M.Z.; Majzner, K.; Kochan, K.; Kaczor, A.; Baranska, M.; Malek, K. Raman and infrared spectroscopy of carbohydrates: A review. *Spectrochim. Acta Part A Mol. Biomol. Spectrosc.* **2017**, *185*, 317–335. [CrossRef] [PubMed]
39. Bellisola, G.; Sorio, C. Infrared spectroscopy and microscopy in cancer research and diagnosis. *Am. J. Cancer Res.* **2012**, *2*, 1–21. [PubMed]
40. Chiang, T.-E.; Lin, Y.-C.; Wu, C.-T.; Yang, C.-Y.; Wu, S.-T.; Chen, Y.-W. Comparison of the accuracy of diagnoses of oral potentially malignant disorders with dysplasia by a general dental clinician and a specialist using the Taiwanese Nationwide Oral Mucosal Screening Program. *PLoS ONE* **2021**, *16*, e0244740. [CrossRef] [PubMed]
41. Tilakaratne, W.M.; Jayasooriya, P.R.; Jayasuriya, N.S.; De Silva, R.K. Oral epithelial dysplasia: Causes, quantification, prognosis, and management challenges. *Periodontology 2000* **2019**, *80*, 126–147. [CrossRef] [PubMed]
42. Schultz, C.P.; Mantsch, H.H. Biochemical imaging and 2D classification of keratin pearl structures in oral squamous cell carcinoma. *Cell. Mol. Biol. (Noisy-Le-Grand Fr.)* **1998**, *44*, 203–210.
43. Schultz, C.P.; Liu, K.Z.; Kerr, P.D.; Mantsch, H.H. In situ infrared histopathology of keratinization in human oral/oropharyngeal squamous cell carcinoma. *Oncol. Res.* **1998**, *10*, 277–286.
44. Fukuyama, Y.; Yoshida, S.; Yanagisawa, S.; Shimizu, M. A study on the differences between oral squamous cell carcinomas and normal oral mucosas measured by Fourier transform infrared spectroscopy. *Biospectroscopy* **1999**, *5*, 117–126. [CrossRef]
45. Bruni, P.; Conti, C.; Giorgini, E.; Pisani, M.; Rubini, C.; Tosi, G. Histological and microscopy FT-IR imaging study on the proliferative activity and angiogenesis in head and neck tumours. *Faraday Discuss.* **2004**, *126*, 19–26, discussion 77–92. [CrossRef]
46. Pallua, J.D.; Pezzei, C.; Zelger, B.; Schaefer, G.; Bittner, L.K.; Huck-Pezzei, V.A.; Schoenbichler, S.A.; Hahn, H.; Kloss-Brandstaetter, A.; Kloss, F.; et al. Fourier transform infrared imaging analysis in discrimination studies of squamous cell carcinoma. *Analyst* **2012**, *137*, 3965–3974. [CrossRef]
47. Wong, P.T.; Wong, R.K.; Caputo, T.A.; Godwin, T.A.; Rigas, B. Infrared spectroscopy of exfoliated human cervical cells: Evidence of extensive structural changes during carcinogenesis. *Proc. Natl. Acad. Sci. USA* **1991**, *88*, 10988–10992. [CrossRef]
48. Banerjee, S.; Pal, M.; Chakrabarty, J.; Petibois, C.; Paul, R.R.; Giri, A.; Chatterjee, J. Fourier-transform-infrared-spectroscopy based spectral-biomarker selection towards optimum diagnostic differentiation of oral leukoplakia and cancer. *Anal. Bioanal. Chem.* **2015**, *407*, 7935–7943. [CrossRef]
49. Naurecka, M.L.; Sierakowski, B.M.; Kasprzycka, W.; Dojs, A.; Dojs, M.; Suszyński, Z.; Kwaśny, M. FTIR-ATR and FT-Raman Spectroscopy for Biochemical Changes in Oral Tissue. *Am. J. Anal. Chem.* **2017**, *8*, 180–188. [CrossRef]
50. Rai, V.; Mukherjee, R.; Routray, A.; Ghosh, A.K.; Roy, S.; Ghosh, B.P.; Mandal, P.B.; Bose, S.; Chakraborty, C. Serum-based diagnostic prediction of oral submucous fibrosis using FTIR spectrometry. *Spectrochim. Acta—Part A: Mol. Biomol. Spectrosc.* **2018**, *189*, 322–329. [CrossRef] [PubMed]
51. Sabbatini, S.; Conti, C.; Rubini, C.; Librando, V.; Tosi, G.; Giorgini, E. Infrared microspectroscopy of Oral Squamous Cell Carcinoma: Spectral signatures of cancer grading. *Vib. Spectrosc.* **2013**, *68*, 196–203. [CrossRef]
52. Bunaciu, A.A.; Aboul-Enein, H.; Fleschin, Ş. Vibrational Spectroscopy in Clinical Analysis. *Appl. Spectrosc. Rev.* **2015**, *50*, 176–191. [CrossRef]
53. Kimber, J.A.; Kazarian, S.G. Spectroscopic imaging of biomaterials and biological systems with FTIR microscopy or with quantum cascade lasers. *Anal. Bioanal. Chem.* **2017**, *409*, 5813–5820. [CrossRef] [PubMed]

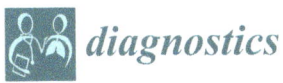

Article

Deep Learning for Caries Detection and Classification

Luya Lian, Tianer Zhu, Fudong Zhu * and Haihua Zhu *

Stomatology Hospital, School of Stomatology, Zhejiang University School of Medicine, Clinical Research Center for Oral Diseases of Zhejiang Province, Key Laboratory of Oral Biomedical Research of Zhejiang Province, Cancer Center of Zhejiang University, Hangzhou 310006, China; 3100102358@zju.edu.cn (L.L.); zhutianer@zju.edu.cn (T.Z.)
* Correspondence: zfd@zju.edu.cn (F.Z.); zhuhh403@zju.edu.cn (H.Z.)

Abstract: Objectives: Deep learning methods have achieved impressive diagnostic performance in the field of radiology. The current study aimed to use deep learning methods to detect caries lesions, classify different radiographic extensions on panoramic films, and compare the classification results with those of expert dentists. Methods: A total of 1160 dental panoramic films were evaluated by three expert dentists. All caries lesions in the films were marked with circles, whose combination was defined as the reference dataset. A training and validation dataset (1071) and a test dataset (89) were then established from the reference dataset. A convolutional neural network, called nnU-Net, was applied to detect caries lesions, and DenseNet121 was applied to classify the lesions according to their depths (dentin lesions in the outer, middle, or inner third D1/2/3 of dentin). The performance of the test dataset in the trained nnU-Net and DenseNet121 models was compared with the results of six expert dentists in terms of the intersection over union (IoU), Dice coefficient, accuracy, precision, recall, negative predictive value (NPV), and F1-score metrics. Results: nnU-Net yielded caries lesion segmentation IoU and Dice coefficient values of 0.785 and 0.663, respectively, and the accuracy and recall rate of nnU-Net were 0.986 and 0.821, respectively. The results of the expert dentists and the neural network were shown to be no different in terms of accuracy, precision, recall, NPV, and F1-score. For caries depth classification, DenseNet121 showed an overall accuracy of 0.957 for D1 lesions, 0.832 for D2 lesions, and 0.863 for D3 lesions. The recall results of the D1/D2/D3 lesions were 0.765, 0.652, and 0.918, respectively. All metric values, including accuracy, precision, recall, NPV, and F1-score values, were proven to be no different from those of the experienced dentists. Conclusion: In detecting and classifying caries lesions on dental panoramic radiographs, the performance of deep learning methods was similar to that of expert dentists. The impact of applying these well-trained neural networks for disease diagnosis and treatment decision making should be explored.

Keywords: deep learning methods; caries diagnosis; dental panoramic images; radiography

Citation: Lian, L.; Zhu, T.; Zhu, F.; Zhu, H. Deep Learning for Caries Detection and Classification. *Diagnostics* 2021, 11, 1672. https://doi.org/10.3390/diagnostics11091672

Academic Editor: Jae-Hong Lee

Received: 25 July 2021
Accepted: 9 September 2021
Published: 13 September 2021

Publisher's Note: MDPI stays neutral with regard to jurisdictional claims in published maps and institutional affiliations.

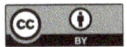

Copyright: © 2021 by the authors. Licensee MDPI, Basel, Switzerland. This article is an open access article distributed under the terms and conditions of the Creative Commons Attribution (CC BY) license (https://creativecommons.org/licenses/by/4.0/).

1. Introduction

Dental caries are common causes of tooth pain and tooth loss, despite being preventable and treatable. Comprehensive and early detection of dental caries can be critical for timely and appropriate treatment. Large, clearly visible tooth cavities induced by caries can be easily detected by using visual inspection and probing with the use of a dental probe and a handheld mirror. These conventional caries detection methods are also effective for partially obscured but accessible caries [1]. X-ray radiography, as an aid for the diagnosis of hidden or inaccessible lesions, is irreplaceable. Panoramic, periapical, and bitewing X-rays are three common types of radiographs that are widely used in clinical practice. Bitewing and periapical X-rays concentrate on the details of the mouth area, such as one or more teeth, whereas panoramic X-rays capture all the teeth and other hard tissues of the maxillofacial region [2]. Although bitewing radiography is the most widely used approach to detect caries lesions and assess their depth, which comes with high sensitivity and specificity [3], it could not perform comprehensive lesions detection of the full mouth in one attempt. Furthermore, panoramic films are taken outside the mouth and have better patient acceptance, a lower infection rate, and a lower radiation exposure [4]. Due to its relative cost effectiveness and diagnostic evidence, panoramic imaging is considered to be the most common and important radiological tool for clinical dental disease screening, diagnosis, and treatment evaluation.

During the diagnosis and treatment of oral diseases, dentists need to interpret panoramic radiographs and record specific symptoms of diseased teeth in the medical records. New dentists require extensive training and time to perform accurate X-ray film interpretations [5]. An X-ray analysis showed that more experienced dentists are almost four times more likely to make a correct assessment of caries lesions than less experienced dentists [6]. Therefore, considerable attention has been given to interpreting panoramic X-rays with dental caries automatically. In recent decades, scientists have tried to deploy machine learning techniques to detect dental diseases. As in the conventional method, operators or experts perform lesion detection and evaluation on radiographs manually and objectively. This task is tedious when facing large amounts of image data and may lead to misinterpretations. Previous efforts have successfully applied convolutional neural network (CNN)-based deep learning models in computer vision. Deep learning methods do not depend on well-designed manual features and have high generalization capabilities. These models have achieved high accuracy and sensitivity and are the most advanced technology for a wide range of applications. The increased interest in deep learning methods has also led to their applications in medical imaging interpretation and in diagnostic assistance systems, for instance, Helicobacter pylori infection detection in gastrointestinal endoscopy [7], skin cancer screenings [8], and coronavirus disease 2019 (COVID-19) detection in computed tomography images [9].

In dentistry, Ronneberger employed U-Net to achieve dental structure segmentation on bitewing radiographs since 2015 [10]. Subsequently, CNNs have been employed with high accuracy to detect alveolar bone loss in periapical X-rays and panoramic X-rays and to identify apical cysts and caries lesions in periapical X-rays [11]. To date, multiple deep learning methods have been used for caries detection in bitewings [12–14] and periapical radiographs [14,15] and other auxiliary testing images such as near-infrared light transillumination images [13,16]. Most previous studies have been limited to lesion segmentation analysis of deep learning models [12–15]. Subsequently, recent research aimed to compare the caries detection performance of deep learning methods and dentists [12,17]. However, there are few studies on neural networks' performance of caries lesions with different radiographic depths. The latter is of great importance to health economic perspectives and treatment decision making, since dental caries treatments, such as remineralization, cavity filling, root canal therapy, and tooth extraction, vary with lesion depth. As for this purpose, Cantus applied U-Net to classify caries depth on 3686 bitewing radiographs and concluded that a deep neural network was more accurate than dentists when detecting caries on bitewing radiographs [12]. However, no study has yet investigated caries lesions segmentation along with classification on panoramic films, which are of great importance in caries screening and diagnosis in primary hospitals. A previous study suggested that dentinal involvement, indicating operative treatment, had a cutoff value of 3 according to a modified International Caries Detection and Assessment System (ICDAS II). For all ICDAS II, the relative dentinal depth of a lesion was expressed as the percentage of the total length of the coronal dentin in histological and radiographic assessments. We focused on dentinal carious decay and divided the entire caries depth into four levels.

In this study, to achieve accurate segmentation of dental caries and diagnosis of lesion extensions, we used nnU-Net and DenseNet121. First, we applied nnU-Net to perform caries lesion segmentation. This segmentation model was based on a deep learning method and inspired by the structure of U-Net, which allowed us to optimally configure the model. This feature allows the model to perform outstandingly in any new task [10]. Second, we proposed DenseNet121 to identify caries stages. This 121-layer connected network alleviated the vanishing gradient issue and strengthened feature propagation by joining all proceeding layers into subsequent layers [18]. Finally, to ensure that the structure attains the best possible performance, we added a dropout mechanism and label softening to the model to address the overfitting phenomenon during model training. Moreover, we compared the caries detection results of dentists and the model to search for a better way to clinically diagnose caries lesions.

Accordingly, the main contributions of our study are threefold: (1) we built a new dataset that was strictly verified by dental experts, (2) we addressed automatic caries lesion segmentation by nnU-Net and applied DenseNet121 to automatically clarify lesion extensions into four levels, (3) we also compared the results of our model with those of a group of experienced dentists to confirm the hypothesis that a combined panoramic interpretation by the model and dentists is more sufficient and accurate than separate interpretations by a dentist or by the model.

2. Materials and Methods

2.1. Study Design

In the current study, the performances of a group of individual dentists and two deep learning methods in identifying caries lesions and their extensions in panoramic images were compared in different dimensions. This study followed the guidelines of the Standards for Reporting of Diagnostic Accuracy Studies (STARD) [19].

Before the study, our group successfully performed automated tooth segmentation, which is the cornerstone of automated diagnostic methodologies for dental films. In the present study, we first applied nnU-Net, which is well known for its state-of-the-art performance on 23 public datasets; nnU-Net is a deep learning-based segmentation method that has been broadly used for medical imaging segmentation tasks and has been proven to surpass countless prevailing approaches without manual intervention [20].

Second, we used the DenseNet121 classification model to identify carious lesions with different degrees of severity, which were previously labeled by three independent dentists. DenseNet [18] was proposed by Huang to solve the vanishing gradient problem of CNN structures, and its performance exceeded the best performance of ResNet in 2016. The key concept of DenseNet is the "skip connection", and it has a CNN structure with dense connections. In this network, all preceding layers' outputs are combined and input into the next layer. Moreover, to prevent losing information during layer-to-layer transmission and to overcome the vanishing gradient problem, the feature map learned by the exact layer is directly transmitted to all the following layers as output. With this model, each pixel that belongs to a radiograph can be distributed into a propriate class; in our study, there were the following four classes: "D0" sound; "D1" caries radiolucency in enamel or in the outer third of dentin; "D2" caries radiolucency in the middle third of dentin; and "D3" caries radiolucency in the inner third of dentin with or without apparent pulp involvement (Table 1).

Table 1. Criterion of caries extension and their stage.

Caries Stage	Caries Extension
D0	Sound
D1	Caries radiolucency in enamel or in the outer third of dentin
D2	Caries radiolucency in the middle third of dentin
D3	Caries radiolucency in the inner third of dentin with or without apparent pulp involvement

To evaluate the performance of trained models, it is necessary to define metrics in the automated approach to measure the level of congruency between the predicted regions and the truly affected regions. Intersection over union (IoU) was the first metric that we leveraged in the present study. It is a widely used parameter that measures the difference between the ground truth region and the predicted region, as it calculates the ratio of the intersection and union of the two areas. To be more accurate, the Dice coefficient was applied to focus on the overlap of the predicted region with the ground truth region to obtain pixel accuracy. To focus on medical significance, other metrics (mainly at the tooth level) were adopted in the current study and are described below.

2.2. Reference Dataset

A set of 1160 panoramic images that originated from dental treatments and routine care were provided by the Affiliated Stomatology Hospital, Zhejiang University School of Medicine. A representative sample was drawn from 2015 and 2020. Panoramic images and metadata, i.e., sex, age, and image creation date, were available. However, the metadata were only allowed for descriptive analyses. The data collection process of the study was ethically approved by the Chinese Stomatological Association ethics committee. Only panoramic images of permanent teeth were included, and those of primary teeth or blurred images were excluded. The mean age (SD, min–max) of the patients included in the dataset was 42.8 (15.3, 18–68) years. Approximately 58% of the patients were male, and 42% of the patients were female. The radiographic data were all generated with radiographic machines from Dentsply Sirona (Bensheim, Germany), Orthophos XG 5OS Ceph.

Three dental experts independently labeled the images in triplicate by using the annotation tool itksnap. Each annotation was further classified into four stages according to the caries lesion depth in the radiographic films by three independent dentists. No clinical records were obtained or assessed in the procedure. For a single image, a consensus of the expert dentists was required to determine the final label, i.e., the experts were asked to repeatedly evaluate caries extensions regarding different opinions, and then, a fourth expert reviewed and revised all of the labels, including addition, deletion, and confirmation operations. All expert dentists were employed at the Affiliated Stomatology Hospital, Zhejiang University School of Medicine and had clinical experience of 3–15 years. A handbook that indicated how to mark caries lesions and annotate their stages with an annotation tool was used to guide the experts. All annotated areas on an image ultimately constructed the reference dataset (the "ground truth"), which consists of 1166 D1 lesions, 1039 D2 lesions, and 1635 D3 lesions.

2.3. Segmentation and Classification Model

The deep learning model applied in dental caries segmentation is nnU-Net, which is different from other improved U-Net-based models. It automatically configures itself, including preprocessing, network architecture, training, and postprocessing, for any new task, to achieve the best performance. The nnU-Net automated method configuration begins with extracting the dataset fingerprint and then executing heuristic rules. A set of fixed parameters, empirical decisions, and interdependent rules are modeled in this process [20]. Similar to other U-Net-derived architectures, a U-shaped configuration of convolutional network layers with skip connections is designed. The network architecture consists of an encoder (the falling part of the "U") and a corresponding decoder (the rising part of the "U"). The encoder network increases the contextual information, condenses the input sequence, and decreases the exact positional information. With the skip connection between the falling and the rising part of the "U", the decoder network expands the contextual information and combines it with precise information about the object locations [21]. The details of the model architecture are provided in Figure 1.

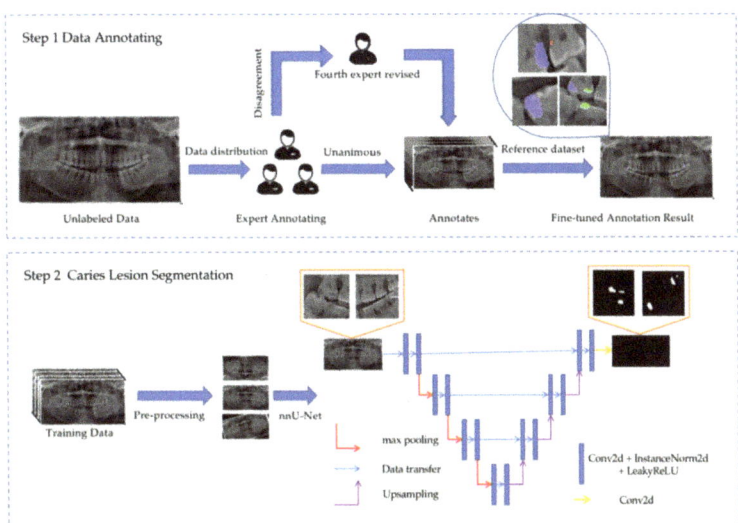

Figure 1. Details of nnU-Net architecture and implementation details in caries segmentation. In step 1, three dental experts were trained to implement dental caries labels and annotations, and a fourth expert revised any controversial results. Purple circle indicates D3 lesions, green circle indicates D2 lesions and red circle indicates D1 lesions. Step 2 shows nnU-Net and how it works in caries lesion segmentation.

The DenseNet model is a CNN and is applied in caries classification. All features used in the previous layers of the architecture are reused in the current layer, and this heavy feature reuse characteristic in each block makes the network focus on efficiency. Due to this structure, the number of parameters in the DenseNet model is reduced, and the feature maps are significantly smaller, as the number of feature maps increases linearly with the growth rate. Moreover, compression layers are applied between dense blocks to keep the feature map sizes small. In addition, the network uses bottlenecks to reduce the number of parameters and the computational effort [18]. The details of the model architecture and the implementation details are presented in Figure 2.

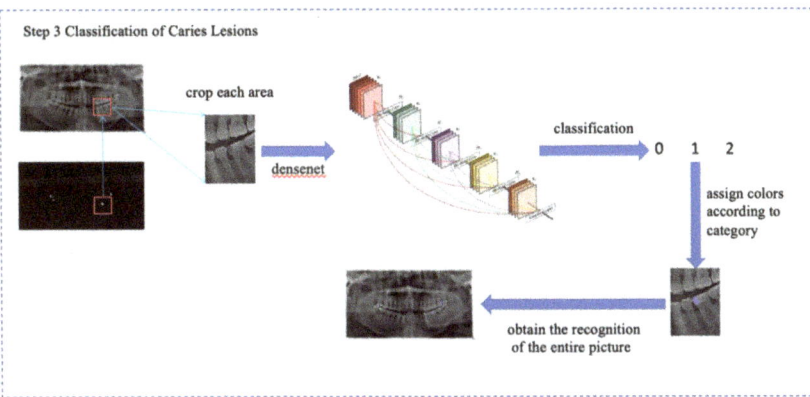

Figure 2. Description of how caries lesions were classified into D1/D2/D3 lesions. First, caries lesions were identified by the model as 3 types, which were represented by the code 0/1/2. Code 0 indicates D1 lesions (which are shown as red circles), Code 1 indicates D2 lesions (which are shown as green circles) and Code 3 indicates D3 lesions (which are shown as purple circl.

The model was implemented by using Ubuntu (version 18.04), pytorch1.6, CUDA10.1, and CUDNN8.0.5.

2.4. Model Training and Data Preparation

2.4.1. Data Preparation

According to caries labeling, a 300 × 400 region-of-interest (ROI) image for each caries area was cut from the panoramic radiographs to form a caries classification dataset. Then, the classification data were divided into the training set and the test set. Horizontal flip, vertical flip, horizontal vertical flip, and random rotation data enhancement operations were adopted for the training set data, and the rotation angle was within 0 and 15 degrees.

2.4.2. Model Training

DenseNet121 was proposed to identify caries lesion extensions. To overcome the small size of the dataset, we used transfer learning during model training. The introduction of transfer learning is reported to save computation time and resources and enable a rapid convergence for the model. To use transfer learning, the pretrained DenseNet121 network transfers parameters to the target DenseNet121 model, which prevents overfitting. We first trained DenseNet121 on the ImageNet dataset and then used the caries dataset to fine-tune the pretrained DenseNet121 to complete caries extension classification.

Overfitting is a common problem that occurs when a CNN with a large number of learnable parameters is trained on a relatively small dataset. As the learned weights are designed mostly for the training set and lack the ability to be generalized to unseen data, the model is prone to obtaining poor performance on the test data not included in the training set. The overfitting problem is believed to be caused by the complex coadaptation of neurons, which is why deep neural networks depend on their joint response rather than favoring each neuron to perform valuable feature learning [22]. Imposing a stochastic behavior in the forward data propagation phase of the network is a commonly used method to enhance the generalization ability of CNNs [23]. Examples of such methods include label smoothing and dropout. We choose dropout [24] to randomly shut down some features and enhance the model's generalization ability; moreover, each time before the activation function is applied, batch normalization is applied to further improve the effect. Label smoothing is another simple but successful regularization approach applied in the study. This method is widely used for multiclass classification tasks, where the CE error is adopted as the standard loss function, and the so-called one-hot encoding is presented in an annotation format. Label smoothing is designed to replace hard labels with smoothed versions; furthermore, label smoothing can prevent overconfident models when calculating the loss value and has been reported to increase the learning speed and benefit the overall accuracy [25]. Label smoothing has been proven to improve model calibration and out-of-distribution detection [26]. Label softening is equivalent to reducing the weight of the category of the real sample label when calculating the loss function and finally has the effect of suppressing overfitting.

2.5. Comparator Dentists

A group of six dentists who worked at Affiliated Stomatology Hospital, Zhejiang University School of Medicine, for 3–15 years were defined as the comparable group. They were enlisted to gauge the performance of the expert dentists against the performance of the neural networks. Each of the participants performed caries segmentation and severity classification tasks on a set of 89 panoramic films (test dataset), which included films of 40 D1 lesions, 53 D2 lesions, and 103 D3 lesions and images without lesions.

2.6. Evaluation Metrics

2.6.1. Performance of nnU-Net in Caries Segmentation

The nnU-Net segmentation model was evaluated, and its performance was compared with that of the doctors. Two distinct metrics, the IoU and the Dice coefficient metrics, were used to evaluate the performance of different dimensions. Despite the similarity of the two metrics, a single instance of bad segmentation was penalized much more in the IoU than in the Dice coefficient. For certain algorithms, the vast majority of instances are correct, but incorrect decisions are made in a few instances. The model Dice coefficient score will be much higher than the corresponding IoU score, which means that the Dice coefficient reflects the average performance better and is not overly sensitive to a few bad results. Both the IoU and the Dice coefficient are calculated by the mean value in a performance assessment. The Dice coefficients indicate the mean value of individual Dice coefficients on the validation and test data. Dice coefficient and IoU values of 1 indicate an ideal algorithm that matches the reference labels 100%. In contrast, the reference and predicted label masks with no overlap will result in two metric values equal to 0.

2.6.2. Performance of DenseNet121 in the Classification of Caries Severity

DenseNet121 was applied for caries severity classification, its performance was evaluated and compared with that of dentists combined with a neural network, and the precision of both was evaluated at the caries level. An ensemble of six different metrics was deployed to capture different aspects of the classification performance of the model and the dentists, including accuracy, recall, specificity, precision, F1-score, and negative predicted value (NPV). The F1-score parameter is the harmonic average of precision and recall. The chi-square test was used to compare the performances of the model and the dentists. A p-value with $p < 0.05$ was considered significant.

3. Results

Table 2 shows the distribution of caries lesions and their extensions in the reference dataset. The image ratio of the training set versus the test set was 982:89. Table 3 shows the segmentation performances of nnU-Net and of the dentists in the test set. Table 4 summarizes the performances of DenseNet121 and of the dentists in stratifying lesions to different extensions in the test set.

Table 2. Reference dataset.

Dataset	D1	D2	D3
Training set	1126	986	1532
Test set	40	53	103
Overall	1166	1039	1635

Table 3. Segmentation performances of nnU-Net and the dentists with the test set.

	Accuracy	Sensitivity	Specificity	Precision	NPV	F1	IoU	Dice
Model	0.986	0.821	1.000	1.000	0.985	0.902	0.785	0.663
Dentists (mean)	0.955	0.773	0.971	0.705	0.981	0.733	0.696	0.570
Dentists (min)	0.933	0.730	0.949	0.554	0.977	0.632	0.711	0.587
Dentists (max)	0.972	0.852	0.992	0.883	0.987	0.802	0.717	0.594

Table 4. Classification performances of DenseNet121 and the dentists with the test set.

Parameter	DenseNet121			Dentists (Mean; Min–Max)		
	D1	D2	D3	D1	D2	D3
Accuracy	0.957	0.832	0.863	0.915; 0.886–0.940	0.792; 0.720–0.828	0.858; 0.783–0.903
Precision	0.812	0.732	0.865	0.798; 0.667–1.000	0.601; 0.458–0.677	0.847; 0.737–0.884
Sensitivity	0.765	0.652	0.918	0.464; 0.250–0.647	0.536; 0.290–0.630	0.947; 0.881–0.988
NPV [1]	0.972	0.867	0.860	0.926; 0.891–0.956	0.847; 0.773–0.878	0.895; 0.745–0.966
F1-score	0.788	0.690	0.891	0.570; 0.400–0.645	0.564; 0.355–0.630	0.892; 0.844–0.929

[1] NPV: negative predictive value. Please see the main text for the definitions of the metrics.

First, the binary classification results of nnU-Net and the dentists are presented. The overall accuracy of the model was 0.986, and the mean accuracy of the dentists was lower than that of the model but not significantly at 0.955 (min–max: 0.933–0.972; CI: 95%; $p > 0.05$). The IoU scores of the model and the dentists were 0.785 and 0.696 (min–max: 0.711–0.717; CI: 95%; $p > 0.05$), respectively. The Dice coefficient scores of the model and the dentists were 0.663 and 0.570 (min–max: 0.587–0.594; CI: 95%; $p > 0.05$), respectively. The model yielded a better accuracy, precision, recall, specificity, NPV, F1-score, IoU, and Dice scores than the dentists, while the results of all metrics showed no significant difference between the model and the dentists (CI: 95%; $p > 0.05$)).

Second, we considered multiclass classification for DenseNet121 and analyzed the performances of the dentists and of deep learning methods for dental caries stage diagnosis. For D1 lesions, the recall rate of the model was 0.765, while it was 0.466 for the dentists (CI: 95%; $p > 0.05$). For D2 lesions, the recall rate of the model was 0.652, while it was 0.539 for the dentists (CI: 95%; $p > 0.05$). For D3 lesions, the recall rate of the model was 0.918, while it was 0.954 for the dentists (CI: 95%; $p > 0.05$). Although there were no significant differences between the sensitivity scores of the dentists and those of the model for all caries stages, the model seemed to be more sensitive in detecting D1 and D2 lesions. The same results were found for accuracy, specificity, precision, NPV, and F1-score metrics. Even though no significant differences were found in the previous metrics, the model yielded higher scores in terms of all metrics for D1 and D2 lesions than the dentists. The recall, NPV, and F1-score values of the dentists for D3 lesions were slightly higher than those of the model.

4. Discussion

Due to the varying accuracy and sensitivity of individual dentists in the detection of caries lesions and their depth, inconsistent treatment decisions and suboptimal care are quite common. High-throughput diagnostic assistance provided by computer-assisted analysis tools could support dentists with these procedures. To date, panoramic films, as the main auxiliary diagnostic method for oral disease screening, have been gradually interpreted by deep learning. However, deep learning has very rarely been used in caries depth classification. Furthermore, the performance of these models is not regularly compared with that of dentists in caries lesion segmentation or classification [27]. The latter (lesion stage-specific classification performance) is of vital importance in clinical decision making. Enamel caries can be treated by remineralization, and dentin caries in the outer space are commonly treated by cavity filling. For deep dentin caries that approach the dental pulp, pulp capping or root canal therapy is required. From this perspective, the automatic and accurate panoramic interpretation of dental caries lesion staging can provide comprehensive treatment recommendations for individuals. This study aimed to design an intelligence-assisted diagnosis method based on a combined nnU-net and DenseNet121 model to replace the manual interpretation of caries lesions and their extensions. We achieved these goals by constructing caries panoramic datasets for four-stage caries extensions. Furthermore, the segmentation performance of nnU-net and the classification performance of DenseNet121 were evaluated individually and in combination with dentist diagnoses to carry out a comparative analysis.

Our results suggest that nnU-Net can be used for the automated interpretation of panoramas to facilitate caries diagnosis. The accuracy of the model was higher than that of models in previous studies [12,28] and yielded a score of 0.986. The performances of the model and of the experienced dentists showed no significant difference in caries lesion segmentation. However, nnU-Net seems to be more efficient and achieved reliable and objective results.

In our study, DenseNet121 proved to be effective in lesion extension classification. Combining transfer learning with simplified image preprocessing improved the classification accuracy and recall of the neural network. It is prudent to conclude that this method allows us to automatically learn the differences among the caries types in caries extension image features and attain valid interpretations.

The results indicate that the model that we used in the study can automatically learn the differences among caries depths in caries extension image features and achieve effective interpretations. Although the chi-square tests of accuracy, recall, specificity, precision, NPV, F1-score, IoU, and Dice metrics between the model and the dentists showed no significant differences (CI: 95%; $p > 0.5$), the model yielded better scores than the dentists for D1 and D2 lesions. Moreover, the model seemed to be more efficacious and reliable than the dentists, since the six experienced dentists did not show good consistency and stability, the 95% confidence interval for the ICC population values of the dentists was 0.595 (0.537 < ICC < 0.653), and the model was much faster and more accurate in lesion classification. Further research needs to be conducted with a larger dataset and different experienced dentists.

In this study, DenseNet121 seemed to be more sensitive in classifying D1 and D2 lesions and had similar recall rates when compared to dentists in classifying D3 lesions, which is consistent with our hypothesis. Notably, in clinical radiograph interpretation, D3 lesions have a larger range of transmission images in panoramic films and are easier to detect with the naked eye. Caries in the D1 and D2 stages are more likely to be missed or have lesion boundaries that are difficult to determine. However, the recall rates of the dentists and the model were not significantly different according to the chi-squared test. The result was as expected. The dentists involved for the comparison were all experienced experts, and their results were used to set the "ground truth". However, larger tests involving more dentists from different departments and with different experience levels may obtain different results in further studies. For better performance, a combination of dentists' diagnoses and the model's results to detect caries and perform classification is recommended.

Nevertheless, it is challenging to achieve satisfying segmentation results due to the slight difference in the gray levels between tooth structures and bone on panoramic films [29]. Complicated changes in the pixel intensity of overlapping skeletal structures in panoramic films are a particular obstacle to overcome. These structures include the nasal area, maxillary sinus, teeth, and surrounding bone [30]. Moreover, our targets (caries lesions) are quite small when compared to the whole image. For these reasons, we enlarged the radiographs to 1:5 when labeling. However, some boundaries of the lesions were undefinable in overlapping two-dimensional images. Moreover, we have constantly increased the dataset and have now built a dataset with 3840 caries verified by experts.

This study has some strengths and limitations. First, we built a large dataset relative to other datasets in the dental field. Since there is no open dataset related to caries stages in relevant research fields, 1160 panoramic X-rays were meticulously collected, and blurred images were excluded. Three expert dentists were trained to label and annotate the dental caries, and a fourth expert revised any controversial results. Second, the predicted caries were output as highlighted areas by nnU-Net and presented in three different colors according to their depths obtained by DenseNet121. Third, the aforementioned performance comparison between dental experts and nnU-Net and DenseNet121 was carried out on a test dataset. As a limitation, our panoramic films were made on the equipment of one company and we excluded the blurred ones (90 out of 1250) before training the models, which means that the reference dataset underlying our research is not fully generalizable. It is essential to verify our neural networks on an external test set in the next steps. Furthermore, we applied no gold standard in the study such as micro-CT and histology of extracted teeth. However, dentists with different experiences and professional backgrounds are required for comparison, which may provide more valuable information. Second, labeling in the constructed reference test was not sufficiently precise, as it was not triangulated with the gold standard (histology). Even without a hard gold standard, "fuzzy" labeling should be verified with data from other diagnostic approaches, such as visual, tactile, or transillumination inspection, if possible. Finally, nnU-Net and DenseNet121 have not been executed or implemented in an auxiliary diagnosis system until now. It is difficult to infer whether the model will have a positive impact when it is actually deployed in patient care [31].

Accordingly, we recommend that further studies use well-trained neural networks in random and prospective designs. The accuracy of neural networks and the correct usage of these tools in the clinic should be explored. This correct usage includes how dentists adopt and interact with the tools, how the diagnostic procedure improves, and how the tools change the treatment decision-making protocol. Before entering clinical care, all deep learning methods are recommended to be reviewed according to the standards of evidence-based practice, and then, a comprehensive set of results should be obtained in various environments to ensure their robustness, universality, and clinical consequences.

5. Conclusions

Accordingly, the well-trained neural network performed similarly to experienced dentists in detecting caries lesions and classifying them according to depth within our limited study. Notably, although the dentists and the neural network seemed to have a similar performance, the neural network might have better sensitivity and accuracy in classifying caries extensions in the outer dentin. The impact of using the network on the accurate diagnosis of diseases and treatment decision making should be further explored.

Author Contributions: Conceptualization, F.Z. and H.Z.; methodology, L.L.; software, T.Z.; validation, T.Z. and L.L.; formal analysis, L.L.; investigation, H.Z.; data curation, T.Z.; writing—original draft preparation, L.L.; writing—review and editing, H.Z.; supervision, F.Z.; project administration, H.Z. All authors have read and agreed to the published version of the manuscript.

Funding: This research was funded by the Natural Science Foundation of Zhejiang Province, grant number LZY21F030002, The Fundamental Research Funds for the Zhejiang Provincial Universities, grant number 2021XZZX033, and China Oral Health Foundation under grand: A2021-008.

Institutional Review Board Statement: The study was approved by the Institutional Review Board (or Ethics Committee) of the Chinese Stomatological Association (protocol code ChiCTR2100044897 and date of approval: 31 December 2020).

Informed Consent Statement: Due to the retrospective nature of the survey and the use of anonymous patient data, consent of patients was not requested by the Ethics Committee of ZJUSS, (approval no. ChiCTR2100044897 and date of approval: 31 December 2020).

Acknowledgments: The authors want to thank the Radiology Department and Electronic Information Department for their cooperation and help.

Conflicts of Interest: The authors declare no conflict of interest. The funders had no role in the design of the study; in the collection, analyses, or interpretation of data; in the writing of the manuscript, or in the decision to publish the results.

References

1. Gill, J. Dental Caries: The Disease and its Clinical Management, Third Edition. *Br. Dent. J.* **2016**, *221*, 443. [CrossRef]
2. Kaur, R.; Sandhu, R.S. Edge detection in digital panoramic dental radiograph using improved morphological gradient and MATLAB. In Proceedings of the 2017 International Conference on Smart Technologies for Smart Nation (SmartTechCon), Bengaluru, India, 17–19 August 2017.
3. Schwendicke, F.; Tzschoppe, M. Radiographic caries detection: A systematic review and meta-analysis. *J. Dent.* **2015**, *43*, 924–933. [CrossRef]
4. Rushton, V. The quality of panoramic radiographs in a sample of general dental practices. *Br. Dent. J.* **1999**, *186*, 630–633. [CrossRef] [PubMed]
5. Wirtz, A.; Mirashi, S.G. *Automatic Teeth Segmentation in Panoramic X-ray Images Using a Coupled Shape Model in Combination with a Neural Network*; Springer: Cham, Switzerland, 2018.
6. Geibel, M.A.; Carstens, S.; Braisch, U.; Rahman, A.; Herz, M.; Jablonski-Momeni, A. Radiographic diagnosis of proximal caries-influence of experience and gender of the dental staff. *Clin. Oral Investig.* **2017**, *21*, 2761–2770. [CrossRef] [PubMed]
7. Min, J.K.; Kwak, M.S. Overview of Deep Learning in Gastrointestinal Endoscopy. *Gut Liver* **2019**, *13*, 388–393. [CrossRef] [PubMed]
8. Esteva, A.; Kuprel, B. Dermatologist-level classification of skin cancer with deep neural networks. *Nature* **2017**, *542*, 115–118. [CrossRef]

9. Wang, S.; Zha, Y.; Li, W.; Wu, Q.; Li, X.; Niu, M.; Wang, M.; Qiu, X.; Li, H.; Yu, H.; et al. A fully automatic deep learning system for COVID-19 diagnostic and prognostic analysis. *Eur. Respir J.* **2020**, *56*, 2000775. [CrossRef]
10. Ronneberger, O.; Fischer, P. *U-Net: Convolutional Networks for Biomedical Image Segmentation*; Springer: Cham, Switzerland, 2015.
11. Prajapati, S.A.; Nagaraj, R. Classification of dental diseases using CNN and transfer learning. In Proceedings of the 2017 5th International Symposium on Computational and Business Intelligence (ISCBI), Dubai, United Arab Emirates, 11–14 August 2017.
12. Cantu, A.G.; Gehrung, S. Detecting caries lesions of different radiographic extension on bitewings using deep learning. *J. Dent.* **2020**, *100*, 103425. [CrossRef]
13. Bayraktar, Y.; Ayan, E. Diagnosis of interproximal caries lesions with deep convolutional neural network in digital bitewing radiographs. *Clin. Oral Investig.* **2021**, 1–10. [CrossRef]
14. Lee, S.; Oh, S.I. Deep learning for early dental caries detection in bitewing radiographs. *Sci. Rep.* **2021**, *11*, 16807. [CrossRef]
15. Lin, X.J.; Zhang, D. Evaluation of computer-aided diagnosis system for detecting dental approximal caries lesions on periapical radiographs. *Chin. J. Stomatol.* **2020**, *55*, 654–660.
16. Schwendicke, F.; Elhennawy, K. Deep learning for caries lesion detection in near-infrared light transillumination images: A pilot study. *J. Dent.* **2020**, *92*, 103260. [CrossRef]
17. You, W.; Hao, A. Deep learning-based dental plaque detection on primary teeth: A comparison with clinical assessments. *BMC Oral Health* **2020**, *20*, 141. [CrossRef] [PubMed]
18. Huang, G.; Liu, Z. Densely Connected Convolutional Networks. In Proceedings of the IEEE Conference on Computer Vision and Pattern Recognition, Honolulu, HI, USA, 21–26 July 2017.
19. Bossuyt, P.M.; Reitsma, J.B. STARD 2015: An updated list of essential items for reporting diagnostic accuracy studies. *BMJ* **2015**, *351*, 1446–1452.
20. Isensee, F.; Jaeger, P.F. nnU-Net: A self-configuring method for deep learning-based biomedical image segmentation. *Nat. Methods* **2021**, *18*, 203–211. [CrossRef]
21. Tan, M.; Le, Q.V. EfficientNet: Rethinking Model Scaling for Convolutional Neural Networks. In Proceedings of the International Conference on Machine Learning, Rome, Italy, 11–13 March 2022.
22. Hinton, G.E.; Srivastava, N. Improving neural networks by preventing co-adaptation of feature detectors. *Comput. Sci.* **2012**, *3*, 212–223.
23. Schmidhuber, J. Deep Learning in Neural Networks: An Overview. *Neural Netw.* **2015**, *61*, 85–117. [CrossRef] [PubMed]
24. Srivastava, N.; Hinton, G. Dropout: A Simple Way to Prevent Neural Networks from Overfitting. *J. Mach. Learn. Res.* **2014**, *15*, 1929–1958.
25. Szegedy, C.; Vanhoucke, V. Rethinking the Inception Architecture for Computer Vision. In Proceedings of the IEEE Conference on Computer Vision and Pattern Recognition, Las Vegas, NV, USA, 26 June–1 July 2016.
26. He, K.; Zhang, X. Deep Residual Learning for Image Recognition. In Proceedings of the IEEE Conference on Computer Vision and Pattern Recognition, Las Vegas, NV, USA, 26 June–1 July 2016.
27. Prados-Privado, M.; García Villalón, J. Dental Caries Diagnosis and Detection Using Neural Networks: A Systematic Review. *J. Clin. Med.* **2020**, *9*, 3579. [CrossRef] [PubMed]
28. Albahbah, A.A.; El-Bakry, H.M. Detection of Caries in Panoramic Dental X-ray Images using Back-Propagation Neural Network. *Int. J. Electron. Commun. Comput. Eng.* **2016**, *7*, 250.
29. Hasan, M.M.; Ismail, W. Automatic segmentation of jaw from panoramic dental X-ray images using GVF snakes. In Proceedings of the 2016 World Automation Congress (WAC), Rio Grande, Puerto Rico, 31 July–4 August 2016.
30. Noujeim, M.; Prihoda, T. Pre-clinical evaluation of a new dental panoramic radiographic system based on tomosynthesis method. *Dentomaxillofac. Radiol.* **2015**, *40*, 42–46. [CrossRef] [PubMed]
31. Nagendran, M.; Chen, Y. Artificial intelligence versus clinicians: Systematic review of design, reporting standards, and claims of deep learning studies. *BMJ* **2020**, *368*, 689. [CrossRef] [PubMed]

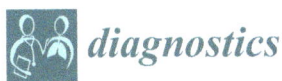

Article

Artificial Intelligence Model to Detect Real Contact Relationship between Mandibular Third Molars and Inferior Alveolar Nerve Based on Panoramic Radiographs

Tianer Zhu [1], Daqian Chen [2], Fuli Wu [2], Fudong Zhu [1,*] and Haihua Zhu [1,*]

[1] Stomatology Hospital, School of Stomatology, Zhejiang University School of Medicine, Clinical Research Center for Oral Disease of Zhejiang Province, Key Laboratory of Oral Biomedical Research of Zhejiang Province, Cancer Center of Zhejiang University, Hangzhou 310006, China; zhutianer@zju.edu.cn

[2] School of Computer Science and Technology, Zhejiang University of Technology, Hangzhou 310006, China; 2111912004@zjut.edu.cn (D.C.); fuliwu@zjut.edu.cn (F.W.)

* Correspondence: zfd@zju.edu.cn (F.Z.); zhuhh403@zju.edu.cn (H.Z.)

Citation: Zhu, T.; Chen, D.; Wu, F.; Zhu, F.; Zhu, H. Artificial Intelligence Model to Detect Real Contact Relationship between Mandibular Third Molars and Inferior Alveolar Nerve Based on Panoramic Radiographs. *Diagnostics* **2021**, *11*, 1664. https://doi.org/10.3390/diagnostics11091664

Academic Editor: Jae-Hong Lee

Received: 29 July 2021
Accepted: 8 September 2021
Published: 11 September 2021

Publisher's Note: MDPI stays neutral with regard to jurisdictional claims in published maps and institutional affiliations.

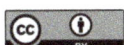

Copyright: © 2021 by the authors. Licensee MDPI, Basel, Switzerland. This article is an open access article distributed under the terms and conditions of the Creative Commons Attribution (CC BY) license (https://creativecommons.org/licenses/by/4.0/).

Abstract: This study aimed to develop a novel detection model for automatically assessing the real contact relationship between mandibular third molars (MM3s) and the inferior alveolar nerve (IAN) based on panoramic radiographs processed with deep learning networks, minimizing pseudo-contact interference and reducing the frequency of cone beam computed tomography (CBCT) use. A deep-learning network approach based on YOLOv4, named as MM3-IANnet, was applied to oral panoramic radiographs for the first time. The relationship between MM3s and the IAN in CBCT was considered the real contact relationship. Accuracy metrics were calculated to evaluate and compare the performance of the MM3–IANnet, dentists and a cooperative approach with dentists and the MM3–IANnet. Our results showed that in comparison with detection by dentists (AP = 76.45%) or the MM3–IANnet (AP = 83.02%), the cooperative dentist–MM3–IANnet approach yielded the highest average precision (AP = 88.06%). In conclusion, the MM3-IANnet detection model is an encouraging artificial intelligence approach that might assist dentists in detecting the real contact relationship between MM3s and IANs based on panoramic radiographs.

Keywords: deep learning network; YOLOv4; mandibular third molar; inferior alveolar nerve; contact relationship; panoramic radiograph

1. Introduction

The high impaction rate of mandibular third molars (MM3s) makes the extraction of third molars a common surgical procedure [1] that can result in multiple complications. Inferior alveolar nerve (IAN) injury is one of the most severe complications, resulting in hypoesthesia and numbness of the lower lip or chin [2]. The incidence of IAN injury ranges from 0.4~6% and IAN injury occurs most frequently when MM3s are closely related to the IAN [3,4]. There are various reasons for IAN injury after the extraction of MM3s, including direct trauma, indirect compression, or lack of bone cortex around the IAN [5]. The risk of IAN injury after tooth extraction increases when MM3s anatomically touch the IAN [6]. When the dental roots are in contact with the IAN, the bone cortex around the IAN may appear absent or discontinuous [7]. When the elevator is inserted into the periodontal ligament space of MM3s, a compressive load is generated in the apical region of the molar; the compressive load will act on the IAN during extraction and lead to IAN injury. Therefore, it is necessary to predict the contact relationship between MM3s and the IAN with radiographic examination before tooth extraction, which contributes to preoperatively predicting surgical difficulty and the possibility of complications [8,9], thereby developing a more minimally invasive extraction strategy and reducing the risk of IAN injury.

In radiographic examination, panoramic radiographs are most commonly used and aid dentists in determining the relationship between MM3s and the IAN canal because it can provide clinical dental image with short scan-time and low radiation dose [10]. However, panoramic radiographs have many shortcomings, such as anatomical noise, superimposition, and geometric distortion effect [11]. It can be difficult to distinguish the real contact relationship between MM3s and the IAN based on panoramic radiographs, especially when dental roots are located in the buccolingual direction of the IAN [12]. Pseudo-contact occurs frequently, which indicates that MM3s contact the IAN in panoramic radiographs, but this contact does not occur in cone beam computed tomography (CBCT). The visual detection of the relationship between MM3s and the IAN by dentists based on panoramic radiographs can thus be limited and unreliable [13]. Currently, the use of CBCT can reflect the three-dimensional structure of a tooth and the IAN to accurately distinguish the contact relationship between the dental roots and the IAN, which contributes to facilitating preoperative planning and reducing the risk of IAN injury [14]. However, CBCT is not used as a routine inspection method because it will significantly increase the patient costs and radiation dose [15,16], which doesn't match the standard dose recommended in some countries [17]. Therefore, it is important to determine whether the real contact relationship can be precisely determined depending on panoramic radiographs, avoiding pseudo-contact issues and reducing the frequency of CBCT use.

Researchers have focused on the issue of pseudo-contact on panoramic radiographs. Studies have shown that when panoramic radiographs exhibit "darkening of the root", "interruption of the radiopaque border of the mandibular canal", and "inferior alveolar neural tube diversion" [18], the dental roots and IAN may display a close relationship, and the probability of IAN injury after extraction increases. However, the technique requires considerable training for dentists, and judgments with these methods are still not sufficiently accurate [19,20], especially for dental roots in the buccolingual direction. Overall, it is difficult but necessary to reliably detect the real relationship between MM3s and the IAN based on panoramic radiographs. Therefore, in this study, we use an artificial intelligence technique to aid in the diagnosis.

Deep learning networks have played an important role in medical image research, which can identify many complex image structures in modern medicine and have been used in various fields, such as multiple organ segmentation for the abdomen [21]. In stomatology, deep learning has also been applied in the detection of caries, periodontal disease, root development staging and other issues [22–24]. In terms of impacted teeth, few studies have focused on the relationship between impacted teeth and the IAN using deep learning. In previous studies, the researchers segmented and identified images of MM3s and IANs based on panoramic radiographs with a deep learning network called U-Net [25], but the accuracy of existing methods remains to be improved and the pseudo-contact of MM3s and the IAN in panoramic radiographs has not been mentioned. Within the limited scope of our knowledge, there has been no research on diagnostic models involving the real contact relationship between MM3s and the IAN with a deep learning network.

Therefore, in this study, we established a novel detection model for automatically assessing the real contact relationship between MM3s and the IAN based on panoramic radiographs and deep learning networks, named as MM3–IANnet. With this model, we sought to achieve two results: (1) minimizing interference from pseudo-contacts in panoramic radiographs, thereby reducing the frequency of CBCT use and (2) assisting dentists in more accurately identifying contact relationships, thereby estimating the risk of IAN injury more accurately before tooth extraction.

2. Materials and Methods

This study (ChiCTR2100044897) was approved by the Medical Ethics Committee of Stomatology Hospital, School of Stomatology, Zhejiang University School of Medicine, and was conducted in compliance with the ICH-GCP principles and the Declaration of Helsinki (2013).

2.1. Image Data Set

The study was conducted at Stomatology Hospital, School of Stomatology, Zhejiang University School of Medicine. The inclusion criteria for panoramic radiographs were as follows: (1) at least one mandibular third molar with fully developed dental roots must be present; (2) panoramic radiographs and CBCT scans less than 3 months apart from the panoramic radiographs must be available; and (3) patients must be older than 18 years old. Panoramic radiographs with buccolingual impacted of MM3s, incomplete panoramic radiographs, or panoramic radiographs of poor quality were not included in the study. All panoramic radiographs were acquired with a Dentsply Sirona (Bensheim, Germany) and an Orthophos XG 5OS Ceph.

All panoramic radiograph datasets were evaluated by three independent dentists who collected and categorized the results with kappa > 0.8. In total, 503 panoramic radiographs (915 MM3s) obtained between January 2016 and January 2021 were selected (age range of patients: 18 to 68 years old). The contact relationship between MM3s and the IAN canal in CBCT was considered the real contact relationship. Based on the real contact relationship between MM3s and the IAN in CBCT, these molars were divided into contact and non-contact groups. For individuals in the contact group, the dental roots of their molars were in contact with the IAN in CBCT, and vice versa for individuals in the non-contact group (Figure 1). The details of the two groups are shown in Table 1. The criteria for contact were as follows: (1) MM3s contacted with the mandibular canal with a defective white line and (2) MM3s penetrated the mandibular canal.

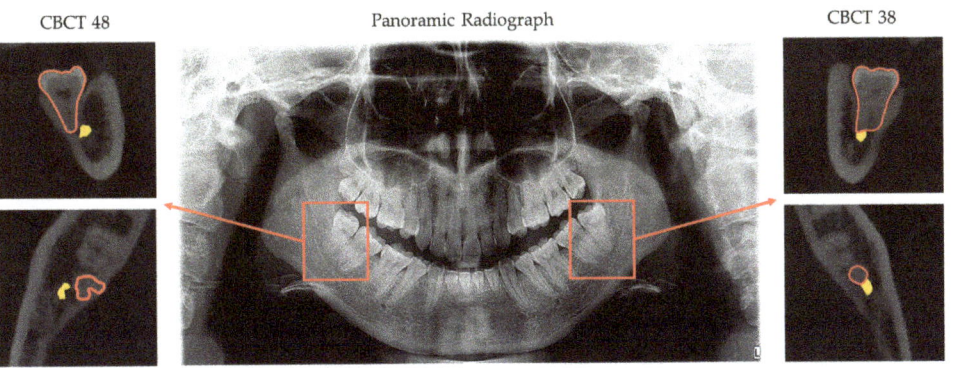

Figure 1. Panoramic view of a patient with corresponding CBCT results. Tooth position was recorded using the Federation Dentaire International system. Forty-eight showed that the dental roots were in contact with the IAN in the panoramic radiograph but not in contact in CBCT, so 48 was classified into the non-contact group. Thirty-eight showed the dental roots in contact with the IAN in both the panoramic radiograph and the CBCT result, so 38 was classified into the contact group.

Table 1. Results for Contact and Non-contact Group Categories.

Categories	Non-Contact Group	Contact Group
MM3 Number	530	328

2.2. Deep Learning Network Construction and Training

The core mechanism of contact detection revolved around a deep learning network called YOLOv4, which had been verified to provide high accuracy and a fast analysis speed in the detection of ROIs [26]. We named our detection model as MM3–IANnet.

We used 80 percent of the images for training, 10 percent for validation and 10 percent for testing. The workflow of the model could be divided into four steps (Figure 2).

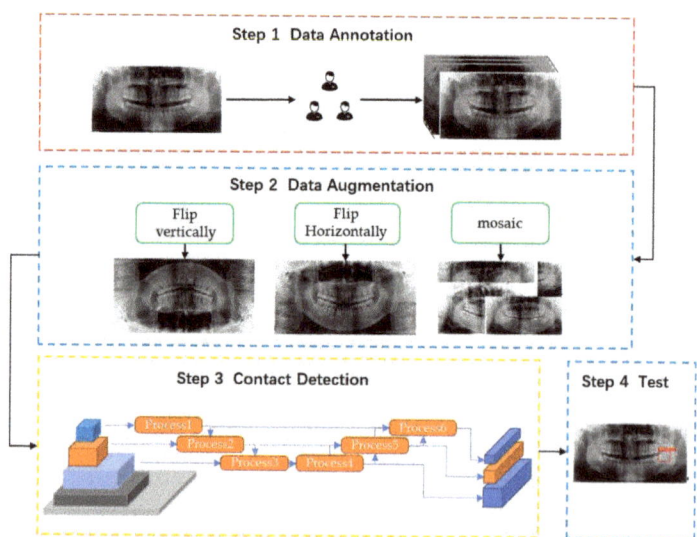

Figure 2. Model of MM3–IANnet system architecture. In step 3, process 1–process 3 was the upper sampling operation and process 4–process 6 was the lower sampling operation.

The first step was data annotation. In this step, all panoramic radiographs were resized to 1440 × 2976 pixels. When MM3s contacted the IAN canal in CBCT images, namely, MM3 were divided into contact group, the MM3s were labeled "touch" with the open-source software LabelImg. In total, 915 MM3s were included, with 549 for training, 183 for validation and 183 for network testing.

The second step was data augmentation. After labeling, we used three methods, namely, horizontal flipping, vertical flipping, and mosaicking, to enhance the data, which effectively expanded the number of datasets and improved training convergence.

The third step was touch detection. Images were input into YOLOv4. In this step, the workflow could be divided into three parts. The first part involved CSPDarkNet53, which was used to extract abundant feature information from the input images. Then SPP + PAN (space pyramid pooling module + path aggregation network) was used to generate feature pyramids. A feature pyramid could enhance the identification and detection of objects with different scales and sizes. YoloHead was used for the final test. The final output vector with class probability, object score, and bounding box information was the output.

The fourth step included inputting test data.

2.3. Diagnostic Performance Analysis

To compare the accuracy between the automated detection models MM3–IANnet and dentists, we randomly selected 188 MM3 as the testing dataset, and three dentists with 3 years of experience (Dentist 1, Dentist 2, and Dentist 3) and two dentists with 1 year of experience (Dentist 4 and Dentist 5) were asked to assess the dataset. Dentists were given background information about the study and the detection task. Furthermore, dentists were required to work cooperatively with the MM3–IANnet. We designed a voting experiment in which we set the weight of each dentist to 1 and the weight of the MM3–IANnet to 2. Firstly, the dentists and MM3-IANnet made independent judgements regarding the relationship between MM3s and the IAN based on the panoramic radiographs, and we then calculated the final test result according to the weighted results.

Based on the results for detection, the metrics were calculated to compare the performance of the deep learning network, the subjective assessments of dentists and the cooperative dentist–MM3–IANnet approach.

2.4. Statistical Analysis

Diagnostic accuracy was calculated using precision (TP/(TP + FP)), recall (TP/(TP + FN)), F1 score (2Precision*Recall/(Precision + Recall)) and average precision (AP = $\int_0^1 p(r)dr$) (Table 2). A Chi-square test was used to compare the assessment results. Statistical analyses were performed with IBM SPSS Statistics 24.0, and the statistical level of significance was set to $p < 0.05$.

Table 2. Confusion matrix.

		Actual Performance	
		1	0
Predicted Performance	1	True Positive (TP)	False Positive (FP)
	0	False Negative (FN)	True Negative (TN)

3. Results

3.1. Deep Learning Network Accuracy

After training, validation, and testing of 915 MM3s, the deep learning network YOLOv4, i.e., MM3-IANnet, yielded an average precision of 85.05%, a precision of 87.18%, a recall of 82.93% and a F1-score of 84.99%. Table 3 showed the detailed accuracy metrics of the new diagnosis model with YOLOv4 for detecting the real contact relationship between MM3s and the IAN based on panoramic radiographs.

Table 3. Accuracy metrics of the MM3-IANnet for detecting real contact relationship.

Parameter	MM3-IANnet
Average precision	85.05%
Precision	87.18%
Recall	82.93%
F1-score	84.99%

3.2. Diagnostic Performance Analysis

Five dentists yielded an average precision of 76.45% ± 8.60%, a precision of 89.85% 6.81%, a recall of 83.00% ± 9.76% and a F1-score of 85.82% ± 5.06%. The mean average precision of dentists with 3 years of work experience (Dentist 1, Dentist 2, and Dentist 3) was 75.30% ± 11.02% (mean ± SD), and that of dentists with 1 year of work experience (Dentist 4 and Dentist 5) was 78.18% ± 6.57%. The intraclass correlation coefficient (ICC) of the five dentists was 0.302. Table 4 showed the detailed accuracy metrics for detections by dentists.

Table 4. Detailed accuracy metrics of detecting ability of dentists.

Parameter	Dentist 1	Dentist 2	Dentist 3	Dentist 4	Dentist 5	Mean ± SD
Average precision	66.82%	71.33%	87.75%	73.53%	82.82%	76.45% ± 8.60%
Precision	95.45%	90.91%	97.22%	82.35%	83.33%	89.85% ± 6.81%
Recall	70.00%	76.92%	89.74%	84.00%	94.34%	83.00% ± 9.76%
F1-score	80.77%	83.33%	93.33%	83.17%	88.50%	85.82% ± 5.06%

After testing of 188 MM3s, based on a comparison of diagnostic performance, MM3–IANnet yielded an average precision of 83.02%, a recall of 91.67% and a F1-score of 90.16%, which were higher than the mean average precision (76.45%), recall (83.00%), and F1-score (85.82%) of the five dentists. The cooperation between dentists and the MM3–IANnet, i.e., the voting experiment, yielded the highest average precision (88.06%), precision (93.88%), recall (92.00%), and F1-score (92.93%). The Chi-square test showed that the dentist–MM3–IANnet approach and MM3–IANnet were not statistically superior to the dentists-based assessment method (Figure 3 and Table 5; $p > 0.05$).

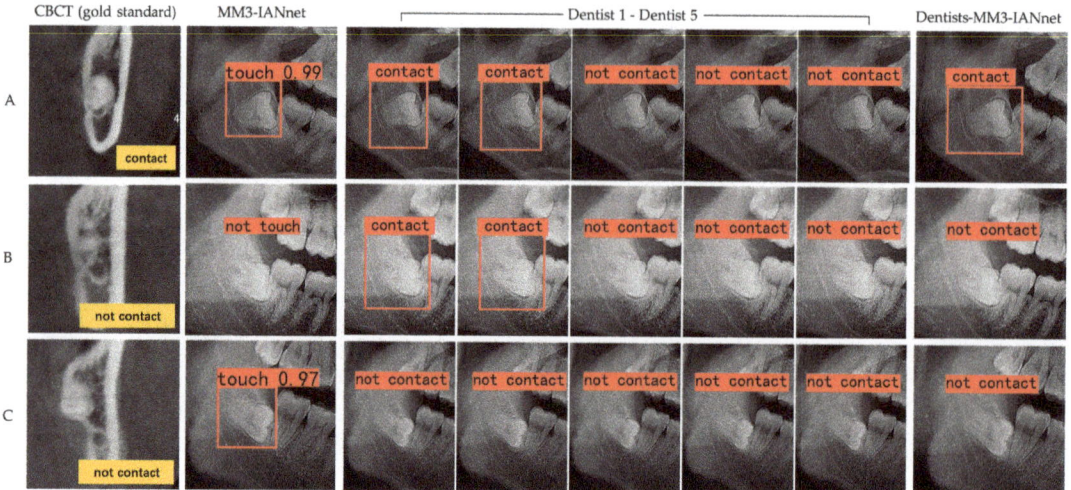

Figure 3. Output results of MM3–IANnet, dentists and cooperative dentist–MM3–IANnet approach. Three typical examples are presented. (**A**) According to the contact relationship in CBCT images (gold standard), the MM3 and IAN were divided into the contact group. The test result of MM3–IANnet was the contact. Two of the five dentists considered the case a contact, and the other three did not. The test result of dentist–MM3–IANnet (voting experiment) was a contact. (**B**) The MM3 and IAN were divided into the non-contact group. The test result of MM3–IANnet was the non-contact, and two of the five dentists considered the case a contact, while the other three did not. The test result of dentists–MM3–IANnet was the non-contact. (**C**) The MM3 and IAN were divided into the non-contact group. The test result of MM3-IANnet was a contact, five dentists considered the case non-contact, and the test result of dentist–MM3–IANnet was non-contact.

Table 5. Performance comparison between the MM3–IANnet, dentists and cooperative dentist-MM3–IANnet approach.

Parameter	MM3-IANnet	Dentists (Mean)	Dentists-MM3-IANnet
Average precision	83.02%	76.45%	88.06%
Precision	88.71%	89.85%	93.88%
Recall	91.67%	83.00%	92.00%
F1-score	90.16%	85.82%	92.93%

4. Discussion

The performance of a MM3–IANnet in detecting the real contact relationship between MM3s and the IAN based on panoramic radiographs was assessed in this paper, and the results were compared to those obtained by five dentists. We assumed the MM3–IANnet based on YOLOv4 yielded higher detection accuracy and reliability than the dentists, and the dentist–MM3–IANnet combination for detection was superior to the MM3–IANnet or dentists alone. Our findings partially support the original hypothesis that the MM3–IANnet yielded higher average precision, recall, and F1 score values than dentists, and the dentist–MM3–IANnet combination, i.e., the voting experiment, produced the highest average precision, precision, recall, and F1 score. However, statistical analysis showed the MM3-IANnet result and dentist–MM3–IANnet result were not statistically significant and superior to that of dentists.

In clinical practice, dentists often rely on experience to evaluate the contact relationship between MM3s and the IAN with the naked eye based on panoramic radiographs. Therefore, many studies have evaluated the predictive value of panoramic radiographs in assessing the relationship between MM3s and the IAN. Studies have shown that among the existing panoramic radiograph-based prediction methods, deflection of the root, narrowing of the root, dark and bifid apex of the root, and narrowing of the canal provide low predictive value, while the presence of a canal diversion, the interruption of the white line of the canal, and darkening of the root in panoramic radiographs could be routinely used to identify high-risk cases [19]. Still, the positive predictive value of these indicators was low and not sufficiently accurate [20]. Moreover, our results indicated that the average precision of the real contact relationship between MM3s and the IAN detected by dentists was only 76.45% ± 8.60%, which suggested that the accuracy was not high. Since there are limits to human assessment capabilities, artificial intelligence may be helpful in this field to identify the three-dimensional CBCT data in two-dimensional panoramic radiographs.

In our experiment, we applied YOLOv4 for detection with oral panoramic radiographs for the first time. YOLOv4, released in April 2020, is a new high-performance detection network that was developed based on the optimization of the previous convolutional neural network and has been applied in modern medicine [26,27]. YOLOv4 has a faster target detection speed and higher accuracy than other convolutional neural networks and has displayed excellent performance in many applications [28,29]. In YOLOv4, the only required input for the neural network to produce detection results is an image, and complex detection process can be avoided. Therefore, the detection speed for given targets is greatly improved. Moreover, YOLOv4 can avoid background errors, prevent false positives, and learn the general characteristics of target objects, thereby improving the detection accuracy. In our experiment, the core of model-based detection was YOLOv4, which performed rapid, real-time, lightweight, and accurate target identification under the premise of ensuring accuracy. Thus, this model could assist dentists in assessing the real contact relationship between MM3s and the IAN and improve the efficiency and accuracy of diagnoses. Therefore, this approach has excellent application potential in clinical practice.

Our study showed that with the application of MM3-IANnet, the predictive accuracy was increased, which in turn might decrease the frequency of CBCT use and IAN risk. The model of the real contact relationship detection between MM3s and the IAN based on panoramic radiographs was generally successful, as the total average precision of the MM3–IANnet was 85.05%. In the human–machine comparison experiment, the results showed that the mean precision of the five dentists was 89.85% ± 6.81%, indicating that the dentists had a certain ability to identify the contact relationship between the dental roots and the IAN from the panoramic radiographs, and their accuracy was acceptable when the dentists believed dental roots contacted the IAN; that is, the probability of dental roots and the IAN being in contact was high based on CBCT. However, the mean recall of dentists was 83.00% ± 9.76%, indicating that when the dental roots were judged by dentists to not be in contact with the IAN based on panoramic radiographs, there was still a high probability of contact based on CBCT. Therefore, the overall average precision of dentists was not high (76.45% ± 8.60%), suggesting that it was difficult for experienced dentists to accurately and comprehensively assess the real contact relationship between dental roots and the IAN in long-term clinical work. In the human–machine contrast experiment, although statistical analysis showed the MM3–IANnet result and dentist–MM3–IANnet result were not statistically significant and superior to that of dentists, the recall, F1 score, and average precision of the MM3–IANnet were numerically higher than those for dentists and the precision was close to that for dentists, indicating that MM3–IANnet at least possessed close ability to the dentists in detecting vague contact states of MM3s and IAN and might be superior to the dentists in accuracy.

In addition, the ICC of five dentists was 0.302 in our experiment, indicating that the five dentists' judgments regarding the real contact relationship between MM3s and the IAN based on the same panoramic radiograph were in poor agreement. Some studies have shown that neither senior nor junior doctors could accurately assess the difficulty of wisdom tooth extraction based on panoramic radiographs, and even panoramic radiographs might hamper decision-making [9], which agreed with our results.

Our findings also suggested that in comparison to detection by dentists or MM3–IANnet independently, the approach in which YOLOv4 was combined with dentist assessment exhibited the highest average precision, precision, recall, and F1 score. The voting experiment was used to set the MM3–IANnet weights, thus enhancing MM3–IANnet accuracy while attenuating the effect of low detection consistency by the dentists. This finding indicated that the combination of the two methods yielded the most accurate results. Therefore, this approach could be clinically practical and has important application prospects.

However, this study had some limitations. The training dataset used in the model was not big enough, and not enough dentists were tested in the experiments. These factors might lead to deviations in the conclusions drawn, and further experimental verification is needed.

In addition to examining the real contact relationship between MM3s and the IAN based on panoramic radiographs, deep learning network can be used to mine more information from panoramic radiographs. The literature suggests that in anatomical studies of MM3s and the IAN, the dental roots are likely to be in close contact with IAN when the roots are buccal to the mandibular IAN, and the risk of nerve injury is high after tooth extraction [4,30]. Moreover, when MM3s are in the tooth germ state, the dental roots are far from the IAN, and the risk of IAN injury after tooth extraction is relatively low. If deep learning network can predict the contact relationship and anatomical position relationship between dental roots and the IAN when an MM3 is in the tooth germ stage, the result will provide important guidance in clinical practice.

5. Conclusions

In conclusion, this study applied a novel artificial intelligence detection model based on YOLOv4, named as MM3–IANnet, which might assist dentists in assessing the real contact relationship between MM3s and the IAN based on panoramic radiographs.

Author Contributions: Conceptualization, H.Z., F.Z. and F.W.; methodology, H.Z., F.Z. and F.W.; software, T.Z., D.C.; validation, D.C.; formal analysis, T.Z.; investigation, T.Z.; resources, T.Z.; data curation, T.Z., D.C.; writing—original draft preparation, T.Z.; writing—review and editing, T.Z., D.C., H.Z., F.Z. and F.W.; visualization, T.Z.; supervision, H.Z., F.Z. and F.W.; project administration, H.Z., F.Z. and F.W.; funding acquisition, H.Z., F.Z. and F.W. All authors have read and agreed to the published version of the manuscript.

Funding: The research was supported by Natural Science Foundation of Zhejiang Province under grand LZY21F030002, the Fundamental Research Funds for the Zhejiang Provincial Universities under grand 2021XZZX033 and China Oral Health Foundation under grand A2021-008.

Informed Consent Statement: Informed consent was obtained from all subjects involved in the study.

Data Availability Statement: The data are not publicly available due to privacy. The data presented in this study are available on request from the corresponding author.

Conflicts of Interest: The authors declare no conflict of interest. The funders had no role in the design of the study; in the collection, analyses, or interpretation of data; in the writing of the manuscript, or in the decision to publish the results.

References

1. Alvira-González, J.; Figueiredo, R.; Valmaseda-Castellón, E.; Quesada-Gómez, C.; Gay-Escoda, C. Predictive factors of difficulty in lower third molar extraction: A prospective cohort study. *Med. Oral Patol. Oral Y Cir. Bucal* **2017**, *22*, e108–e114. [CrossRef]
2. Luo, Q.; Diao, W.; Luo, L.; Zhang, Y. Comparisons of the Computed Tomographic Scan and Panoramic Radiography Before Mandibular Third Molar Extraction Surgery. *Med. Sci. Monit. Int. Med. J. Exp. Clin. Res.* **2018**, *24*, 3340–3347. [CrossRef]
3. Kim, J.W.; Cha, I.H.; Kim, S.J.; Kim, M.R. Which risk factors are associated with neurosensory deficits of inferior alveolar nerve after mandibular third molar extraction? *J. Oral Maxillofac. Surg. Off. J. Am. Assoc. Oral Maxillofac. Surg.* **2012**, *70*, 2508–2514. [CrossRef]
4. Gu, L.; Zhu, C.; Chen, K.; Liu, X.; Tang, Z. Anatomic study of the position of the mandibular canal and corresponding mandibular third molar on cone-beam computed tomography images. *Surg. Radiol. Anat. SRA* **2018**, *40*, 609–614. [CrossRef]
5. Liu, W.; Yin, W.; Zhang, R.; Li, J.; Zheng, Y. Diagnostic value of panoramic radiography in predicting inferior alveolar nerve injury after mandibular third molar extraction: A meta-analysis. *Aust. Dent. J.* **2015**, *60*, 233–239. [CrossRef]
6. Gomes, A.C.; Vasconcelos, B.C.; Silva, E.D.; Caldas Ade, F., Jr.; Pita Neto, I.C. Sensitivity and specificity of pantomography to predict inferior alveolar nerve damage during extraction of impacted lower third molars. *J. Oral Maxillofac. Surg. Off. J. Am. Assoc. Oral Maxillofac. Surg.* **2008**, *66*, 256–259. [CrossRef]

7. Kubota, S.; Imai, T.; Nakazawa, M.; Uzawa, N. Risk stratification against inferior alveolar nerve injury after lower third molar extraction by scoring on cone-beam computed tomography image. *Odontology* **2020**, *108*, 124–132. [CrossRef]
8. Sánchez-Torres, A.; Soler-Capdevila, J.; Ustrell-Barral, M.; Gay-Escoda, C. Patient, radiological, and operative factors associated with surgical difficulty in the extraction of third molars: A systematic review. *Int. J. Oral Maxillofac. Surg.* **2020**, *49*, 655–665. [CrossRef]
9. Barreiro-Torres, J.; Diniz-Freitas, M.; Lago-Méndez, L.; Gude-Sampedro, F.; Gándara-Rey, J.M.; García-García, A. Evaluation of the surgical difficulty in lower third molar extraction. *Med. Oral Patol. Oral Y Cir. Bucal* **2010**, *15*, e869–e874. [CrossRef]
10. Kim, S.; Ra, J.B. Dynamic focal plane estimation for dental panoramic radiography. *Med. Phys.* **2019**, *46*, 4907–4917. [CrossRef]
11. Nardi, C.; Calistri, L.; Grazzini, G.; Desideri, I.; Lorini, C.; Occhipinti, M.; Mungai, F.; Colagrande, S. Is Panoramic Radiography an Accurate Imaging Technique for the Detection of Endodontically Treated Asymptomatic Apical Periodontitis? *J. Endod.* **2018**, *44*, 1500–1508. [CrossRef]
12. Sedaghatfar, M.; August, M.A.; Dodson, T.B. Panoramic radiographic findings as predictors of inferior alveolar nerve exposure following third molar extraction. *J. Oral Maxillofac. Surg. Off. J. Am. Assoc. Oral Maxillofac. Surg.* **2005**, *63*, 3–7. [CrossRef]
13. Komerik, N.; Muglali, M.; Tas, B.; Selcuk, U. Difficulty of impacted mandibular third molar tooth removal: Predictive ability of senior surgeons and residents. *J. Oral Maxillofac. Surg. Off. J. Am. Assoc. Oral Maxillofac. Surg.* **2014**, *72*, 1062.e1–1062.e6. [CrossRef]
14. Selvi, F.; Dodson, T.B.; Nattestad, A.; Robertson, K.; Tolstunov, L. Factors that are associated with injury to the inferior alveolar nerve in high-risk patients after removal of third molars. *Br. J. Oral Maxillofac. Surg.* **2013**, *51*, 868–873. [CrossRef]
15. Matzen, L.H.; Berkhout, E. Cone beam CT imaging of the mandibular third molar: A position paper prepared by the European Academy of DentoMaxilloFacial Radiology (EADMFR). *Dento Maxillo Facial Radiol.* **2019**, *48*, 20190039. [CrossRef] [PubMed]
16. Ghaeminia, H.; Gerlach, N.L.; Hoppenreijs, T.J.; Kicken, M.; Dings, J.P.; Borstlap, W.A.; de Haan, T.; Bergé, S.J.; Meijer, G.J.; Maal, T.J. Clinical relevance of cone beam computed tomography in mandibular third molar removal: A multicentre, randomised, controlled trial. *J. Cranio-Maxillo-Facial Surg. Off. Publ. Eur. Assoc. Cranio-Maxillo-Facial Surg.* **2015**, *43*, 2158–2167. [CrossRef] [PubMed]
17. Estrela, C.; Bueno, M.R.; Leles, C.R.; Azevedo, B.; Azevedo, J.R. Accuracy of cone beam computed tomography and panoramic and periapical radiography for detection of apical periodontitis. *J. Endod.* **2008**, *34*, 273–279. [CrossRef] [PubMed]
18. Miclotte, A.; Van Hevele, J.; Roels, A.; Elaut, J.; Willems, G.; Politis, C.; Jacobs, R. Position of lower wisdom teeth and their relation to the alveolar nerve in orthodontic patients treated with and without extraction of premolars: A longitudinal study. *Clin. Oral Investig.* **2014**, *18*, 1731–1739. [CrossRef] [PubMed]
19. Su, N.; van Wijk, A.; Berkhout, E.; Sanderink, G.; De Lange, J.; Wang, H.; van der Heijden, G. Predictive Value of Panoramic Radiography for Injury of Inferior Alveolar Nerve After Mandibular Third Molar Surgery. *J. Oral Maxillofac. Surg. Off. J. Am. Assoc. Oral Maxillofac. Surg.* **2017**, *75*, 663–679. [CrossRef]
20. Tolstunov, L. The quest for causes of inferior alveolar nerve injury after extraction of mandibular third molars. *J. Oral Maxillofac. Surg. Off. J. Am. Assoc. Oral Maxillofac. Surg.* **2014**, *72*, 1644–1646. [CrossRef]
21. Ma, J.; Zhang, Y.; Gu, S.; Zhang, Y.; Zhu, C.; Wang, Q.; Liu, X.; An, X.; Ge, C.; Cao, S.-C.; et al. AbdomenCT-1K: Is Abdominal Organ Segmentation A Solved Problem? *IEEE Trans. Pattern Anal. Mach. Intell.* **2021**. Epub ahead of print. [CrossRef]
22. Krois, J.; Ekert, T.; Meinhold, L.; Golla, T.; Kharbot, B.; Wittemeier, A.; Dörfer, C.; Schwendicke, F. Deep Learning for the Radiographic Detection of Periodontal Bone Loss. *Sci. Rep.* **2019**, *9*, 8495. [CrossRef]
23. Banar, N.; Bertels, J.; Laurent, F.; Boedi, R.M.; De Tobel, J.; Thevissen, P.; Vandermeulen, D. Towards fully automated third molar development staging in panoramic radiographs. *Int. J. Leg. Med.* **2020**, *134*, 1831–1841. [CrossRef]
24. Lee, J.H.; Kim, D.H.; Jeong, S.N.; Choi, S.H. Detection and diagnosis of dental caries using a deep learning-based convolutional neural network algorithm. *J. Dent.* **2018**, *77*, 106–111. [CrossRef]
25. Vinayahalingam, S.; Xi, T.; Bergé, S.; Maal, T.; de Jong, G. Automated detection of third molars and mandibular nerve by deep learning. *Sci. Rep.* **2019**, *9*, 9007. [CrossRef]
26. Tack, A.; Preim, B.; Zachow, S. Fully automated Assessment of Knee Alignment from Full-Leg X-Rays employing "a YOLOv4 And Resnet Landmark regression Algorithm" (YARLA): Data from the Osteoarthritis Initiative. *Comput. Methods Programs Biomed.* **2021**, *205*, 106080. [CrossRef]
27. Kumar, N.S.; Goel, A.K.; Jayanthi, S. A Scrupulous Approach to Perform Classification and Detection of Fetal Brain using Darknet YOLO v4. In Proceedings of the 2021 International Conference on Advance Computing and Innovative Technologies in Engineering (ICACITE), New Delhi, India, 4–5 March 2021; pp. 578–581.
28. Bochkovskiy, A.; Wang, C.-Y.; Liao, H.J.A. YOLOv4: Optimal Speed and Accuracy of Object Detection. *arXiv* **2020**, arXiv:2004.10934.
29. Abdurahman, F.; Fante, K.A.; Aliy, M. Malaria parasite detection in thick blood smear microscopic images using modified YOLOV3 and YOLOV4 models. *BMC Bioinform.* **2021**, *22*, 112. [CrossRef] [PubMed]
30. Ghaeminia, H.; Meijer, G.J.; Soehardi, A.; Borstlap, W.A.; Mulder, J.; Bergé, S.J. Position of the impacted third molar in relation to the mandibular canal. Diagnostic accuracy of cone beam computed tomography compared with panoramic radiography. *Int. J. Oral Maxillofac. Surg.* **2009**, *38*, 964–971. [CrossRef] [PubMed]

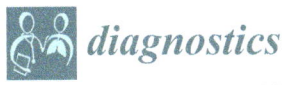

Communication

Automatized Detection and Categorization of Fissure Sealants from Intraoral Digital Photographs Using Artificial Intelligence

Anne Schlickenrieder [1], Ole Meyer [2], Jule Schönewolf [1], Paula Engels [1], Reinhard Hickel [1], Volker Gruhn [2], Marc Hesenius [2] and Jan Kühnisch [1,*]

1. Department of Conservative Dentistry and Periodontology, University Hospital, Ludwig-Maximilians University Munich, 80336 Munich, Germany; anne.schlickenrieder@t-online.de (A.S.); juleschoenewolf@web.de (J.S.); paula.engels@icloud.com (P.E.); hickel@dent.med.uni-muenchen.de (R.H.)
2. Institute for Software Engineering, University of Duisburg-Essen, 45147 Essen, Germany; ole.meyer@uni-due.de (O.M.); gruhn@adesso.de (V.G.); marc.hesenius@uni-due.de (M.H.)
* Correspondence: jkuehn@dent.med.uni-muenchen.de; Tel.: +49-89-4400-59301

Citation: Schlickenrieder, A.; Meyer, O.; Schönewolf, J.; Engels, P.; Hickel, R.; Gruhn, V.; Hesenius, M.; Kühnisch, J. Automatized Detection and Categorization of Fissure Sealants from Intraoral Digital Photographs Using Artificial Intelligence. *Diagnostics* 2021, 11, 1608. https://doi.org/10.3390/diagnostics11091608

Academic Editor: Jae-Hong Lee

Received: 2 August 2021
Accepted: 1 September 2021
Published: 3 September 2021

Publisher's Note: MDPI stays neutral with regard to jurisdictional claims in published maps and institutional affiliations.

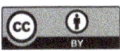

Copyright: © 2021 by the authors. Licensee MDPI, Basel, Switzerland. This article is an open access article distributed under the terms and conditions of the Creative Commons Attribution (CC BY) license (https://creativecommons.org/licenses/by/4.0/).

Abstract: The aim of the present study was to investigate the diagnostic performance of a trained convolutional neural network (CNN) for detecting and categorizing fissure sealants from intraoral photographs using the expert standard as reference. An image set consisting of 2352 digital photographs from permanent posterior teeth (461 unsealed tooth surfaces/1891 sealed surfaces) was divided into a training set (n = 1881/364/1517) and a test set (n = 471/97/374). All the images were scored according to the following categories: unsealed molar, intact, sufficient and insufficient sealant. Expert diagnoses served as the reference standard for cyclic training and repeated evaluation of the CNN (ResNeXt-101-32x8d), which was trained by using image augmentation and transfer learning. A statistical analysis was performed, including the calculation of contingency tables and areas under the receiver operating characteristic curve (AUC). The results showed that the CNN accurately detected sealants in 98.7% of all the test images, corresponding to an AUC of 0.996. The diagnostic accuracy and AUC were 89.6% and 0.951, respectively, for intact sealant; 83.2% and 0.888, respectively, for sufficient sealant; 92.4 and 0.942, respectively, for insufficient sealant. On the basis of the documented results, it was concluded that good agreement with the reference standard could be achieved for automated sealant detection by using artificial intelligence methods. Nevertheless, further research is necessary to improve the model performance.

Keywords: pit and fissure sealants; caries assessment; visual examination; clinical evaluation; artificial intelligence; convolutional neural networks; deep learning; transfer learning

1. Introduction

The availability of artificial intelligence (AI) methods has aroused increasing interest in developing convolutional neural networks (CNNs) for automated detection and categorization of diagnostic images in medicine and dentistry to objectify the classification of pathological findings [1]. In dentistry, radiographs are mostly used as image sources for CNNs to identify pathologies. Specifically, caries detection has been trained on bitewings [2–7], apical radiographs [8] or panoramic X-rays [9]. By contrast, there have been few attempts to apply AI technology to assess clinical images, which can be interpreted as a machine-readable equivalent for visual inspection. This study is the first report of automatic detection and categorization of dental caries [10–13] or dental plaque [14] from clinical photographs. When considering the broad spectrum of pathological findings on dental hard tissue, e.g., caries, erosion or developmental disorders, as well as dental interventions, e.g., sealants, dental restorations or prosthodontic measures, it is evident that CNNs need to be trained separately for each of the aforementioned categories. The aim of this pioneering project on the automated detection of dental materials was to identify and categorize opaque sealants, which is primarily justified by the frequent use of these sealants in dental health services of industrialized nations [15]. Second, sealant materials constitute a uniform group of materials that are typically white and easily visually detectable on posterior teeth compared to other dental restorations. Consequently, it can be hypothesized that the learning of a CNN for detecting sealants from dental photographs represents a first step before considering other types of dental restorations. Therefore, in this diagnostic study, the ability of a CNN to detect and categorize fissure sealants was investigated (as a test method) using digital photographs of posterior teeth, and the diagnostic outcome was compared with expert evaluation (the reference standard).

2. Materials and Methods

2.1. Study Design

The reporting of this study followed the recommendations of the Standard for Reporting of Diagnostic Accuracy Studies (STARD) steering committee [16] and topic-related recommendations [17].

2.2. Photographic Images

All the images were taken for use in previous studies, as well as for clinical or teaching purposes, by an experienced dentist (J.K.). All the images were photographed using a professional single reflex lens camera (Nikon D300, D7100 or D7200 with a Nikon Micro 105-mm lens; Nikon, Tokyo, Japan) and Macro Flash EM-140 DG (Sigma, Rödermark, Germany) after tooth cleaning and drying. Molar teeth were photographed indirectly using intraoral mirrors (Reflect-Rhod, Hager and Werken, Duisburg, Germany) that were heated before being positioned in the oral cavity to prevent condensation on the mirror surface.

To ensure the best possible image quality, deficient photographs, e.g., out-of-focus images or images with saliva contamination, were excluded. Furthermore, duplicate photos from identical teeth or surfaces were removed from the dataset. This selection step ensured there were no repetitions in the included clinical photographs. All jpeg images (RGB format, resolution 1200 × 1200 pixel, no compression) were cropped to an aspect ratio of 1:1 and/or rotated in a standard manner using professional image editing software (Affinity Photo, Serif, Nottingham, UK) until, finally, the tooth surface filled most of the frame. Considering the study aim, images from healthy teeth or sealed surfaces were also included. Photographs with (additional) cavitated caries lesions or other hard tissue defects, e.g., enamel hypomineralization, hypoplasia, extensive tooth wear, and direct and indirect restorations, were excluded. Finally, 2352 anonymized, high-quality clinical photographs from permanent posterior teeth and the corresponding occlusal surfaces were included.

2.3. Categorization of Sealants (Reference Standard)

Each image was examined on a computer to detect and categorize fissure sealants using well-accepted international classification systems [18,19]. The following categories were used: 0—occlusal surfaces with no sealant; 1—occlusal surfaces with a clinically intact fissure sealant (up to one third loss of material in the periphery of the fissure pattern); 2—occlusal surface with a sufficient fissure sealant (retention of the material in the main fissure or loss of material exceeding one third of the fissure pattern); 3—insufficient (nearly complete loss of material and re-exposure of the main fissures) (Figure 1). Each of the given diagnostic categories is typically linked with different treatment modalities in daily dental practice and, in consequence, the quality staging appears of clinical relevance and justifies its scientific consideration in the present study. All the images were prelabeled by a group of three graduated dentists and subsequently independently counterchecked by an experienced examiner (J.K., >20 years of clinical practice and scientific experience). In the case of divergent opinions, each image was discussed until a consensus was reached. Each diagnostic decision—one per image—served as a reference standard for cyclic training and repeated evaluation of the deep-learning-based CNN.

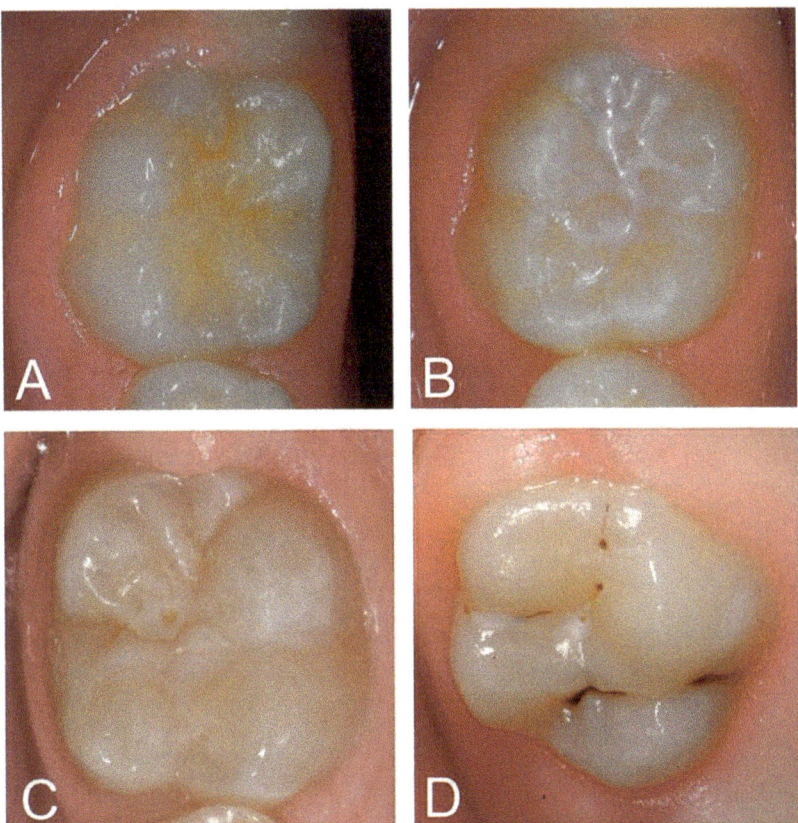

Figure 1. Example clinical images for each category: unsealed molar (**A**) and intact (**B**), sufficient (**C**) and insufficient fissure sealant (**D**).

All the annotators (A.S., J.S., P.E.) were trained during a 2-day workshop by the principal investigator (J.K.) and calibrated before beginning the study. The intra- and inter-examiner reproducibility was determined using 60 photographs, and the corresponding Kappa values showed at least a substantial capability for detecting and categorizing fissure sealants. The intra-/inter-examiner reproducibilities were 0.784/0.753 (A.S.), 0.779/0.752 (J.S.) and 0.779/0.752 (P.E.).

2.4. Programming and Configuration of the Deep-Learning-Based CNN for Sealant Detection and Categorization (Test Method)

The CNN was trained stepwise using a pipeline of established procedures, mainly image augmentation and transfer learning. Before training, the entire image set (2352 images/461 unsealed tooth surfaces/1891 sealed surfaces) was divided into a training set ($n = 1881/364/1517$) and a test set ($n = 471/97/374$). The latter was never made available to the CNN as training material and served as an independent test set.

Image augmentation was used to provide a large number of variable images to the CNN on a recurring basis. For this purpose, the randomly selected images (batch size = 16) were multiplied by a factor of ~5, altered by image augmentation (random center and margin cropping by up to 30% each, random deletion up to 30%, random affine transformation up to 180 degrees, random perspective transformation up to a distortion of 0.5, and random changes in brightness, contrast and saturation up to 10%) and resized (to 300 × 300 pixels) by using torchvision (version 0.9.1, https://pytorch.org) in conjunction with the PyTorch library (version 1.8.1, https://pytorch.org). All the images were normalized to compensate for under- and overexposure.

ResNeXt-101–32x8d [20] was used as the basis for the continuous adaptation of CNN for sealant detection and categorization. The CNN was trained using backpropagation to determine the gradient for learning. Backpropagation was repeated iteratively for images and labels using the abovementioned batch size and parameters. Overfitting was prevented by first selecting a low learning rate (0.00005) and then performing dropout (at a rate of 0.5) on the final linear layers as a regularization technique [21]. To train the CNN, this step was repeated for 10 epochs. The cross entropy loss as an error function and the Adam optimizer (Betas 0.9 and 0.999, Epsilon 10^{-8}) were applied.

To accelerate the training process of the CNN, an open-source neural network with pretrained weights was employed (ResNeXt-101-32x8d pretrained on ImageNet., Stanford Vision and Learning Lab, Stanford University, Palo Alto, CA, USA). This step enabled the transfer of existing learning results to increase the efficiency of recognition of basic structures in the existing image set. The training of the CNN was executed on a university-based server with the following specifications: RTX A6000 48 GB (Nvidia, Santa Clara, CA, USA), i9 10850K 10x3.60 GHz (Intel Corp., Santa Clara, CA, USA) and 64 GB RAM.

2.5. Statistical Analysis

The data were analyzed using Python (http://www.python.org, version 3.8). The overall diagnostic accuracy (ACC = (TN + TP)/(TN + TP + FN + FP)) was determined by calculating the number of true positives (TP), false positives (FP), true negatives (TN) and false negatives (FN) after using 25%, 50%, 75% and 100% of the images of the training data set. The sensitivity (SE), specificity (SP), positive and negative predictive values (PPV and NPV, respectively), and the area under the receiver operating characteristic (ROC) curve (AUC) were computed for the selected types of teeth and surfaces [22]. Saliency maps were plotted to identify image areas that are important for the CNN to make individual decisions. We calculated the saliency maps [23] by backpropagating the CNN prediction and visualized the gradient of the input of the resized images (300 × 300 pixels).

3. Results

The trained deep-learning-based CNN detected sealants correctly in 98.7% of all the test cases, corresponding to an AUC of 0.996 (Table 1, Figure 2). Additionally, the SE (96.9), SP (99.2), PPV (96.9) and NPV (99.2) were documented to be close to perfect (Table 1). By comparison, the model diagnostic performance was lower for the sealant subcategories (Table 1, Figure 2). Here, the AUC values were highest for the identification of intact sealants (0.951), followed by insufficient sealants (0.942) and sufficient sealants (0.888). These numbers, as well as the other performance data (Table 1), indicate that the automated identification of the subcategories in the present stage was less accurate than the simple detection of opaque sealant material from clinical photographs. The detailed case distribution was obtained from the confusion matrix (Figure 3). Here, the majority of incorrect decisions by the CNN occurred for categories other than the true classification, which indicates there were no major misclassifications. Most incorrect decisions were made for sufficient sealants. This observation is in line with the diagnostic parameters shown in Table 1. In addition to the descriptive and explorative data presentation, saliency maps (Figure 4) were plotted to illustrate the parts of each image that were used by the CNN for decision making.

Table 1. Overview of the diagnostic performance of the developed convolutional neural network (CNN), where the independent test set (n = 471) was compared against independent expert evaluation of the caries detection level. The calculations were performed for different types of teeth, surfaces and training steps. In this context, the overall diagnostic accuracy (ACC), sensitivity (SE), specificity (SP), negative predictive value (NPV), positive predictive value (PPV) and area under the receiver operating characteristic curve (AUC).

Diagnostic Categories	True Positives (TP)		True Negatives (TN)		False Positives (FP)		False Negatives (FN)		Diagnostic Performance					
	n	%	n	%	n	%	n	%	ACC	SE	SP	NPV	PPV	AUC
Overall sealant detection	94	20.0	371	78.8	3	0.6	3	0.6	98.7	96.9	99.2	99.2	96.9	0.996
Identification of intact sealants	141	29.9	281	59.7	33	7.0	16	3.4	89.6	89.8	89.5	94.6	81.0	0.951
Identification of sufficient sealants	99	21.0	293	62.2	33	7.0	46	9.8	83.2	68.3	89.9	86.4	75.0	0.888
Identification of insufficient sealants	52	11.0	383	81.3	16	3.4	20	4.3	92.4	72.2	96.0	95.0	76.5	0.942

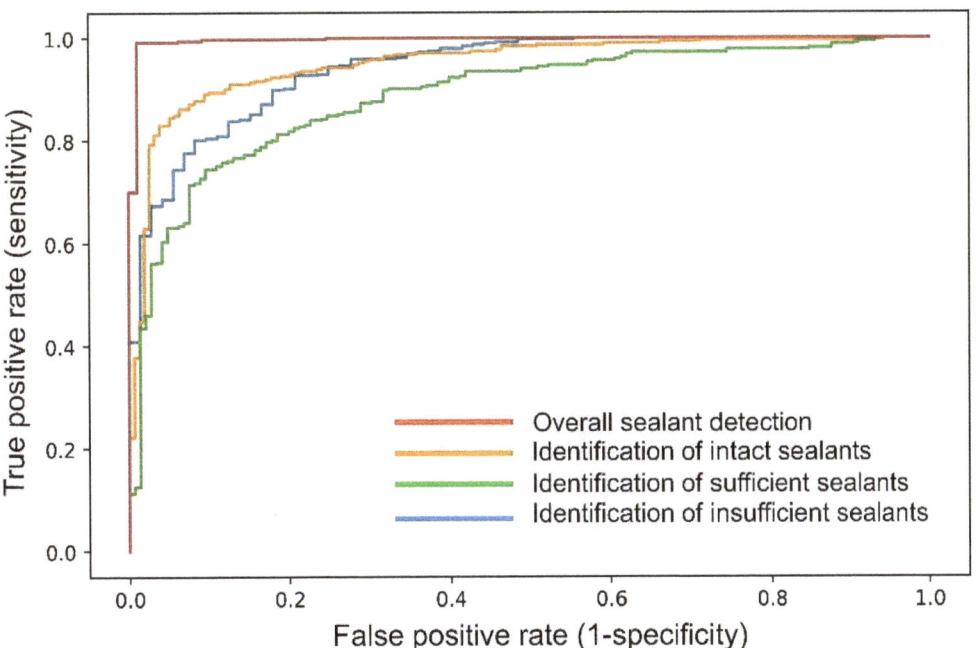

Figure 2. The ROC curves illustrate the model performance of the developed CNN for overall and categorical sealant detection.

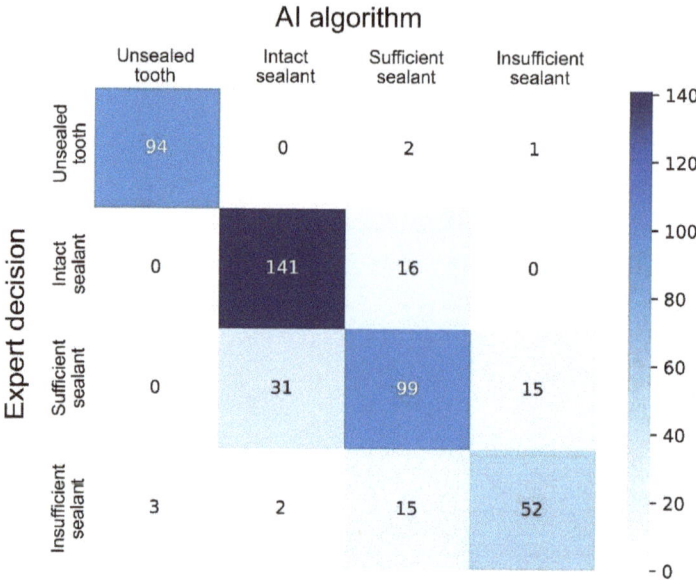

Figure 3. Confusion matrix showing the CNN classification performance for the test sample.

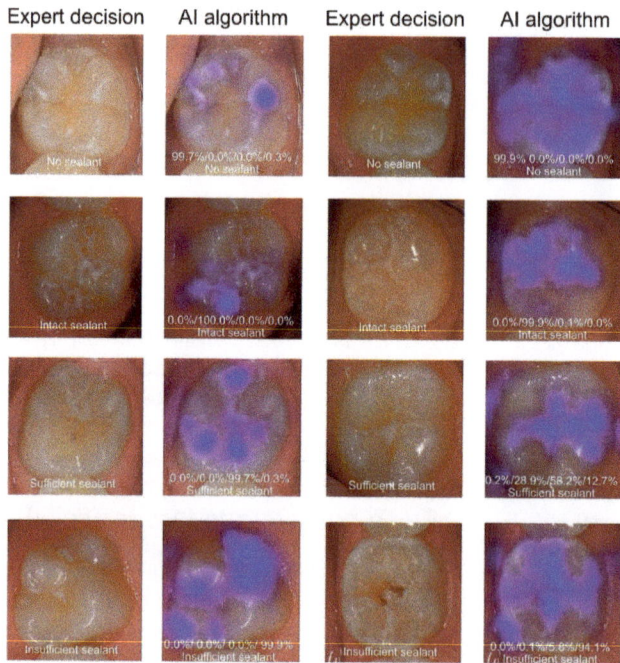

Figure 4. Examples of clinical images showing the reference decision and paired images with saliency maps visualizing the image areas (in blue) used in decision making by the AI method. The corresponding test results by the AI method are given for each example (unsealed tooth/intact fissure sealant/sufficient sealant/insufficient sealant).

4. Discussion

The results of the present diagnostic study demonstrated that AI algorithms can detect and categorize sealants from machine-readable intraoral photographs. A high diagnostic accuracy of 98.7% and AUC of 0.996 were found (Table 1). Unlike this promising result, the CNN classified subcategories less accurately. Here, a diagnostic performance of approximately 90% accuracy was achieved (Table 1). In particular, sufficiently sealed occlusal surfaces were identified less reliably than the two other categories, which illustrates that further improvement is needed.

In addition, it can be concluded that the developed CNN can be used in future software applications and can identify sealants accurately with a high probability from intraoral photographs. To our knowledge, no comparable studies have been carried out thus far on the evaluation of fissure sealants using artificial intelligence, which should be recognized as a unique feature of our study. The current diagnostic performance data fit into the overall context of existing dental studies. For example, studies with a similar methodology have documented an accuracy of up to 90% for the detection of caries lesions from clinical images [10,11] or radiographs [2–9]. Considering earlier published data from methodologically similar projects, it can be concluded that our most recent results (Table 1, Figures 2 and 3) are in line with an expected outcome. Our data need to be critically assessed from different methodological perspectives. First, it should be highlighted that the pipeline used for image augmentation, transfer learning and the chosen CNN architecture (ResNeXt-101-32x8d) represents an up-to-date approach that may have enhanced the documented results. Second, as our study was performed on good quality professional clinical photographs, the results may have been be positively influenced by this factor. None of the images used were overexposed or underexposed, and the teeth investigated were mostly free of plaque, calculus and saliva. All the images were normalized, cropped and standardized before processing. Third, only unsealed posterior teeth and sealed teeth of varying quality were included in the study materials. Cases with caries lesions, developmental defects, and direct or indirect dental restorations were excluded from the project to enable unbiased learning of the CNN. Another methodological advantage in this context appears to be the use of single tooth images, because interfering information from adjacent teeth or margins was mostly excluded. Consequently, it can be expected that the use of other image formats, e.g., clinical images with multiple teeth or the whole jaw, will result in a lower model performance. The number of available clinical photographs is a limitation that must be critically examined. Here, several thousand images at best should be includable, as the number of images is a crucial consideration for this type of study. In the present analysis, we were able to include 2352 clinical images, which should be interpreted as the minimum number. This fact should not be underestimated, because increasing the number of images will extend the training of the CNN and could improve the CNN precision. Further improvements in the model performance can be expected by extending the number of image samples and using the image segmentation technique. The latter approach results in precise image labeling and could be considered as the method of choice to reach the long-term goal of almost perfect detection and assessment of fissure sealants from clinical photographs by AI methods.

5. Conclusions

The clinical application of AI methods in software applications may be feasible but fundamental dental research needs to be performed first. The results of the present study show that a trained CNN detected sealant intraoral photographs with an agreement of 98.7% with reference decisions. The categorical classification into intact, sufficient and insufficient sealants was performed with a diagnostic accuracy of approximately 90%. Considering the complexity of intraoral findings, it can be concluded that further training of AI-based detection, as well as categorization of prevalent and less-prevalent dental diseases and all types of restorations, is required before clinical use can be recommended.

Author Contributions: J.K., R.H., O.M., V.G. and M.H. designed the study protocol. J.K. provided all the intraoral photographs. A.S., J.S., P.E. and J.K. performed all the examinations. O.M. and M.H. programmed the CNN and conducted the statistical analyses. All the authors drafted the manuscript, contributed equally to the interpretation of data and approved the final manuscript version. All authors have read and agreed to the published version of the manuscript.

Funding: No funding was received for this study.

Institutional Review Board Statement: This study was approved by the Ethics Committee of the Medical Faculty of the Ludwig-Maximilians-University of Munich (project number 020-798, approved on 8 October 2020).

Informed Consent Statement: All procedures performed in studies involving human participants were in accordance with the ethical standards of the institutional and/or national research committee and with the 1964 Helsinki declaration and its later amendments or comparable ethical standards.

Data Availability Statement: The datasets used and analyzed during the current study are available from the corresponding author on reasonable request.

Conflicts of Interest: The authors declare no potential conflict of interest with respect to the authorship and publication of this article, including financial interests and the provision of study materials by the manufacturer for free or at a discount.

References

1. Schwendicke, F.; Samek, W.; Krois, J. Artificial Intelligence in Dentistry: Chances and Challenges. *J. Dent. Res.* **2020**, *99*, 769–774. [CrossRef] [PubMed]
2. Bejnordi, B.E.; Litjens, G.; van der Laak, J.A. Machine learning compared with pathologist assessment-reply. *JAMA* **2018**, *319*, 1726. [CrossRef] [PubMed]
3. Cantu, A.G.; Gehrung, S.; Krois, J.; Chaurasia, A.; Rossi, J.G.; Gaudin, R.; Elhennawy, K.; Schwendicke, F. Detecting caries lesions of different radiographic extension on bitewings using deep learning. *J. Dent.* **2020**, *100*, 103425, online ahead of print. [CrossRef] [PubMed]
4. Geetha, V.; Aprameya, K.S.; Hinduja, D.M. Dental caries diagnosis in digital radiographs using back-propagation neural network. *Health Inf. Sci. Syst.* **2020**, *8*, 8, (eCollection Dec). [CrossRef] [PubMed]
5. Khan, H.A.; Haider, M.A.; Ansari, H.A.; Ishaq, H.; Kiyani, A.; Sohail, K.; Muhammad, M.; Khurram, S.A. Automated feature detection in dental periapical radiographs by using deep learning. *Oral Surg. Oral Med. Oral Pathol. Oral Radiol.* **2020**, *131*, 711–720. [CrossRef] [PubMed]
6. Lee, J.H.; Kim, D.H.; Jeong, S.N.; Choi, S.H. Diagnosis and prediction of periodontally compromised teeth using a deep learning-based convolutional neural network algorithm. *J. Periodontal Implant Sci.* **2018**, *48*, 114–123. [CrossRef] [PubMed]
7. Park, W.J.; Park, J.B. History and application of artificial neural networks in dentistry. *Eur. J. Dent.* **2018**, *12*, 594–601. [CrossRef]
8. Lee, J.H.; Kim, D.H.; Jeong, S.N.; Choi, S.H. Detection and diagnosis of dental caries using a deep learning-based convolutional neural network algorithm. *J. Dent.* **2018**, *77*, 106–111. [CrossRef]
9. Vinayahalingam, S.; Kempers, S.; Limon, L.; Deibel, D.; Maal, T.; Hanisch, M.; Bergé, S.; Xi, T. Classification of caries in third molars on panoramic radiographs using deep learning. *Sci. Rep.* **2021**, *11*, 12609. [CrossRef] [PubMed]
10. Askar, H.; Krois, J.; Rohrer, C.; Mertens, S.; Elhennawy, K.; Ottolenghi, L.; Mazur, M.; Paris, S.; Schwendicke, F. Detecting white spot lesions on dental photography using deep learning: A pilot study. *J. Dent.* **2021**, *107*. online ahead of print. [CrossRef]
11. Kühnisch, J.; Meyer, O.; Hesenius, M.; Hickel, R.; Gruhn, V. Caries detection on intraoral images using artifical intelligence. *J. Dent. Res.* **2021**. online ahead of print. [CrossRef] [PubMed]
12. Moutselos, K.; Berdouses, E.; Oulis, C.; Maglogiannis, I. Recognizing Occlusal Caries in Dental Intraoral Images Using Deep Learning. *Annu. Int. Conf. IEEE Eng. Med. Biol. Soc.* **2019**, *2019*, 1617–1620. [CrossRef] [PubMed]
13. Zhang, X.; Liang, Y.; Li, W.; Liu, C.; Gu, D.; Sun, W.; Miao, L. Development and evaluation of deep learning for screening dental caries from oral photographs. *Oral Dis.* **2020**, *26*. online ahead of print. [CrossRef]
14. You, W.; Hao, A.; Li, S.; Wang, Y.; Xia, B. Deep learning-based dental plaque detection on primary teeth: A comparison with clinical assessments. *BMC Oral Health* **2020**, *20*, 141. [CrossRef] [PubMed]
15. Jordan, R.A.; Micheelis, W. *Fünfte Deutsche Mundgesundheitsstudie (DMS V)*; Institut der deutschen Zahnärzte (IDZ): Köln, Germany, 2016; ISBN 978-3-7691-0020-4.
16. Bossuyt, P.M.; Reitsma, J.B.; Bruns, D.E.; Gatsonis, C.A.; Glasziou, P.P.; Irwig, L.; Lijmer, J.G.; Moher, D.; Rennie, D.; de Vet, H.C.; et al. STARD Group. STARD 2015: An updated list of essential items for reporting diagnostic accuracy studies. *BMJ* **2015**, *351*, h5527. [CrossRef] [PubMed]
17. Schwendicke, F.; Singh, T.; Lee, J.H.; Gaudin, R.; Chaurasia, A.; Wiegand, T.; Uribe, S.; Krois, J.; IADR e-oral health network and the ITU WHO focus group AI for Health. Artificial intelligence in dental research: Checklist for Authors, Reviewers, Readers. *J. Dent.* **2021**, *107*.[CrossRef] [PubMed]

18. Heinrich-Weltzien, R.; Kühnisch, J. Häufigkeit und Qualität der Fissurenversiegelung bei 8- und 14-jährigen. *Prophyl. Impuls* **1999**, *3*, 6–14.
19. Simonsen, R.J. Retention and effectiveness of dental sealants after 15 years. *JADA* **1991**, *122*, 34–42. [CrossRef] [PubMed]
20. Xie, S.; Girshick, R.; Dollár, P.; Tu, Z.; He, K. Aggregated residual transformations for deep neural networks. *IEEE Conf. Comput. Vis. Pattern Recognit.* **2017**, 5987–5995. [CrossRef]
21. Srivastava, N.; Hinton, G.; Krizhevsky, A.; Sutskever, I.; Salakhutdinov, R. Dropout: A Simple Way to Prevent Neural Networks from Overfitting. *JMLR* **2014**, *15*, 1929–1958.
22. Matthews, D.E.; Farewell, V.T. *Using and Understanding Medical Statistics*, 5th ed.; Karger: Basel, Switzerland, 2015; ISBN 3318054585.
23. Simonyan, K.; Vedaldi, A.; Zisserman, A. Deep Inside Convolutional Networks: Visualising Image Classification Models and Saliency Maps. Available online: https://arxiv.org/pdf/1312.6034.pdf (accessed on 26 July 2021).

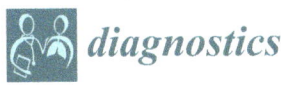

Review

Application and Performance of Artificial Intelligence Technology in Oral Cancer Diagnosis and Prediction of Prognosis: A Systematic Review

Sanjeev B. Khanagar [1,2], Sachin Naik [3], Abdulaziz Abdullah Al Kheraif [3], Satish Vishwanathaiah [4], Prabhadevi C. Maganur [4], Yaser Alhazmi [5], Shazia Mushtaq [6], Sachin C. Sarode [7], Gargi S. Sarode [7], Alessio Zanza [8], Luca Testarelli [8] and Shankargouda Patil [5,*]

1. Preventive Dental Science Department, College of Dentistry, King Saud Bin Abdulaziz University for Health Sciences, Riyadh 11481, Saudi Arabia; sanjeev.khanagar76@gmail.com
2. King Abdullah International Medical Research Center, Ministry of National Guard Health Affairs, Riyadh 11481, Saudi Arabia
3. Dental Biomaterials Research Chair, Dental Health Department, College of Applied Medical Sciences, King Saud University, Riyadh 11433, Saudi Arabia; snaik@ksu.edu.sa (S.N.); aalkhuraif@ksu.edu.sa (A.A.A.K.)
4. Department of Preventive Dental Sciences, Division of Pedodontics, College of Dentistry, Jazan University, Jazan 45142, Saudi Arabia; drvsatish77@gmail.com (S.V.); prabhadevi.maganur@gmail.com (P.C.M.)
5. Department of Maxillofacial Surgery and Diagnostic Sciences, Division of Oral Pathology, College of Dentistry, Jazan University, Jazan 45142, Saudi Arabia; dr.y.alhazmi@gmail.com
6. College of Applied Medical Sciences, Dental Health Department, King Saud University, Riyadh 12372, Saudi Arabia; smushtaqdr@gmail.com
7. Department of Oral and Maxillofacial Pathology, Dr. D.Y. Patil Dental College and Hospital, Dr. D. Y. Patil Vidyapeeth, Pimpri, Pune 411018, India; drsachinsarode@gmail.com (S.C.S.); gargi14@gmail.com (G.S.S.)
8. Department of Maxillo and Oro-Facial Sciences, University of Rome La Sapienza, 00185 Rome, Italy; ale.zanza@gmail.com (A.Z.); luca.testarelli@uniroma1.it (L.T.)
* Correspondence: dr.ravipatil@gmail.com

Abstract: Oral cancer (OC) is a deadly disease with a high mortality and complex etiology. Artificial intelligence (AI) is one of the outstanding innovations in technology used in dental science. This paper intends to report on the application and performance of AI in diagnosis and predicting the occurrence of OC. In this study, we carried out data search through an electronic search in several renowned databases, which mainly included PubMed, Google Scholar, Scopus, Embase, Cochrane, Web of Science, and the Saudi Digital Library for articles that were published between January 2000 to March 2021. We included 16 articles that met the eligibility criteria and were critically analyzed using QUADAS-2. AI can precisely analyze an enormous dataset of images (fluorescent, hyperspectral, cytology, CT images, etc.) to diagnose OC. AI can accurately predict the occurrence of OC, as compared to conventional methods, by analyzing predisposing factors like age, gender, tobacco habits, and bio-markers. The precision and accuracy of AI in diagnosis as well as predicting the occurrence are higher than the current, existing clinical strategies, as well as conventional statistics like cox regression analysis and logistic regression.

Keywords: artificial intelligence; artificial neural networks; oral cancer diagnosis; machine learning; oral cancer prediction

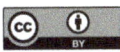

1. Introduction

Oral cancer (OC) is one of the most common lethal diseases and has been a major public health concern around the world. OC is a subdivision of head and neck cancers with 275,000 fresh cases per year worldwide. The survival rate of the early stage (Stage I) disease is around 80%, whereas for the late stage disease (Stage II and III), it is less than 20% [1,2].

Among OC, squamous cell carcinoma (OSCC) of the oral cavity is the most common type and comprises 90% of the disease [3]. Early diagnosis of OC is significant, however, most patients are diagnosed at a late stage of the disease, leading to a poor prognosis. The clinical appearance of OC is not a sufficient parameter for identifying the status, analysis, or dysplastic level, therefore, the treatment selection based on the clinical appearance of the disease is not sufficient. OC is associated with multiple factors, and the survival rate after treatment is also unpredictable [4,5].

Potentially malignant lesions like leukoplakia, erythroplakia, and oral submucous fibrosis are also prevalent among the risk population. Differentiating these lesions from the malignant lesions are also important. Risk factors like age, gender, and tobacco habits may affect the prognosis of OC [6].

Understanding the refinements of innovations like Artificial Intelligence (AI) could relieve potential clinical entanglements [7,8]. Application of AI in the oral malignant growths can improve the current challenges in the disease diagnosis, as well as in predicting the prognosis. AI, which mimics human cognitive functions, is a forward leap in innovation, and has enamored the minds of scientists over the globe [9]. Its use in dentistry has begun recently, which has led to extraordinary accomplishments. History goes back to as early as 400 BC; Plato visualized an essential model of brain function. AI system is a framework that takes u information, discovers designs, uses data to train itself, and yields results [9–11].

AI works in two phases—the first phase, which involves "training" and the second phase which is "testing". The model set uses the training data to set the parameters. The model uses the data from past examples, like data from patients or data with different examples, retrospectively. These parameters are then applied on the test sets. Various studies that have described the prognostic factors of OC are detected through AI by different biomarkers. Early diagnosis of the malignant lesion is good for patient survival rate and proper treatment therapy [12–16]. Many studies have been conducted using image analysis to smartphone-based OC detectors, based on AI algorithms. The AI technology facilitates the diagnosis, treatment, and management of patients with OC. AI reduces workload, complex data, and fatigue among physicians, for easy diagnosis [4,17]. The present systematic review intends to report on the application and role of AI-based technology in diagnosis and prediction of OC occurrence.

2. Materials and Methods

2.1. Search Strategy

In this systematic review, we followed the guidelines given by preferred reporting items for systematic reviews and meta-analyses extension, for the diagnostic test accuracy (PRISMA-DTA) [18]. Data search was mainly carried out through an electronic search in several renowned databases, which mainly included PubMed, Google Scholar, Scopus, Embase, Cochrane, Web of Science, and the Saudi Digital Library for articles that were published between January 2000 to March 2021. Index words like "artificial intelligence; oral cancer diagnosis; oral cancer prediction; oral cancer prognosis; deep learning; and machine learning" were used for searching the articles. Boolean operators (AND, OR) with language filters for English were used for searching articles in most electronic databases.

Simultaneously, a manual search for the research articles was also conducted along with the electronic search. A search for articles was carried out for the relevant citations from the reference list of previously retrieved articles in department and college libraries, where hard copies of the journals were available.

PICO (problem/patient, intervention/indicator, comparison, and outcome) elements were used for searching data on this topic (Table 1).

Table 1. Description of the PICO (P = Population, I = Intervention, C = Comparison, O = Outcome) elements.

Research question	What are the applications and performance of the artificial intelligence models that have been widely used in oral cancer diagnosis, and predicting the prognosis.
Population	Patients, clinical images, radiographs, datasets, and histological images.
Intervention	AI-based models for oral cancer diagnosis and predicting prognosis.
Comparison	Expert opinions and reference standards.
Outcome	Measurable or predictive outcomes such as accuracy, sensitivity, specificity, ROC = Receiver Operating Characteristic curve, AUC = Area Under the Curve, ICC = Intra-class Correlation Coefficient, PPV = Positive Predictive Values, and NPV = Negative Predictive Values.

2.2. Study Selection

The electronic database search yielded 620 articles that were followed by hand searching, which yielded another 8 articles, which made a total of 628 articles. Initially, the articles chosen were based on relevance in the area of research, the title, and the abstract. Later, the articles were also manually checked for duplication by 2 members who were not involved in the preliminary search, which further eliminated 288 duplicated articles. Following this, 340 full-text articles were selected for data selection. The following eligibility criteria were applied at the next stage.

2.3. Inclusion and Exclusion Criteria

The articles were included according to the following inclusion criteria—(a) the article must be original research and must report on the AI technology; (b) quantifiable values that can be evaluated/analyzed should be mentioned in the article; and (c) the data used in evaluating these AI-based models should be mentioned. There was no limit set for the study design for inclusion in this systematic review.

The articles excluded were—(a) the articles in which AI innovation were not mentioned; (b) unpublished articles or conference papers that were uploaded online; (c) articles where full-text versions were not available; and (d) articles available in languages other than English.

2.4. Data Extraction

After applying the inclusion criteria, we filtered 12 articles out of the total. These 12 articles were considered to be potentially eligible articles for this systematic review, and were critically analyzed by the entire team. The details of the journal were covered before circulating them for critical analysis among authors. The QUADAS-2 tool was used for assessing the quality of the studies reporting on diagnostic accuracy. It has four domains which are assessed in terms of risk of bias and applicability concerns. The domains are patient selection, index test, reference standard, and flow and timing [18]. The authors disagreed with including 3 articles in this systematic review, as there was no mention of the reasonable data supporting the results and conclusions. Following this, the articles were further reduced to 16. The selection of the articles for qualitative synthesis for this systematic review is represented in the flow chart (Figure 1). The articles were further quantified with regards to the year of publication, to report on the trends in research that has been conducted on OC diagnosis and the prediction of prognosis, using the AI technology.

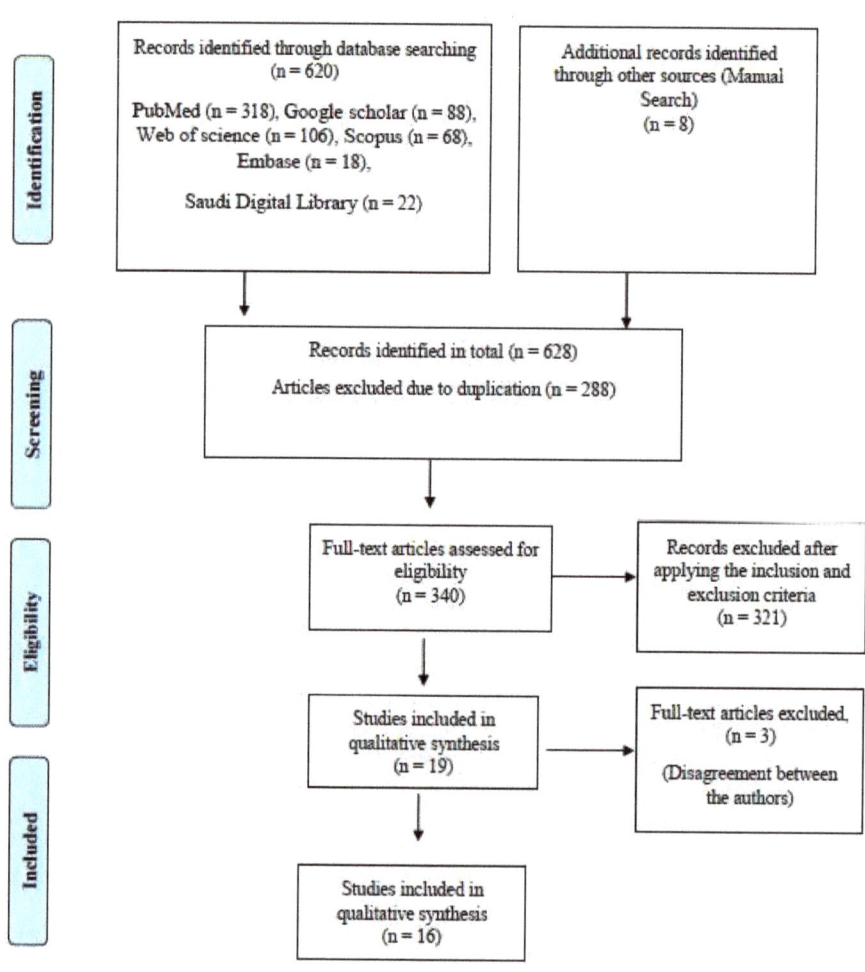

Figure 1. Flow chart for screening and selection of articles.

3. Results

Finally, 9 articles were critically analyzed for the extraction of the quantitative data. Most studies reported in the literature revealed that these studies were reported over the last 15 years. The trend showed a gradual increase in the studies reporting on the application of AI for OC diagnosis and the prediction of prognosis.

3.1. Qualitative Synthesis of the Included Studies

AI technology has been mainly applied for differentiating between normal, premalignant, and malignant conditions [19–23], predicting the likelihood of oral cancer incidence [24–26], prognosis, early detection of pre-cancerous and cancerous lesions [27–30], predicting the risk of recurrence [31,32], predicting the possibility of disease development from potential malignant lesion, and predicting the survival of patients [33,34].

In this systematic review, 4 studies were reported using convolutional neural networks (CNNs), and another 4 studies were reported using artificial neural networks (ANNs). These neural networks were mainly designed for assessing patient datasets, high-resolution cytology images, hyperspectral images, autofluorescence images (AFI), and white light imaging (WLI) (Table 2).

Table 2. Details of the studies that have used AI-based models for oral cancer diagnosis and predicting the prognosis.

Sr. No.	Authors	Year of Publication	Algorithm Architecture	Study Design	Objective of the Study	No. of Images/Photographs for Testing	Study Factor	Modality	Comparison, If Any	Evaluation Accuracy/Average Accuracy	Results (+) Effective, (−) Non Effective (N) Neutral	Outcomes	Authors Suggestions/Conclusions
1	Nayak et al. [19]	2005	ANNs	Cross sectional study	Discriminating normal, potentially malignant, and malignant conditions using principal component analysis (PCA) and artificial neural network (ANN)	50	Differentiating normal, potentially malignant, and malignant	Recorded spectra	Principal component analysis (PCA)	Accuracy 98.3%, specificity of 100% and sensitivity 96.5%	(+) Effective	ANN is found to be slightly better than PCA	This model is efficient for real-time application.
2	Tseng et al. [27]	2015	ANNs	Cohort study	ANN for predicting oral cancer prognosis	-	Determining the differences between the symptoms shown in past cases	Datasets	Decision tree (DT)	Not Mentioned	(+) Effective	Both decision tree and artificial neural network models showed superiority to the traditional statistical model.	Decision tree models are relatively easier to interpret compared to artificial neural network models.
3	Uthoff et al. [28]	2017	CNN's	Crossectional study	AI-based deep (CNNs) for early detection of pre-cancerous and cancerous lesions	170	Detection of pre-cancerous and cancerous lesions	Autofluorescence imaging (AFI) and white light imaging (WLI)	Specialist's diagnosis	Sensitivities 85%, specificities 88.75% positive predictive values 87.67%, and negative predictive values 85.49	(+) Effective	CNN achieving high values of sensitivity, specificity, PPV, and NPV compared to the on-site specialist gold standard.	Performance should increase as additional images are collected.
4	Shams et al. [31]	2017	CNN's	Cross sectional comparative study	Deep Neural Network (DNN) for predicting the possibility of oral cancer development in Oral potentially malignant lesion patients	10	Oral cancer development in Oral potentially malignant lesion patients	Datasets	Support Vector Machine (SVM), Regularized Least Squares (RLS), Multi-Layer Perception (MLP)	High accuracy 96%	(+) Effective	The results show high accuracy using DNN than SVM and MLP	None
5	Jeyaraj et al. [30]	2019	CNN's	Cross sectional comparative study	Deep learning algorithm for an automated, computer-aided oral cancer-detecting system	100	Detection of pre-cancerous as benign and post cancerous as malignant region	Hyperspectral images	The traditional medical image classification algorithm	Accuracy of 91.4%, sensitivity 94% and a specificity of 91%	(+) Effective	The quality of diagnosis is increased by proposed regression-based partitioned CNN learning algorithm for a complex medical image of oral cancer diagnosis	This deep learning the algorithm can be easily deployed for providing an automatic medical image classifier without expert knowledge.
6	Fahed Jubair et al. [20]	2020	CNN's	Crossectional study	Develop a lightweight deep CNN using EfficientNet B0 transfer model CNN for binary classification of oral lesions into benign and malignant or potentially malignant using standard real-time clinical images	716	Detecting oral cancer	Clinical images	None	accuracy was 85.0%, specificity, 84.5%, sensitivity 86.7%	(+) Effective	AI can improve the quality and reach of oral cancer screening and early detection.	This model of being small in size and need small computation power and memory capacity.
7	Sunny et al. [29]	2019	ANNs	Cross sectional comparative study	Artificial Neural Network (ANN) based risk-stratification model for early detection of oral potentially malignant (OPML)/malignant lesion.	82	Oral potentially malignant (OPML)/malignant lesion.	High-resolution cytology images	Conventional cytology and histology	84–86% Accuracy Sensitivity 93%	(+) Effective	ANN-based risk stratification model improved the detection sensitivity of malignant lesions (93%) and high-grade OPML (73%), increasing the overall accuracy by 30%.	This model can be an invaluable Point-of-Care (POC) tool for early detection/screening in oral cancer.
8	Jelena Musulin et al. [21]	2021	ANNs	Cross sectional comparative study	Diagnosing OC using the histological image of a biopsy	322	Detecting oral cancer	Histological image	ResNet50, ResNet101 Xception MobileNetv2	Xception and SWT resulted in the highest classification value of 0.96 (σ = 0.042) AUCmacro	(+) Effective	The AI-based system has great potential in the diagnosis of OSCC	This cell shape and size, pathological mitoses, tumor-stroma ratio and the distinction between early and advanced-stage OSCCs

Table 2. Cont.

Sr. No.	Authors	Year of Publication	Algorithm Architecture	Study Design	Objective of the Study	No. of Images/Photographs for Testing	Study Factor	Modality	Comparison, If Any	Evaluation Accuracy/Average Accuracy	Results (+) Effective, (-) Non Effective (N) Neutral	Outcomes	Authors Suggestions/Conclusions
9	M. Praveena Kirubabai et al. [22]	2021	CNN	Cross sectional study	To classify the oral images into either normal or abnormal images and diagnosed into 'Mild' or 'Severe' using a deep learning algorithm	160	Detecting oral cancer	Oral images	None	accuracy was 99.7%, 98.6% of sensitivity, 99.1% of specificity, and 99.7%	(+) Effective	CNN has high accuracy in detecting OC	None
10	Jyoti Rathod et al. [23]	2019	CNN's	Cross sectional comparative study	Classify different stages of oral cancer using machine learning techniques	-	Diagnosing and classifying the premalignant lesion	Data set	SVM, KNN, MLP RSF, and Logistic Regression	DT 90.68%, RSF 91%, SVM 88%, KNN 85%, MLP 81% and Logistic Regression gives 80% of accuracy	(+) Effective	DT and RSF produced the same accuracy results	classification of oral cancer can be classified efficiently with help of Random Forest and Decision Tree
11	Alabi et al. [33]	2019	ANNs	Cross sectional comparative study	Comparing the performance of four machine learning Models (ML) for Predicting Risk of recurrence of oral tongue squamous cell carcinoma (OTSCC)	311	Prediction of reoccurrence	Patient datasets	5 Prognostic significance of the depth of invasion (DOI).	Accuracy of 68% for Support Vector Machine (SVM), 70% Naive Bayes (NB), 81% Boosted Decision Tree (BDT) and 78% Decision Forest (DF)	(+) Effective	Best classification accuracy was achieved with the boosted decision tree algorithm. These models outperformed the DOI-based approach	Machine algorithms should be considered in medical applications.
12	Kim et al. [35]	2019	CNNs	Retrospective study	Deep learning-based survival prediction method in oral squamous cell carcinoma (SCC) patients	255	Survival prediction	Datasets	Random Survival Forest (RSF) and the Cox proportional hazard model (CPH)	c-index of testing sets reaching 0.781	(+) Effective	This AI model displayed the best performance among the three models	This model can be effective in predicting, with higher accuracy and can guide clinicians both in choosing treatment options and avoiding unnecessary treatments
13	Anwar Alhazmi et al. [25]	2020	ANNs	Crosssectional study	To develop (ANN) based model in predicting OC	73	Predicting risk of developing OC	Datasets	None	Accuracy of 78.95%	(+) Effective	ANN could perform well in estimating the probability of malignancy	More cohort studies are required based on this model
14	Chui S. Chu et al. [26]	2021	CNN's	Cross sectional comparative study	To evaluate the ability of supervised machine learning models to predict disease outcome	467	Predicting risk of developing OC	Clinicopathological data	linear regression (LR), DT, SVM, and k-nearest neighbors (KNN) models	70.59% accuracy (AUC 0.67), 41.98% sensitivity, and a high specificity of 84.12%.	(+) Effective	CNN's DT model was most successful in identifying "true positive" progressive disease	AI models in this study have shown promise in predicting progressive OSCC disease outcomes
15	Rosma et al. [24]	2010	ANNs	Cross sectional comparative study	Performances of the two artificial Intelligent prediction models when compared with a group of oral cancer clinicians.	171	Predicting the likelihood of an individual developing oral cancer	Datasets	27 oral cancer clinicians	Mean accuracy, sensitivity, and specificity of the models were 59.9, 45.5, and 85.3 for fuzzy neural network models; 63.1, 54.2, and 78.6 for oral cancer clinicians predictions and 67.5, 69.0 and 64.7 for fuzzy regression prediction models.	(+) Effective	Fuzzy regression and fuzzy neural network performed better than oral cancer clinicians	These neural network models provide a suitable alternative to human expert prediction in predicting oral cancer susceptibility.
16	Omar A. Karadaghy et al. [32]	2019	CNN's	Crosssectional study	To develop a prediction DT model using machine learning for 5-year overall survival among patients with OSCC	33,065	Predicting OSCC	Dataset	None	accuracy was 71%, precision was 71%	(+) Effective	AI better in predicting OSCC	AI learning may play in individual patient risk estimation in the era of big data.

ANNs: Artificial Neural Networks, CNNs: Convolutional Neural Networks, DNNs: Deep Neural Networks, and c-index: concordance index.

3.2. Risk of Bias Assessment and Applicability Concerns

The QUADAS-2 assessment tool was used for assessing the quality and risk of bias of the included studies (Table S1). Most studies involved using photographic data as an input to the CNNs and ANNs, and hence, 76.47% of the included studies reported a low risk of bias for the patient-selection domain. However, in four studies, the patient-selection method was unclear. Since the data feeding in AI technology was highly standardized and there was no effect of flow and time frame on the final output, both the factors were categorized in a low-risk group. Nayak et al. used histopathology as the gold standard and studies by Tseng et al., Alabi et al., and Kim et al., were based on the prognostic outcome of the OSCC patients [19,27,33,34]. Hence, the reference standard in this situation was graded as low risk. Reference standard and the flow and timing domain were unclear in 17.64% and 29.41%, respectively. Hence, in this paper, a low risk of bias was reported in the index test (100%) and (70.58%) the inflow and timings. Under the risk of a bias arm of the QUADAS-2 tool, the applicability concern arms also showed 88.23% and 47.05% low risk of bias in the index test and the reference standard. However, patient selection and index test domain were unclear for 35.29% and 11.76% (Table S2, and Figures 2 and 3).

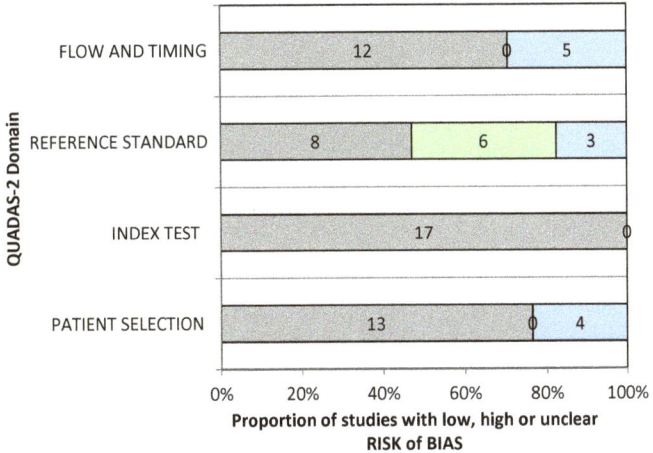

Figure 2. QUADAS-2 assessment of the individual risk of bias domains.

☐ Low ☐ High ☐ Unclear

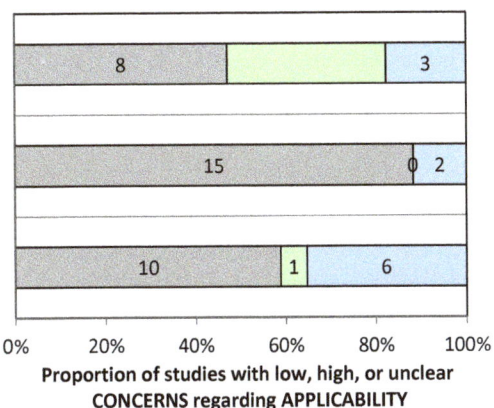

Figure 3. QUADAS-2 assessment of applicability concerns.

4. Discussion

Oral cancer is one of the most prevalent cancer with high mortality, and it is a significant public health issue. Late diagnosis and high death rates are attributes of cancer around the world. According to the 2015 statistics of World Health Organization (WHO), cancer is the first or the second driving reason of death in almost 91 of 172 countries. The diagnosis and prediction of the reoccurrence of OC are the challenging factors, as AI involves complex data on etiology and risk factors [35–37].

AI is an exceptionally fresh development with a significant prognostic power, which allows clinicians to select appropriate treatment modalities. AI holds an incredible guarantee to empower clinicians to make noteworthy choices, depending on the immense amount of digitized data. Previous studies have applied machine-learning methods to huge patient datasets for early diagnosis and predicting the risk of occurrence of OC.

AI has a more preferred advantage over existing techniques for detecting OC. It is a versatile innovation and can acquire additional information at any time. As AI calculations get information from new patients, they can merge this information into their dynamic datasets to improve their prescient exhibition and can reduce the burden of treatment and cost for patients [38]. There are two types of AI technologies, artificial neural networks (ANN) and convolution neural networks (CNN). The significant difference between the two is that in CNN, only the last layer of a neuron is completely associated. While in ANN, every neuron is associated with each different neuron [39]. This paper expects to examine the performance of these AI-based models that have reported on the diagnosis and prediction of the risk of occurrence of OC.

4.1. Artificial Intelligence in Detecting and Diagnosing Oral Cancer

As the late-stage disease has poor prognosis, early detection is important in OC patients. The data obtained from cytology images, fluorescent images, CT images, and depth of invasion can be used in AI learning tools, and OC can be diagnosed quickly with more accuracy. From our collected list of articles, 6 articles reported the application of AI-based computerized models for diagnosing OC. Several studies have carried out early detection of the advanced stage of OC and studies have reported that OC arise from different subsites of the oral cavity such as tongue, buccal mucosa, etc. This heterogeneity of oral malignant growth makes it difficult to be analyzed.

Sunny et al. conducted a study by ANN for early detection of OC, using tele cytology (TC), which is digitization of the cytology slides [29]. The efficacy of AI was compared with conventional cytology and histology; 11,981 prepossessed images were loaded for AI analysis, based on the risk stratification model. Results showed an accuracy of 80–84% in diagnosis, with no difference in tele cytology and conventional cytology detection, however, potentially malignant oral lesions were detected with low sensitivity, using tele cytology. The ANN-based model showed improved malignant detection accuracy to 93%, and a potentially malignant lesion to 73%. The study used the brush biopsy method for sample collection, which is less invasive, and this factor should also be considered while detecting cancer.

Jeyaraj et al. conducted a study in which OC was diagnosed based on a regression-based deep-learning algorithm for the characterization of oral malignant growth [30]. A deep-learning algorithm of CNN was developed in a computer-aided OC detecting system and 100 hyperspectral images (HIS) were analyzed. They observed a 91.4% sensitivity in detecting cancerous lesions using the regression-based algorithm, and the results were compared to the traditional algorithm using the same images. The quality of diagnosis was improved for the proposed model of the algorithm, as compared to the conventional.

Uthoff et al. conducted a study on detecting OC by using smartphone-based images and AI technology [28]. Based on the concept of point of care, smartphone-based images were developed. Autofluorescence and white light imaging were added to the pictures, and these pictures were stacked to AI algorithms for recognizing oral malignancy. A sum of 170 autofluoresced pictures was taken. This strategy was very convenient for application, and the accuracy was improved. However, the study needs to be conducted on a large population for further validation. A similar study was done by Nayak et al., using autofluorescent spectral images, and analysis was done using principal component analysis (PCA) and ANN [19]. PCA is computing based on principal components of data and the results from ANN performance was slightly better than the PCA. The advantage of this technique was that fluorescence spectroscopy image uses a minimally invasive technique and there is no need for biopsy [27,40]. In a study conducted by Musulin et al., AI showed better results in detecting OC, by using Histology images [21]. Similarly, in a study conducted by Kirubabai et al., CNN was better at differentiating malignant lesions as mild or severe, by using clinical images of patients [22].

Kann et al. applied deep-learning machines on 106 OC patients for the identification of nodal metastasis and tumor extra-nodal extension involvement [17]. The dataset comprised 2875 CT (computerized tomography) segmented lymph node samples. This study explored the capability of the deep-learning model to assist head and neck cancer patient management. For DNN, the area under the receiver operating characteristic curve (AUC) showed 0.91, which implied a higher accuracy. AUC represents the two-dimensional areas under the receiver operating characteristic curve (ROC). Similarly, Chang et al., reported an AUC of 0.90 for predicting the occurrence of OC, using AI based on genome markers [41]. In this study, logistic regression analysis was used to compare with AI. However, the study was conducted on 31 patients, which is a considerably less sample size, a study on a larger number of patients has to be carried out for better analysis.

4.2. Artificial Intelligence in Predicting the Occurrence of Oral Cancer

Currently, OC is treated with advanced treatment aids, however, the reoccurrence rate of OC is very high. Treatment of oral malignant growth relies on the stage of the disease. Lack of an evidence-on staging system may prompt deficient or pointless treatment. Different prognostic biomarkers and restorative targets have been proposed in ongoing periods, but they are not reproduced in the present cancer staging system. To date traditional statistical methods have been used for predicting OC, for example, cox proportional hazard (CPH), and it is not suitable for predicting conditions like OC.

Considering the complex 'dataset' of oral carcinoma, an AI-based anticipation prediction will give satisfied outcomes. Previous studies that used AI for predicting OC yielded excellent results [34,42,43].

Alabi et al. conducted a study on 311 patients in Brazil which compared four machine-learning algorithms in predicting the risk of reoccurrence of oral tongue squamous cell carcinoma [33]. These different machine-learning AI-based algorithms were based on support vector machine (SVM), naïve Bayes (NB), boosted decision tree (BDT), and decision forest (DF). All these algorithms showed improved accuracy in diagnosis, but the BDT algorithm showed the highest accuracy. However, the study included fewer samples, and more external algorithm data is required.

Shams et al. employed AI with the gene expression profile, to predict the occurrence of OC and also the transformation of oral potentially malignant lesions [31]. The study was conducted on 86 subjects, among them, 51 subjects developed OC and 31 subjects remained without malignancy. The study compared SVM, DNN, and multi-layer perception (MLP). Excellent results were obtained by deep-learning machines with 96.5% accuracy and 94% accuracy was obtained with MLP [43].

Chui et al., predicted the occurrence of cancer, based on clinical, pathological data, and compared linear regression (LR), BDT, SVM, and k-nearest neighbors (KNN) models, and concluded that BDT was the best model [26].

Tseng et al. determined the difference between symptoms exhibited by demised and survived OC patients [27]. The performance was compared between conventional logistic regression, decision tree, and ANN, and was conducted on 674 OC patients. Study used prognostic factors such as survival rate, death, cancer occurrence, and metastasis. The study concluded that the decision tree was easy to interpret and accuracy of the decision tree, and ANN was compared more to conventional logistic regression.

Rosma et al. tested the effectiveness of AI in predicting cancer based on the risk habits and demographic profiles in a Malaysian cohort [24]. Prediction of OC was compared between fuzzy regression model, fuzzy neural network prediction model, and clinician opinion. Fuzzy regression provides means when there is a lack of data and also provides a relationship between explanatory and response variables. The AI-based neural network and fuzzy regression model performed better in accuracy than human opinion, in predicting the OC.

5. Conclusions

AI is more accurate in diagnosing oral cancer as compared to the conventional method of diagnosis. Retrospective clinical data of patients may help in improving the AI-based diagnosis. Additionally, AI-based algorithms showed more accurate results in predicting the OC occurrence. More data and studies are needed to conduct AI-based algorithms to predict OC. The treatment of OC will not be effective if they are diagnosed at a later stage. Subsequently, early recognition techniques are required. The complex etiology and high recurrence rate make the investigation difficult. The patients can be classified as high- and low-risk groups, using accurate data from AI, which helps clinicians in planning and treatment, as compared to conventional methods. Patients can be directed with sensible advice and the clinicians can be guided with informed decisions.

Supplementary Materials: The following are available online at https://www.mdpi.com/article/10.3390/diagnostics11061004/s1, Table S1: Quality assessment (QUADAS 2) summary of the risk of bias; Table S2: Quality assessment (QUADAS 2) summary of applicability concerns.

Author Contributions: Conceptualization, S.B.K., and S.V.; methodology, S.N.; software, S.V.; validation, S.P., L.T. and A.Z.; formal analysis, A.A.A.K.; investigation, P.C.M.; resources, Y.A.; data curation, G.S.S.; writing—original draft preparation, A.A.A.K.; writing—review and editing, S.M.; visualization, S.C.S.; supervision, S.P.; project administration, S.P. All authors have read and agreed to the published version of the manuscript.

Funding: This is a non-funded research and there has been no financial support for this work that could have influenced its outcome.

Data Availability Statement: Data is contained within the article.

Conflicts of Interest: The authors declare no conflict of interest.

References

1. World Health Organization. *WHO Report on Cancer: Setting Priorities, Investing Wisely and Providing Care for All*; Technical Report; World Health Organization: Geneva, Switzerland, 2020.
2. Sinevici, N.; O'sullivan, J. Oral cancer: Deregulated molecular events and their use as biomarkers. *Oral Oncol.* **2016**, *61*, 12–18. [CrossRef]
3. Lewin, F.; Norell, S.; Johansson, H.; Gustavsson, P.; Wennerberg, J.; Biörklund, A.; Rutqvist, L. Smoking Tobacco, Oral Snuff, and Alcohol in the Etiology of Squamous Cell Carcinoma of the Head and Neck: A Population-Based Case-Referent Study in Sweden. *Cancer* **1998**, *82*, 1367–1375. [CrossRef]
4. Ilhan, B.; Lin, K.; Guneri, P.; Wilder-Smith, P. Improving Oral Cancer Outcomes with Imaging and Artificial Intelligence. *J. Dent. Res.* **2020**, *99*, 241–248. [CrossRef] [PubMed]
5. Dhanuthai, K.; Rojanawatsirivej, S.; Thosaporn, W.; Kintarak, S.; Subarnbhesaj, A.; Darling, M.; Kryshtalskyj, E.; Chiang, C.P.; Shin, H.I.; Choi, S.Y.; et al. Oral cancer: A multicenter study. *Med. Oral Patol. Oral Cir. Bucal* **2018**, *23*, e23–e29. [CrossRef] [PubMed]
6. Lavanya, L.; Chandra, J. Oral Cancer Analysis Using Machine Learning Techniques. *Int. J. Eng. Res. Technol.* **2019**, *12*, 596–601.
7. Kearney, V.; Chan, J.W.; Valdes, G.; Solberg, T.D.; Yom, S.S. The application of artificial intelligence in the IMRT planning process for head and neck cancer. *Oral Oncol.* **2018**, *87*, 111–116. [CrossRef] [PubMed]
8. Hamet, P.; Tremblay, J. Artificial intelligence in medicine. *Metabolism.* **2017**, *69*, S36–S40. [CrossRef]
9. Kaladhar, D.; Chandana, B.; Kumar, P. Predicting Cancer Survivability Using Classification Algorithms. Books 1 View project Protein Interaction Networks in Metallo Proteins and Docking Approaches of Metallic Compounds with TIMP and MMP in Control of MAPK Pathway View project Predicting Cancer. *Int. J. Res. Rev. Comput. Sci.* **2011**, *2*, 340–343.

10. Kalappanavar, A.; Sneha, S.; Annigeri, R.G. Artificial intelligence: A dentist's perspective. *Pathol. Surg.* **2018**, *5*, 2–4. [CrossRef]
11. Krishna, A.B.; Tanveer, A.; Bhagirath, P.V.; Gannepalli, A. Role of artificial intelligence in diagnostic oral pathology-A modern approach. *JOMFP* **2020**, *24*, 152–156.
12. Kareem, S.A.; Pozos-Parra, P.; Wilson, N. An application of belief merging for the diagnosis of oral cancer. *Appl. Soft Comput. J.* **2017**, *61*, 1105–1112. [CrossRef]
13. Arbes, S.J. Factors contributing to the poorer survival of black Americans diagnosed with oral cancer (United States). *Cancer Causes Control* **1999**, *10*, 513–523. [CrossRef]
14. de Melo, G.M.; Ribeiro, K.; Kowalski, L.; Deheinzelin, D. Risk Factors for Postoperative Complications in Oral Cancer and Their Prognostic Implications. *Arch. Otolaryngol. Head Neck Surg.* **2001**, *127*, 828–833.
15. Bànkfalvi, A.; Piffkò, J. Prognostic and predictive factors in oral cancer: The role of the invasive tumour front. *J. Oral Pathol. Med.* **2000**, *29*, 291–298. [CrossRef] [PubMed]
16. Schliephake, H. Prognostic relevance of molecular markers of oral cancer—A review. *Int. J. Oral Maxillofac. Surg.* **2003**, *32*, 233–245. [CrossRef] [PubMed]
17. Kann, B.H.; Aneja, S.; Loganadane, G.V.; Kelly, J.R.; Smith, S.M.; Decker, R.H.; Yu, J.B.; Park, H.S.; Yarbrough, W.G.; Malhotra, A.; et al. Pretreatment Identification of Head and Neck Cancer Nodal Metastasis and Extranodal Extension Using Deep Learning Neural Networks. *Sci. Rep.* **2018**, *8*, 1–11. [CrossRef] [PubMed]
18. Whiting, P.F.; Rutjes, A.W.S.; Westwood, M.E.; Mallett, S.; Deeks, J.J.; Reitsma, J.B.; Leeflang, M.M.G.; Sterne, J.A.C.; Bossuyt, P.M.M. Quadas-2: A revised tool for the quality assessment of diagnostic accuracy studies. *Ann. Intern. Med.* **2011**, *155*, 529–536. [CrossRef]
19. Nayak, G.S.; Kamath, S.; Pai, K.M.; Sarkar, A.; Ray, S.; Kurien, J.; D'Almeida, L.; Krishnanand, B.R.; Santhosh, C.; Kartha, V.B.; et al. Principal component analysis and artificial neural network analysis of oral tissue fluorescence spectra: Classification of normal premalignant and malignant pathological conditions. *Biopolymers* **2006**, *82*, 152–166. [CrossRef] [PubMed]
20. Jubair, F.; Al-karadsheh, O.; Malamos, D.; Al Mahdi, S.; Saad, Y.; Hassona, Y. A novel lightweight deep convolutional neural network for early detection of oral cancer. *Oral Dis.* **2021**, 1–8. [CrossRef]
21. Musulin, J.; Štifanić, D.; Zulijani, A.; Ćabov, T.; Dekanić, A.; Car, Z. An enhanced histopathology analysis: An ai-based system for multiclass grading of oral squamous cell carcinoma and segmenting of epithelial and stromal tissue. *Cancers* **2021**, *13*, 1784. [CrossRef]
22. Kirubabai, M.P.; Arumugam, G. View of Deep Learning Classification Method to Detect and Diagnose the Cancer Regions in Oral MRI Images. *Med. Legal Update* **2021**, *21*, 462–468.
23. Rathod, J.; Sherkay, S.; Bondre, H.; Sonewane, R.; Deshmukh, D. Oral Cancer Detection and Level Classification Through Machine Learning. *Int. J. Adv. Res. Comput. Commun. Eng.* **2020**, *9*, 177–182. [CrossRef]
24. Rosma, M.D.; Sameem, A.K.; Basir, A.; Siti Mazlipah, I.; Norzaidi, M.D. The use of artificial intelligence to identify people at risk of oral cancer: Empirical evidence in Malaysian university. *Int. J. Sci. Res. Educ.* **2010**, *3*, 10–20.
25. Alhazmi, A.; Alhazmi, Y.; Makrami, A.; Masmali, A.; Salawi, N.; Masmali, K.; Patil, S. Application of artificial intelligence and machine learning for prediction of oral cancer risk. *J. Oral Pathol. Med.* **2021**, 1–7. [CrossRef]
26. Chu, C.S.; Lee, N.P.; Adeoye, J.; Thomson, P.; Choi, S. Machine learning and treatment outcome prediction for oral cancer. *J. Oral Pathol. Med.* **2020**, *49*, 977–985. [CrossRef] [PubMed]
27. Tseng, W.T.; Chiang, W.F.; Liu, S.Y.; Roan, J.; Lin, C.N. The Application of Data Mining Techniques to Oral Cancer Prognosis. *J. Med. Syst.* **2015**, *39*, 59–66. [CrossRef] [PubMed]
28. Uthoff, R.D.; Song, B.; Sunny, S.; Patrick, S.; Suresh, A.; Kolur, T.; Keerthi, G.; Spires, O.; Anbarani, A.; Wilder-Smith, P.; et al. Point-of-care, smartphone-based, dual-modality, dual-view, oral cancer screening device with neural network classification for low-resource communities. *PLoS ONE* **2018**, *13*, 1–21. [CrossRef] [PubMed]
29. Sunny, S.; Baby, A.; James, B.L.; Balaji, D.; N. V., A.; Rana, M.H.; Gurpur, P.; Skandarajah, A.; D'Ambrosio, M.; Ramanjinappa, R.D.; et al. A smart tele-cytology point-of-care platform for oral cancer screening. *PLoS ONE* **2019**, *14*, 1–16. [CrossRef]
30. Jeyaraj, P.R.; Samuel Nadar, E.R. Computer-assisted medical image classification for early diagnosis of oral cancer employing deep learning algorithm. *J. Cancer Res. Clin. Oncol.* **2019**, *145*, 829–837. [CrossRef] [PubMed]
31. Shams, W.K.; Htike, Z.Z. Oral Cancer Prediction Using Gene Expression Profiling and Machine Learning. *Int. J. Appl. Eng. Res.* **2017**, *12*, 4893–4898.
32. Karadaghy, O.A.; Shew, M.; New, J.; Bur, A.M. Development and Assessment of a Machine Learning Model to Help Predict Survival among Patients with Oral Squamous Cell Carcinoma. *JAMA Otolaryngol. Head Neck Surg.* **2019**, *145*, 1115–1120. [CrossRef] [PubMed]
33. Alabi, R.O.; Elmusrati, M.; Sawazaki-Calone, I.; Kowalski, L.P.; Haglund, C.; Coletta, R.D.; Mäkitie, A.A.; Salo, T.; Almangush, A.; Leivo, I. Comparison of supervised machine learning classification techniques in prediction of locoregional recurrences in early oral tongue cancer. *Int. J. Med. Inform.* **2020**, *136*, 104068. [CrossRef] [PubMed]
34. Kim, D.W.; Lee, S.; Kwon, S.; Nam, W.; Cha, I.H.; Kim, H.J. Deep learning-based survival prediction of oral cancer patients. *Sci. Rep.* **2019**, *9*, 1–10. [CrossRef] [PubMed]
35. Warnakulasuriya, S. Global epidemiology of oral and oropharyngeal cancer. *Oral Oncol.* **2009**, *45*, 309–316. [CrossRef]
36. Gupta, N.; Gupta, R.; Acharya, A.K.; Patthi, B.; Goud, V.; Reddy, S.; Garg, A.; Singla, A. Changing Trends in oral cancer—A global scenario. *Nepal J. Epidemiol.* **2017**, *6*, 613–619. [CrossRef]

37. Dhage, S.N. A Review on Early Detection of Oral Cancer using ML Techniques. *Int. J. Sci. Prog. Res.* **2019**, *158*, 1–5.
38. Chan, C.H.; Huang, T.T.; Chen, C.Y.; Lee, C.C.; Chan, M.Y.; Chung, P.C. Texture-Map-Based Branch-Collaborative Network for Oral Cancer Detection. *IEEE Trans. Biomed. Circuits Syst.* **2019**, *13*, 766–780. [CrossRef]
39. Bur, A.M.; Holcomb, A.; Goodwin, S.; Woodroof, J.; Karadaghy, O.; Shnayder, Y.; Kakarala, K.; Brant, J.; Shew, M. Machine learning to predict occult nodal metastasis in early oral squamous cell carcinoma. *Oral Oncol.* **2019**, *92*, 20–25. [CrossRef]
40. Kan, C.W.; Nieman, L.T.; Sokolov, K.; Markey, M.K. AI in clinical decision support: Applications in optical spectroscopy for cancer detection and diagnosis. *Stud. Comput. Intell.* **2008**, *107*, 27–49. [CrossRef]
41. Chang, S.W.; Abdul-Kareem, S.; Merican, A.F.; Zain, R.B. Oral cancer prognosis based on clinicopathologic and genomic markers using a hybrid of feature selection and machine learning methods. *BMC Bioinform.* **2013**, *14*, 170–185. [CrossRef] [PubMed]
42. Lucheng, Z.; Wenhua, L.; Meng, S.; Hangping, W.; Juan, W.; Xuebang, Z.; Changlin, Z. Comparison between artificial neural network and Cox regression model in predicting the survival rate of gastric cancer patients. *Biomed. Rep.* **2013**, *1*, 757–760. [CrossRef]
43. Zheng, B.; Yoon, S.W.; Lam, S.S. Breast cancer diagnosis based on feature extraction using a hybrid of K-means and support vector machine algorithms. *Expert Syst. Appl.* **2014**, *41*, 1476–1482. [CrossRef]

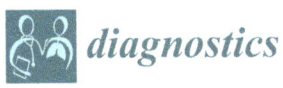

Article

Machine Learning Study in Caries Markers in Oral Microbiota from Monozygotic Twin Children

Esther Alia-García [1], Manuel Ponce-Alonso [2,†], Claudia Saralegui [2,†], Ana Halperin [2], Marta Paz Cortés [1], María Rosario Baquero [1], David Parra-Pecharromán [1,3], Javier Galeano [4,*] and Rosa del Campo [1,2,†]

1. Facultad de Ciencias de la Salud, Universidad Alfonso X El Sabio, Villanueva de la Cañada, 28691 Madrid, Spain; estheraliagarcia@yahoo.es (E.A.-G.); mpazcor@uax.es (M.P.C.); mbaquart@uax.es (M.R.B.); dparrpec@uax.es (D.P.-P.); rosacampo@yahoo.com (R.d.C.)
2. Servicio de Microbiología, Hospital Universitario Ramón y Cajal and Instituto Ramón y Cajal de Investigaciones Sanitarias (IRYCIS), 28034 Madrid, Spain; lugonauta@gmail.com (M.P.-A.); claudiasaralegui1994@gmail.com (C.S.); ana.halperin@gmail.com (A.H.)
3. Departamento de Biología, Servicio de Criminalística, Dirección General de la Guardia Civil, 28003 Madrid, Spain
4. Complex Systems Group, Universidad Politécnica de Madrid, 28040 Madrid, Spain
* Correspondence: javier.galeano@upm.es
† Spanish Network for Research in Infectious Diseases (REIPI)

Citation: Alia-García, E.; Ponce-Alonso, M.; Saralegui, C.; Halperin, A.; Paz Cortés, M.; Baquero, M.R.; Parra-Pecharromán, D.; Galeano, J.; del Campo, R. Machine Learning Study in Caries Markers in Oral Microbiota from Monozygotic Twin Children. *Diagnostics* **2021**, *11*, 835. https://doi.org/10.3390/diagnostics11050835

Academic editor: Jae-Hong Lee

Received: 13 April 2021
Accepted: 3 May 2021
Published: 6 May 2021

Publisher's Note: MDPI stays neutral with regard to jurisdictional claims in published maps and institutional affiliations.

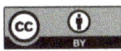

Copyright: © 2021 by the authors. Licensee MDPI, Basel, Switzerland. This article is an open access article distributed under the terms and conditions of the Creative Commons Attribution (CC BY) license (https://creativecommons.org/licenses/by/4.0/).

Abstract: In recent years, the etiology of caries has evolved from a simplistic infectious perspective based on *Streptococcus mutans* and/or *Lactobacillus* activity, to a multifactorial disease involving a complex oral microbiota, the human genetic background and the environment. The aim of this work was to identify bacterial markers associated with early caries using massive 16S rDNA. To minimize the other factors, the composition of the oral microbiota of twins in which only one of them had caries was compared with their healthy sibling. Twenty-one monozygotic twin pairs without a previous diagnosis of caries were recruited in the context of their orthodontic treatment and divided into two categories: (1) caries group in which only one of the twins had caries; and (2) control group in which neither of the twins had caries. Each participant contributed a single oral lavage sample in which the bacterial composition was determined by 16S rDNA amplification and further high-throughput sequencing. Data analysis included statistical comparison of alpha and beta diversity, as well as differential taxa abundance between groups. Our results show that twins of the control group have a closer bacterial composition than those from the caries group. However, statistical differences were not detected and we were unable to find any particular bacterial marker by 16S rDNA high-throughput sequencing that could be useful for prevention strategies. Although these results should be validated in a larger population, including children from other places or ethnicities, we conclude that the occurrence of caries is not related to the increase of any particular bacterial population.

Keywords: machine learning; oral microbiota; LEfSe; PCoA; alloprevotella; prevotella; core microbiota

1. Introduction

The microbial colonization of the oral cavity starts immediately after birth, differencing among early colonizers (*Streptococcus*, *Veillonella* and *Lactobacillus*), constant (*Gemella*, *Granulicatella*, *Haemophilus* and *Rothia*) and late colonizers (*Actinomyces*, *Porphyromonas*, *Abiotrophia* and *Neisseria*) [1–3]. The establishment of this ecosystem and its further composition is influenced by numerous factors as the mode of delivery, diet and antibiotic consumption [4]. Oral health is not only a local stomatological problem, but also an important driver of systemic health, as it has been linked to numerous disorders of the digestive, cardiovascular and genitourinary tracts [5–7].

Caries is the most prevalent human disease worldwide, although its incidence varies according to geography and ethnicity [8], and it has conventionally been attributed to the direct action of acidogenic bacteria such as *Streptococcus mutans*, *Lactobacillus* and *Bifidobacterium* since these microorganisms have been isolated from the lesions. The application of molecular tools based on high-throughput sequencing of the 16S rDNA gene has revealed that microbiota associated to caries is a much more complex ecosystem than expected (http://www.homd.org/, accessed on 5 May 2021) [9]. While traditional studies classified bacteria as pathogens or commensals according to their potential etiological role on diseases, greater focus has been put on the new concepts of eubiosis/dysbiosis and the disbalance of alkalinogenic/acidogenic bacteria in the caries [3,4]. In addition, metatranscriptomic analyses have permitted to extend the cause of oral diseases as periodontitis from the action of a single microorganism to the metabolic activity of the entire ecosystem [10]. Consequently, the number of microorganisms linked to caries has increased considerably in the last decade [11–13], including *Streptococcus, Lactobacillus, Veillonella, Actinomyces, Granulicatella, Leptotrichia, Megasphaera, Olsenella, Shuttleworthia* and, most recently, *Scardovia, Atopobium* and *Selemonas* [14]. One of the major challenges is to identify early markers of caries in order to monitor and prevent this disease during childhood. The exploration of biomarkers in saliva has already demonstrated its usefulness in other pathologies [7,15].

Due to all this complexity in the detection of caries markers, we think that a predictive analysis using machine learning tools can be a good starting point in the study of caries using the oral microbiota. Despite the fact that the implementation of Artificial Intelligence (AI) is still far from being completely common in oral health, some studies highlight the improvements that its use would imply in different areas [16].

The rationale of the present work was to identify bacterial biomarkers in saliva for early caries detection. For this purpose, we explored by massive 16S rDNA sequencing combined with robust bioinformatics tools, statistical analysis and machine learning the oral microbiota of monozygotic twins with and without caries.

2. Materials and Methods

2.1. Patients and Samples

Twenty-one pairs of monozygotic twins were recruited by the first author EAG and divided into two categories: (1) caries group where only one of the twins had caries (22 infants, 73% females, median age of 9 years, range from 6 to 12 years); and (2) control group where neither of them had caries (20 infants, 70% females, median age of 6.7 years, range from 4 to 12 years) (Table 1). Infants were enrolled in 2018 from January to May in four different dental clinics of Madrid (Spain) within the context of their orthodontic treatment. Each child contributed with a single oral lavage sample after 5 min of vigorous rising with 10 mL of sterile water. Samples were immediately frozen after collection and stored at $-80\ °C$ until processing. The inclusion criteria were twins aged 4–12 years whose parents and they accepted to participate in the study. In the caries group kids with clear lesions as well as pre-cavity lesions, mainly white spots, were included, whereas other types of lesions were excluded. All participants were adequately instructed to avoid teeth brushing, food and sugar drinks intake during the 2 h before sampling.

2.2. Oral Microbiota Characterization

Oral lavages were slowly defrosted at $-20\ °C$ during 24 h, followed by another 24 h at $4\ °C$, and centrifuged at 14,000 r.p.m. for 15 min discharging the supernatant. Total DNA was obtained from the pellet with the Speedtools tissue DNA extraction kit (Biotools), determining their concentration and quality by Qubit fluorometer (Thermo Fisher Scientific, MA, USA). DNA samples were sent to FISABIO (Valencia, Spain) for massive sequencing (2×300 bp, MiSeq, Illumina. Cod. 15044223 Rev. A) of the V3 and V4 regions of the 16S rRNA gene, which were amplified with the following primers: Forward Primer: 5'-TCGTCGGCAGCGTCAGATGTGTATAAGAGACAGC CTACGGGNGGCWGCAG; and Reverse Primer: 5'-GTCTCGTGGGCTCGGAGATGTGTATAAGAGACAGGACTACHVGG GT ATCTAATCC. Sequence quality was measured according to the following parameters:

minimum length, 250 bp; trimming quality measure type, mean; trimming quality number from 3' extreme, 30; and trimming quality window, 10 bp. Shannon–Weaver and Chao1 indexes were used for bacterial alpha diversity estimation excluding taxa with three or fewer reads. Taxonomic affiliations were assigned using the Silva 119 database, and reads with an RDP score below 0.8 were assigned to the upper taxonomic rank, leaving the last rank as unidentified. Relative abundance and contingency tables of the operational taxonomic units (OTUs) included singletons and very low-represented taxa.

Table 1. Main characteristics of the 42 participants. C, caries; H, healthy.

Caries Group 22 Infants	Sex	Age
1C/1H	females	12
2C/1H	females	7
3C/1H	females	8
4C/1H	females	6
5C/1H	females	11
6C/1H	males	9
7C/1H	females	8
8C/1H	males	10
9C/1H	females	12
10C/1H	females	9
11C/1H	males	9
Control Group 20 Infants	**Sex**	**Age**
12	females	12
13	females	7
14	males	4
15	females	8
16	females	9
17	females	5
18	females	9
19	males	4
20	females	4
21	males	5

2.3. Statistical Analysis and Machine Learning Modeling

Statistical analysis was performed using R statistical software v3.5.3. Quantitative data of the reads were homogenized using their relative percentage from the total reads of each sample to allow the comparison between samples. Finally, the Galaxy Huttenhower Platform (http://huttenhower.sph.harvard.edu/galaxy, accessed on 5 May 2021) was used to calculate the Linear Discriminant Effect Size Analysis (LEfSe) algorithm to identify which microbial taxa explain significant differences among groups of samples [17]. The PCoA analyses were performed by Past 3.0 software. Raw sequences were deposited in the GenBank database as Bioproject PRJNA643173.

Simultaneously, we carried out a statistical exploratory analysis to later search for a machine learning model for a possible caries prediction. To carry out this analysis, we ruled out bacterial species with fewer than 50 data with non-zero values. Exploratory analysis was performed using own software in Python. Machine Learning models were developed with Orange3 v3.27 [18]. We carried out different classification models in two ways. In the first case, we used healthy, control and cavity sample labels. In the second case, we only used healthy and caries labels to classify our samples. Using k-cross validation (k = 10), we tested five different classification model: Random Forest, Neural Network, Support Vector Machine, KNN model and a logistic regression.

To evaluate the results of the used algorithms, we used:

1. Classification accuracy is the proportion of correctly classified examples.

2. F-1 is a weighted harmonic mean of precision and recall.
3. Precision is the proportion of true positives among instances classified as positive, e.g., the proportion of cavity correctly identified as cavity.
4. Recall is the proportion of true positives among all positive instances in the data, e.g., the number of cavity among all diagnosed as cavity.

3. Results

Both groups of participants were comparable in demographic and anthropometric terms, and all were recruited during their orthodontic treatment without previous suspicion of caries. Oral lavages were processed in a single session and the 16S rDNA massive sequencing was developed successfully, passing the quality filters with adequate negative controls. The numbers of read counts were comparable for all samples. The alpha diversity was analyzed by the Shannon–Weaver and Chao 1 alpha diversity indexes showed no significant differences between groups, but more disperse values were detected in the caries group (Figure 1).

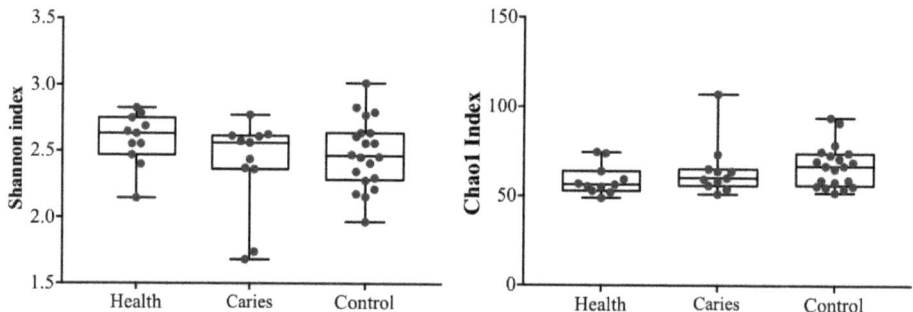

Figure 1. Alpha diversity indexes in all samples. Statistical differences were not detected.

Phyla distributions showed a preserved pattern for each pair of twins, including those from the caries group (Figure 2). Children with caries had a similar phyla distribution to their healthy siblings, whereas controls presented higher proportions of Firmicutes and lower proportions of Proteobacteria.

Up to 119 genera were identified, although 13 of them accounted for 90% of the total abundance [*Streptococcus* (≈30%), *Prevotella* (≈10 %), *Neisseria* (≈9%), *Veillonella* (≈8%), *Gemella* (≈7%), *Haemophilus* (≈6%), *Alloprevotella* (≈5%), *Rothia* (≈5%), *Porphyromonas* (≈2%), *Fusobacterium* (≈2%), *Leptotrichia* (≈2%), *Granucalicatella* (≈2%) and *Actinomyces* (≈2%)]. The remaining genera represented 10% of the abundance, comprising 106 genera with a total population density less than 1 for each one (Figure 3).

To obtain a global overview of the oral microbiome complexity, we designed an interaction network representing all taxa detected for each subject in circles proportional to their frequency and joined the circles, called nodes, proportional to their frequency joining the circles by lines, called links, to build a network per sample. Subsequently, we superimposed all the individual networks to define the core of the microbiome of each condition (caries, health and controls), and the thickness of the links between nodes is the accumulated number of lectures in all samples, representing the stability in the coexistence of the connecting taxa (Figure 4).

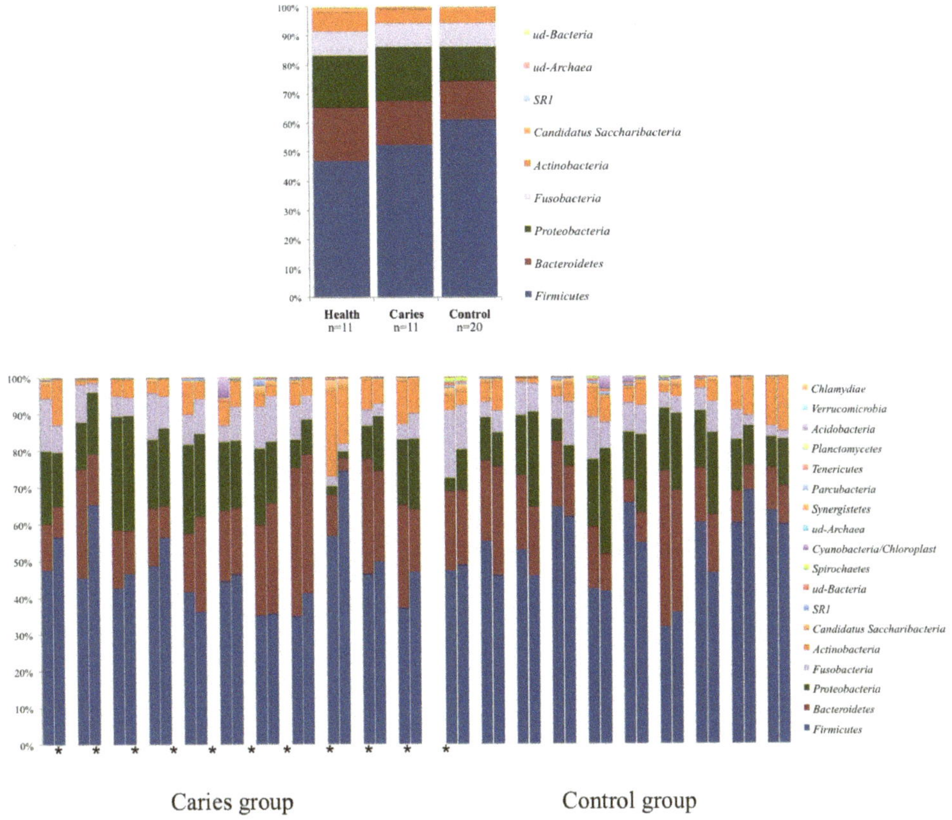

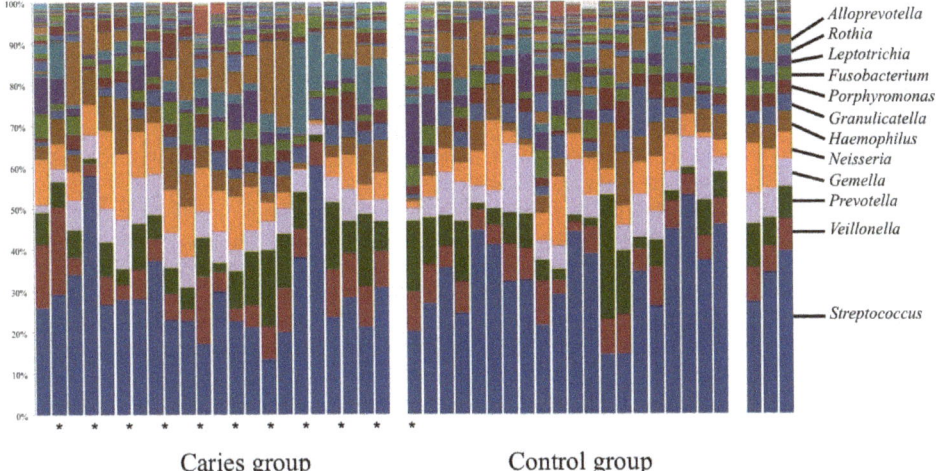

Figure 2. Phyla distribution: (**top**) the median values for each phyla and group; and (**bottom**) all individual values. * Represents Children with caries.

Figure 3. Distribution of the major bacterial genera among all participants.* Represents Children with caries.

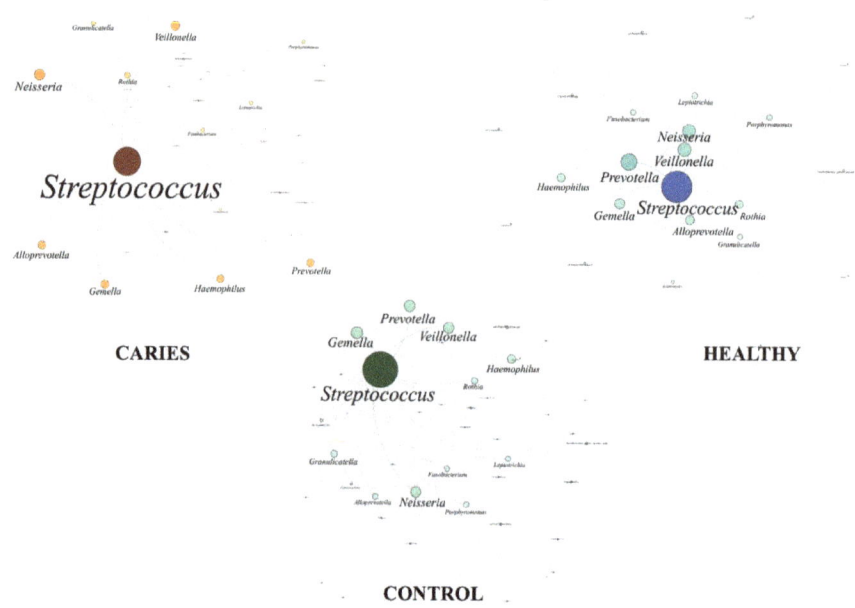

Figure 4. Complex networks core microbiota for the three differenced subjects using Gephi.

PCoA analysis separated the healthy, caries and control groups (Figure 5), showing a higher level of *Veillonella*, *Prevotella* and *Fusobacterium* genera linked to a healthy status, whereas *Alloprevotella* and *Granullicatella* were the most differentiated genera among children with cavities. The control group was allocated in a separate quadrant marked by the abundance of *Capnocytophaga*, *Lautropia* and *Streptobacillus*. Curiously, most of the control group twins were located on the same quadrant (8 out of 10 pairs), three pairs being located in Quadrant 3 (dominated by *Gemella* and *Haemophilus*), three in Quadrant 4 (*Streptococcus* and *Rothia*) and two in Quadrant 1 (*Prevotella* and *Veillonella*). The remaining two pairs of control twins were located on separated coordinates (Quadrants 1–3 and 2–3). Considering the twins of the caries group, only 6 out of the 11 pairs had both children located in the same quadrant: one in Quadrant 1 (*Prevotella* and *Veillonella*), three in Quadrant 2 (*Neisseria*, *Alloprevotela* and *Leptotrichia*), one in Quadrant 3 (*Gemella* and *Haemophilus*) and one in Quadrant 4 (*Streptococcus* and *Rothia*). The remaining five pairs were distributed in separated quadrants: two pairs in Quadrants 1–2, one pair in Quadrants 2–3, one in Quadrants 1–4 and one in Quadrants 1–3.

Furthermore, differential abundance analysis on microbiota composition by LEfSE in relation to the group, age and the sex of children did not obtain any significant result.

Finally, to address the possibility to predict the cavity in patients, we developed five classification models using machine learning tools (Table 2). The model that showed the highest classification accuracy (CA) was the Random Forest model with a value of 0.881 followed by the Neural Network with 0.810. Studying the confusion matrix, from the point of view of caries, the Random Forest model does not produce false positives but does generate quite a few false negatives (54.5%). On the contrary, Neural Network model produce 16.1% false positives but a lower percentage, with respect to the Random Forest, of false negatives (27.3%).

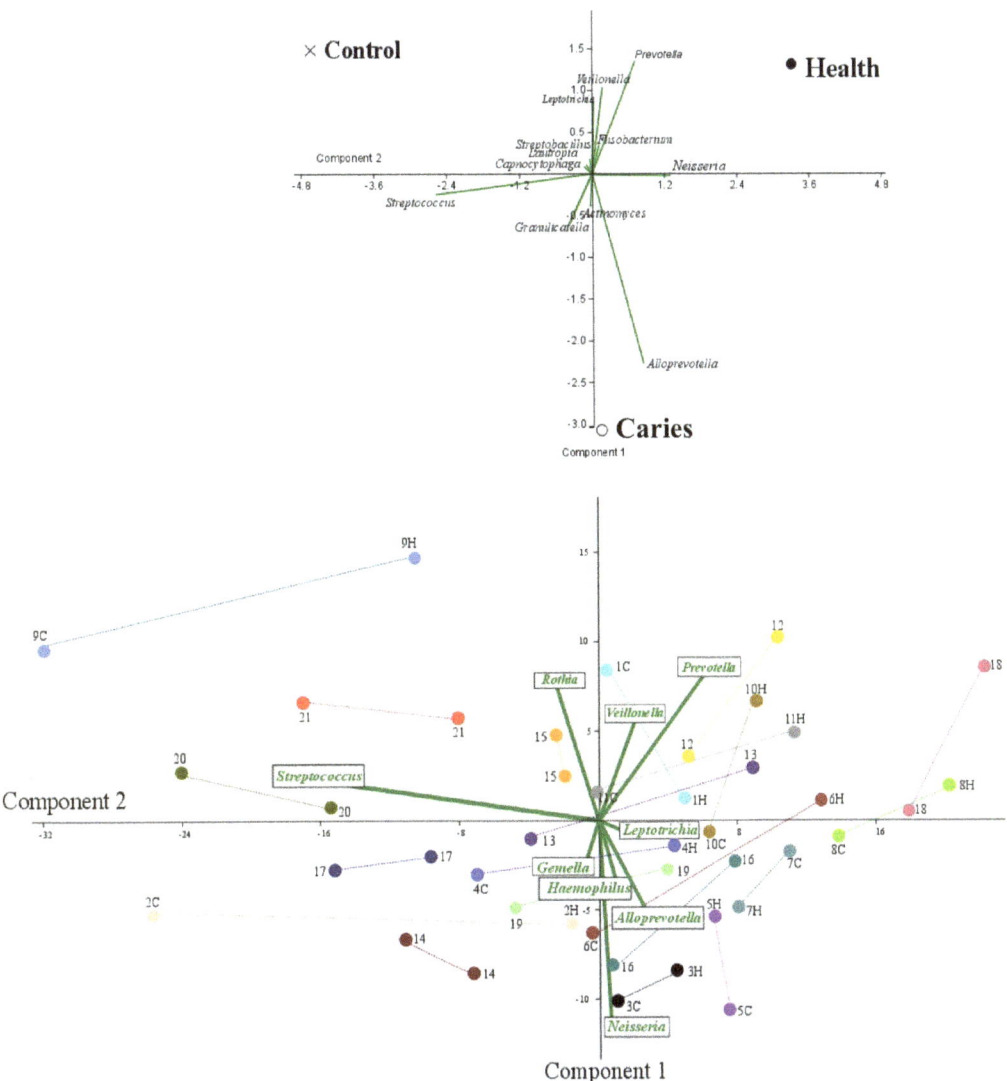

Figure 5. PCoA analysis: (**top**) the median value for the three categories of subjects respect to the abundance bacterial genera; and (**bottom**) the same analysis but considering each of the children and in relation to their sibling. The pairs of twins are linked by colored lines. Random colors are used to highlight the two pairs of twins.

Table 2. Results of the accuracy of the 5 model used in this study. We have used different measures: Classification accuracy (CA), F1, precision, and recall.

Model	CA	F1	Precision	Recall
kNN	0.666	0.655	0.646	0.665
SVM	0.738	0.627	0.545	0.738
Random Forest	0.881	0.874	0.880	0.881
Neural Network	0.810	0.814	0.823	0.810
Logistic Regression	0.595	0.601	0.607	0.595

4. Discussion

In the last years, the etiology of caries has evolved from a simplistic infectious perspective (*S. mutans* and/or *Lactobacillus* colonization) to a multifactorial disease involving oral microbiota, human genetic background and environment [3]. In accordance, research tools have evolved from culturomics to metagenomics, transcriptomics and proteomics. Diet continues to be one of the most decisive factors in caries incidence and accounts for the individual susceptibility in relation to carbohydrates intake and bacterial fermentation [19,20], whereas human genetic background seems to be not so relevant, as previously expected [4,21]. The main objective of our work was twofold, on the one hand, to detect early metagenomic markers based on the abundance of particular genera in the oral microbiota associated with caries in the context of monozygotic twins with the same genetic, dietary and environmental context, and, on the other hand, address a classification model to predict caries using this microbiota of patients. When the participation in the project was offered to children, none of them had been previously diagnosed of caries. The bioinformatic analyses showed a more uniform microbiota in the control twin group, but without statistical significance. We were unable to identify any bacterial taxon exclusive of participants with caries, discarding the contribution of oral bacteria microbiota at the initial cariogenic process.

To obtain a representative sample of the entire oral microbiota, all children refrained from tooth brush and avoided food intake for at least 2 h. Despite the high and continuous contamination of the oral microbiota with foreign environmental microorganisms, intra-individual particularities of saliva microbiota have been postulated as a forensic marker to identify subjects, even for twins [22]. Some studies perform the sampling directly from the lesion or at the supragingival plaque, but we decided to use rinsing of the total oral microbiota as a representative sample easily collected by children with the absence of macroscopically visible lesions, which seems to be the most suitable option for surveillance purposes. Even though saliva and supragingival plaque are different in terms of bacterial composition [23], saliva has been used in similar studies, providing differentiation between subjects with and without caries [24]. The use of saliva in the identification of biomarkers associated to both local and general health was previously validated [7,15].

Previous studies on monozygotic and dizygotic twins reported discordant results regarding the incidence of caries and the oral microbiota composition [4,21,23,25,26], although those studies have been conducted in different age groups and using different microbiological methodologies, which could explain the lack of reproducibility. In the last years, tools for massive sequencing data analysis have been evolving considerably, allowing us to applied some of those novel tools to our data, including LEfSE and network analysis of the ecosystem.

Our PCoA analysis consistently associates a higher abundance of *Alloprevotella* in subjects with cavities, whereas in their healthy counterparts *Prevotella* was the most differential marker. Surprisingly, both genera belong to the same family and might have synonymous metabolic functions, although we cannot rule out synergistic effects of combination of microorganisms [27] and, most notably, the interaction of particular bacterial genera with fungi or virus, which has not been extensively explored. Most of the published studies using the entire oral microbiota with a metagenomic approach failed to find significant differences among healthy and caries status in non-related subjects [4,11,24,28,29]. However, a structural conservation between twins can be observed in our PCoA analysis, where control subjects are also more homogeneous (8/10 in the same quadrant) than the caries group (6/11), suggesting an incipient diversification on the oral microbiome.

As in other human ecosystems, the oral microbiome is usually constant and specific in each individual, but may be influenced by ethnicity [30]. A higher prevalence of caries has been described in a group of subjects from China, with special enrichment of *Scardovia* [24], whereas this genus is not particularly abundant in our population. In the study by Yasunaga et al., individuals without caries had more diverse communities, with a significantly higher proportion of the genus *Porphyromonas*, in particular *Porphyromonas pasteri* [31]. Belstrøm et al. also observed a higher alpha diversity in subjects with caries and an enrichment of *Neisseria*, *Haemophilus* and *Fusobacterium* compared to individuals without caries [29]. In contrast, in our study, both bacterial density and alpha diversity parameters are similar in children of both groups and conditions. An important point is that the composition of the community does not necessarily reflect its metabolic activity [10], particularly in microorganisms represented in low proportions, and it could have essential metabolic activities for the community [5].

Extremely high levels of *S. mutans* have been associated with caries, and, whereas *Streptococcus* was the majoritarian genera, we cannot investigate this point since our metagenomic approach is not able to assign to the level of species, due to the short length of the sequences obtained by massive sequencing. The dominance of *Streptococcus* in the oral cavity can be found in both patients with caries and in controls [29,32], as observed in our case, but being more abundant in the healthy control group than among the cavity group. A protective effect of some streptococcal species has been demonstrated [33], and, beyond the microbiota composition, there is an increasing emphasis on the global ecosystem richness, distribution and functionality [34]. However, in our case, LEfSE analysis failed in the discrimination of children by their cavity status, age, or sex, being the oral microbiota of all participants comparable.

In this study, the classification models showed relatively good precision in predicting caries in our data set (Table 2). The best performing classification models were Random Forest that showed the highest classification accuracy (CA) of a value of 0.881 and closely followed by Neural Networks with an CA of 0.810. One of the most interesting points of the Random Forest model was that it did not produce false positives. However, the worst aspect of these models was the percentage of false negatives (54.5%). On the contrary, the Neural Network model produced 16.1% false positives but a lower percentage, with respect to the Random Forest model, of false negatives (27.3%). This problem could be overcome with a large data-set of caries patients.

The major strength and, at the same time, the major limitation of our study is the inclusive criteria of children, which were enrolled during their orthodontic treatment independently of their caries' status. In fact, all the detected lesions were small and superficial, corresponding probably to the onset of the disease. Of course, we are unable to ascertain if this was also the case of the control group, where caries were not observed in any children but could be closed to appearing. The oral microbiota could be also implicated in the tooth development [8], and likewise the age of the patient might be considered, since different composition of the oral microbiota has been related to it. Finally, our results show that machine learning models could help us in caries prevention using microbiota data, although they are still far from having good accuracy. In summary, our results demonstrate that composition of oral microbiota in twins is highly conserved independently of their cariogenic process. We were unable to find any bacterial marker by 16S rDNA massive sequencing associated to caries; on the contrary, Isola et al. demonstrated a significant relationship between the salivary IL-6 concentration and existence of periodontitis [7,15].

Author Contributions: E.A.-G., M.R.B., D.P.-P. and R.d.C., study design, data analysis and drafting of the paper; M.P.-A., C.S., A.H. and J.G., data analysis and drafting of the paper; and M.P.C., data collection and drafting of the paper. All authors have read and agreed to the published version of the manuscript.

Funding: Claudia Saralegui was financed by a project of the Fundación Mutua Madrileña (grant to Rosa del Campo achieved in 2017 call with reference number AP165902017). This study was supported by Instituto de Salud Carlos III and the European Regional Development Fund (ERDF, 'A way to achieve Europe') (PI17/115 to Rosa del Campo) and Fundación Universidad Alfonso X El Sabio – Santander Universidades (Project number 1.010.811).

Institutional Review Board Statement: The study protocol was approved by the Ethical Committee of the Alfonso X El Sabio University (reference CE2017_0011) approved on 23 February 2017. The research was conducted ethically, in accordance with the World Medical Association Declaration of Helsinki. All participants and their parents/legal guardians signed a written informed consent form. Children received a report of their oral health status and were referred to dental treatment when necessary.

Informed Consent Statement: Informed consent was obtained from all subjects involved in the study.

Data Availability Statement: Data supporting our study can be found in the GenBank database as Bioproject PRJNA643173.

Conflicts of Interest: The authors declare no conflict of interest. The funders had no role in the design of the study; in the collection, analyses, or interpretation of data; in the writing of the manuscript, or in the decision to publish the results

References

1. Dzidic, M.; Collado, M.C.; Abrahamsson, T.; Artacho, A.; Stensson, M.; Jenmalm, M.C.; Mira, A. Oral microbiome development during childhood: An ecological succession influenced by postnatal factors and associated with tooth decay. *ISME J.* **2018**, *12*, 2292–2306. [CrossRef] [PubMed]
2. Fakhruddin, K.S.; Ngo, H.C.; Samaranayake, L.P. Cariogenic microbiome and microbiota of the early primary dentition: A contemporary overview. *Oral Dis.* **2019**, *25*, 982–995. [CrossRef] [PubMed]
3. Lamont, R.J.; Koo, H.; Hajishengallis, G. The oral microbiota: Dynamic communities and host interactions. *Nat. Rev. Microbiol.* **2018**, *16*, 745–759. [CrossRef] [PubMed]
4. Gomez, A.; Nelson, K.E. The oral microbiome of children: Development, disease, and implications beyond oral health. *Microb. Ecol.* **2017**, *73*, 492–503. [CrossRef]
5. Hajishengallis, G.; Darveau, R.P.; Curtis, M.A. The keystone-pathogen hypothesis. *Nat. Rev. Microbiol.* **2012**, *10*, 717–725. [CrossRef]
6. Peres, M.A.; Macpherson, L.M.D.; Weyant, R.J.; Daly, B.; Venturelli, R.; Mathur, M.R.; Listl, S.; Celeste, R.K.; Guarnizo-Herreño, C.C.; Kearns, C.; et al. Oral diseases: A global public health challenge. *Lancet* **2019**, *394*, 249–260. [CrossRef]
7. Isola, G.; Polizzi, A.; Alibrandi, A.; Williams, R.; Leonardi, R. Independent impact of periodontitis and cardiovascular disease on elevated soluble urokinase-type plasminogen activator receptor (suPAR) levels. *J. Periodontol.* **2020**. [CrossRef]
8. Chen, T.; Shi, Y.; Wang, X.; Wang, X.; Meng, F.; Yang, S.; Yang, J.; Xin, H. High-throughput sequencing analyses of oral microbial diversity in healthy people and patients with dental caries and periodontal disease. *Mol. Med. Rep.* **2017**, *16*, 127–132. [CrossRef]
9. Fernández-Escapa, I.; Chen, T.; Huang, Y.; Gajare, P.; Dewhirst, F.E.; Lemon, K.P. New insights into human nostril microbiome from the expanded Human Oral Microbiome Database (eHOMD): A resource for species-level identification of microbiome data from the aerodigestive tract. *mSystems* **2018**, *3*, e00187-18.
10. Solbiati, J.; Frías-Lopez, J. Metatranscriptome of the oral microbiome in health and disease. *J. Dent. Res.* **2018**, *97*, 492–500. [CrossRef]
11. Jiang, W.; Ling, Z.; Lin, X.; Chen, Y.; Zhang, J.; Yu, J.; Xiang, C.; Chen, H. Pyrosequencing analysis of oral microbiota shifting in various caries states in childhood. *Microb. Ecol.* **2014**, *67*, 962–969. [CrossRef]
12. Xu, H.; Tian, J.; Hao, W.; Zhang, Q.; Zhou, Q.; Shi, W.; Qin, M.; He, X.; Chen, F. Oral Microbiome shifts from caries-free to caries-affected status in 3-year-old chinese children: A longitudinal study. *Front. Microbiol.* **2018**, *9*, 2009. [CrossRef]
13. Xu, L.; Chen, X.; Wang, Y.; Jiang, W.; Wang, S.; Ling, Z.; Chen, H. Dynamic alterations in salivary microbiota related to dental caries and age in preschool children with deciduous dentition: A 2-year follow-up study. *Front. Physiol.* **2018**, *9*, 342. [CrossRef]
14. Kressirer, C.A.; Smith, D.J.; King, W.F.; Dobeck, J.M.; Starr, J.R.; Tanner, A.C.R. Scardovia wiggsiae and its potential role as a caries pathogen. *J. Oral Biosci.* **2017**, *59*, 135–141. [CrossRef]
15. Isola, G.; Giudice, A.L.; Polizzi, A.; Alibrandi, A.; Murabiato, P.; Indelicato, F. Identification of the different salivary Interleukin-6 profiles in patients with periodontitis: A cross-sectional study. *Arch. Oral Biol.* **2021**. [CrossRef]
16. Schwendicke, F.; Samek, W.; Krois, J. Artificial Intelligence in Dentistry: Chances and Challenges. *J. Dent. Res.* **2020**, *99*, 769–774. [CrossRef]
17. Segata, N.; Izard, J.; Waldron, L.; Gevers, D.; Miropolsky, L.; Garrett, W.S.; Huttenhower, C. Metagenomic biomarker discovery and explanation. *Genome Biol.* **2011**, *12*, R60. [CrossRef]
18. Demsar, J.; Curk, T.; Erjavec, A.; Gorup, C.; Hocevar, T.; Milutinovic, M.; Mozina, M.; Polajnar, M.; Toplak, M.; Staric, A.; et al. Orange: Data Mining Toolbox in Python. *J. Mach. Learn. Res.* **2013**, *14*, 2349–2353.
19. Ribeiro, A.A.; Azcarate-Peril, M.A.; Cadenas, M.B.; Butz, N.; Paster, B.J.; Chen, T.; Bair, E.; Arnold, R.R. The oral bacterial microbiome of occlusal surfaces in children and its association with diet and caries. *PLoS ONE* **2017**, *12*, e0180621. [CrossRef]
20. Ledder, R.G.; Kampoo, K.; Teanpaisan, R.; McBain, A.J. Oral microbiota in severe early childhood caries in Thai children and their families: A pilot study. *Front. Microbiol.* **2018**, *9*, 2420. [CrossRef]
21. Silva, M.J.; Kilpatrick, N.M.; Craig, J.M.; Manton, D.J.; Leong, P.; Burgner, D.P.; Scurrah, K.J. Genetic and early-life environmental influences on dental caries risk: A twin study. *Pediatrics* **2019**, *143*, e20183499. [CrossRef]

22. Stahringer, S.S.; Clemente, J.C.; Corley, R.P.; Hewitt, J.; Knights, D.; Walters, W.A.; others. Nurture trumps nature in a longitudinal survey of salivary bacterial communities in twins from early adolescence to early adulthood. *Genome Res.* **2012**, *22*, 2146–2152. [CrossRef]
23. Wu, H.; Zeng, B.; Li, B.; Ren, B.; Zhao, J.; Li, M.; Peng, X.; Feng, M.; Li, J.; Wei, H.; et al. Research on oral microbiota of monozygotic twins with discordant caries experience—In vitro and in vivo study. *Sci. Rep.* **2018**, *8*, 7267. [CrossRef]
24. Zhou, J.; Jiang, N.; Wang, S.; Hu, X.; Jiao, K.; He, X.; Li, Z.; Wang, J. Exploration of human salivary microbiomes–insights into the novel characteristics of microbial community structure in caries and caries-free subjects. *PLoS ONE* **2016**, *11*, e0147039. [CrossRef]
25. Lovelina, F.D.; Shastri, S.M.; Kumar, P.D. Assessment of the oral health status of monozygotic and dizygotic twins—A comparative study. *Oral Health Prev. Dent.* **2012**, *10*, 135–139.
26. Zheng, Y.; Zhang, M.; Li, J.; Li, Y.; Teng, F.; Jiang, H.; Du, M. Comparative analysis of the microbial profiles in supragingival plaque samples obtained from twins with discordant caries phenotypes and their mothers. *Front Cell Infect Microbiol.* **2018**, *8*, 361. [CrossRef]
27. Simón-Soro, A.; Mira, A. Solving the etiology of dental caries. *Trends Microbiol.* **2015**, *23*, 76–82. [CrossRef] [PubMed]
28. Jiang, S.; Gao, X.; Jin, L.; Lo, E.C. Salivary microbiome diversity in caries-free and caries-affected children. *Int. J. Mol. Sci.* **2016**, *17*, 1978. [CrossRef] [PubMed]
29. Belstrom, D.; Constancias, F.; Liu, Y.; Yang, L.; Drautz-Moses, D.I.; Schuster, S.C.; Kohli, G.S.; Jakobsen, T.H.; Holmstrup, P.; Givskov, M. Metagenomic and metatranscriptomic analysis of saliva reveals disease-associated microbiota in patients with periodontitis and dental caries. *NPJ Biofilms Microbiomes* **2017**, *3*, 23. [CrossRef] [PubMed]
30. Richards, V.P.; Alvarez, A.J.; Luce, A.R.; Bedenbaugh, M.; Mitchell, M.L.; Burne, R.A.; Nascimento, M.M. Microbiomes of site-specific dental plaques from children with different caries status. *Infect. Immun.* **2017**, *85*. [CrossRef]
31. Yasunaga, H.; Takeshita, T.; Shibata, Y.; Furuta, M.; Shimazaki, Y.; Akifusa, S. Exploration of bacterial species associated with the salivary microbiome of individuals with a low susceptibility to dental caries. *Clin. Oral Investig.* **2017**, *21*, 2399–2406. [CrossRef]
32. Wang, Y.; Zhang, J.; Chen, X.; Jiang, W.; Wang, S.; Xu, L.; Tu, Y.; Zheng, P.; Wang, Y.; Lin, X.; et al. Profiling of oral microbiota in early childhood caries using single-molecule real-time sequencing. *Front. Microbiol.* **2017**, *8*, 2244. [CrossRef]
33. López-López, A.; Camelo-Castillo, A.; Ferrer, M.D.; Simon-Soro, A.; Mira, A. Health-associated niche inhabitants as oral probiotics: the case of Streptococcus dentisani. *Front. Microbiol.* **2017**, *8*, 379. [CrossRef]
34. Kim, B.S.; Han, D.H.; Lee, H.; Oh, B. Association of salivary microbiota with dental caries incidence with dentine involvement after 4 years. *J. Microbiol. Biotechnol.* **2018**, *28*, 454–464. [CrossRef]

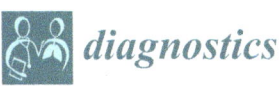

Article

Deep Active Learning for Automatic Segmentation of Maxillary Sinus Lesions Using a Convolutional Neural Network

Seok-Ki Jung [1,†], Ho-Kyung Lim [2,†], Seungjun Lee [3], Yongwon Cho [4,*] and In-Seok Song [3,*]

1. Department of Orthodontics, Korea University Guro Hospital, Seoul 08308, Korea; jgosggg@korea.ac.kr
2. Department of Oral and Maxillofacial Surgery, Korea University Guro Hospital, Seoul 08308, Korea; ungassi@korea.ac.kr
3. Department of Oral and Maxillofacial Surgery, Korea University Anam Hospital, Seoul 02841, Korea; brianlee877@gmail.com
4. Department of Radiology, Korea University Anam Hospital, Seoul 02841, Korea
* Correspondence: dragon1won@korea.ac.kr (Y.C.); densis@korea.ac.kr (I.-S.S.)
† These authors contributed equally to this work.

Abstract: The aim of this study was to segment the maxillary sinus into the maxillary bone, air, and lesion, and to evaluate its accuracy by comparing and analyzing the results performed by the experts. We randomly selected 83 cases of deep active learning. Our active learning framework consists of three steps. This framework adds new volumes per step to improve the performance of the model with limited training datasets, while inferring automatically using the model trained in the previous step. We determined the effect of active learning on cone-beam computed tomography (CBCT) volumes of dental with our customized 3D nnU-Net in all three steps. The dice similarity coefficients (DSCs) at each stage of air were 0.920 ± 0.17, 0.925 ± 0.16, and 0.930 ± 0.16, respectively. The DSCs at each stage of the lesion were 0.770 ± 0.18, 0.750 ± 0.19, and 0.760 ± 0.18, respectively. The time consumed by the convolutional neural network (CNN) assisted and manually modified segmentation decreased by approximately 493.2 s for 30 scans in the second step, and by approximately 362.7 s for 76 scans in the last step. In conclusion, this study demonstrates that a deep active learning framework can alleviate annotation efforts and costs by efficiently training on limited CBCT datasets.

Keywords: active learning; maxillary sinusitis; convolutional neural network; deep learning; segmentation

1. Introduction

Deep learning technology is advancing daily. Previously, it was only used in some areas such as image processing; however, artificial intelligence (AI) technology using deep learning has been used in various fields. In particular, deep learning technology using convolutional neural networks (CNNs) has excellent performance in analyzing image information [1,2]. This is going beyond object detection to find a specific object in an image, object classifications to classify which object it is, and this continues to develop into object segmentation, a technology that finds and separates the area of a specific object. Among them, object segmentation is the most difficult technique [3].

AI technology that analyzes and evaluates images is creating a lot of synergy in the medical field. In particular, this makes a significant contribution to the field of diagnosis [4]. Owing to the characteristics of medical fields, determining whether or not there is a specific disease using X-ray radiographs, computed tomography (CT), and magnetic resonance imaging (MRI) data is the most active field in which artificial intelligence technology is used. Analysis of whether there is a lesion, such as cancer, or what kind of disease the lesion is being performed [5,6]. Similar studies have been conducted in the dental field in recent years [7,8]. Likewise, the dental field is a field where many X-rays and CTs are taken, and the evaluation and diagnosis of the image is essential [9]. It would be nice to be able to obtain the help of highly skilled experts every time, but there is a lot of possibilities that a general practitioner may miss when it comes to difficult diseases. For this, if AI can screen for and inform a specific disease, the general practitioner can be alert to the diagnosis, and if necessary, it can be referred to a higher-level hospital or specialist. Accordingly, many previous studies have analyzed panoramic images to analyze tooth decay and periodontal disease and to detect changes in alveolar bone [10,11]. In addition, lesions for malignant diseases, such as ameloblastoma, are easily detected and not missed so that the patient's disease can be detected early [12].

In the dental field, not only diseases related to the teeth, but also the maxillary sinus is the subject of much interest [13,14]. The maxillary sinus is also an important part of the dental field, such as maxillary molar tooth disease, which causes maxillary sinusitis; if the maxillary molar implant has insufficient bone, maxillary sinus elevation is performed and bone grafts are performed. Accordingly, it is very helpful to accurately diagnose, analyze, and evaluate maxillary sinus diseases. In a two-dimensional panoramic picture, the maxillary sinus area is distorted and overlapped by the vertebrae, which is difficult to evaluate [14]. CT data, which are 3D images, are necessary for the accurate evaluation of the maxillary sinus. Deep learning analysis of 3D images is a much more difficult area than the analysis of 2D images. It is a complex area that needs to be reconstructed and evaluated again after analysis of the 2D slice image. The maxillary sinus is connected to various sinuses, such as the nasal cavity, ethmoid sinus, and frontal sinus, and is adjacent to the orbit and skull in the upper direction; therefore, it is very difficult to separate. Thus, it is even more difficult to segment the disease in the maxillary sinus.

Therefore, we studied a technique for segmenting maxillary sinus diseases using deep learning technology using 3D cone-beam computed tomography (CBCT) data. Segmentation has developed significantly with the development of CNN technology, but it is difficult to obtain sufficient labeled data for training in medical data. In this study, a customized 3D U-Net capable of active learning was used to increase training efficiency with limited data and reduce labeling efforts. This technology improves performance in an organic and dynamic way in which a person evaluates and corrects the result determined by artificial intelligence, and the artificial intelligence reflects and learns it again. The aim of this study was to segment the maxillary sinus into the maxillary bone, air, and lesion, and to evaluate its accuracy by comparing and analyzing the results performed by experts. We also determined whether active learning could improve segmentation accuracy and labeling efficiency.

2. Materials and Methods

2.1. Datasets and Pre-Processing

We used CBCT datasets (103 patients-internal and 20 patients-external) of consecutively patients with various sinuses that were confirmed between January 2018 and May 2020. All CBCT were acquired on the KAVO 3D Exam, Model 17–19 (Imaging Sciences International, Hatfield, PA, USA) for internal data and CS 9300 (Carestream Dental, GA, USA) for external data. In each scan, both bilateral maxillary sinuses were entirely visible. The exclusion criteria were when the radiograph quality was poor due to artifacts, there was an abnormality in the maxillary sinus or a history of surgery in the maxillary sinus.

Maxillary sinus segmentation was performed using CBCT. We randomly selected 83 patients for deep active learning (Table 1). For training, tuning, and testing, all datasets were split into 70:10:20 ratios. The ground truth of 40 cases for the first step with 20-internal Korea University Anam Hospital (KUAH) and 20 external Korea University Ansan Hospital (KUANH) scans for testing were verified by an expert reviewer using the AVIEW software, version 1.0.3 (Coreline Software, Seoul, Korea). In the second and last steps, 64 cases were used for active learning with limited data.

Table 1. Characteristics and acquisition parameters of the study population by group.

Characteristic	Training and Tuning (KUAH) (n = 83)	Internal-Validation (KUAH) (n = 20)	External-Validation KUANH (n = 20)
Age	59.9 ± 17.2	63.1 ± 16.9	40 ± 19.7
Male	44	10	10
Female	39	10	10
Tube voltage (kV)	120	120	90
Tube current (mA)	5	5	4
Scan time (s)	16.8	16.8	14.3
Voxel size (mm)	0.3	0.3	0.3
FOV (mm)	230 × 170	230 × 170	170 × 135
Focal spot (mm)	0.58	0.58	0.70

Note: Internal dataset: Korea University Anam Hospital (KUAH); external dataset—Korea University Ansan Hospital (KUANH); Field-of-view (FOV).

All input volumes were resized to 320 × 320 pixels with intensity normalization using the mean and standard deviation of the pixel on volumes. Third-order spline interpolation was performed by resampling each label separately. Aggressive data augmentation was used with the batch generator framework, involving gamma correction augmentation, random scaling, random rotations, random elastic deformations, and mirroring [15].

2.2. Training Architecture

The 3D U-Net of nnU-Net was used for maxillary sinus segmentation, including air and lesions in CBCT [16,17]. This architecture (customized 3D U-Net) is shown in Figure 1. The architecture comprises an encoder and a decoder network with transposed convolutional layers for backward operations. The left side reduces the dimensionality of the input, and the right side recovers the original dimensionality. The architecture involves 30 convolutional filters in the first layer and max pooling (2 × 2 × 2). The encoder network is similar to a conventional convolution neural network (CNN), which results in the reduction of spatial information and a loss of localization accuracy. In pixel-wise segmentation, both spatial and semantic information are important for training and testing medical images or volumes. The decoder of U-Net exploits deconvolution with a skip connection to maintain spatial information using semantic information from the low vertex. In this study, we replaced the leaky rectified linear unit (ReLU) activation functions with random ReLU of the original 3D nnU-Net and used cross-entropy, dice coefficient, and boundary loss functions. In the low vertex, adaptive layer-instance normalization (AdaLin) was added to help the attention-guided model correspond to the shape transformation [18]. For learning maxillary sinus segmentation on CBCT, the Adam optimization algorithm with an initial learning rate (3×10^{-4}) and l2-weight decay (3×10^{-5}) was used. If the exponential moving average of the training loss did not improve over the previous 30 epochs, the learning rate was reduced by 0.2 times. Training was stopped after exceeding 1000 epochs, or if the learning rate fell below 10^{-6}. The analysis of segmentation was calculated using the dice similarity coefficient (DSC), as defined in Equation (1). The loss functions include dice loss (DLS), boundary loss (BLS), and binary cross-entropy (BCE), which are defined in Equations (2)–(4), respectively [19]. V_{gs} is the volume parameter of the ground truth, and V_{seg} is the CNN segmentation.

$$DSC\left(V_{seg}, V_{gs}\right) = \frac{2|V_{seg} \cap V_{gs}|}{|V_{seg}| + |V_{gs}|}, \quad (1)$$

$$DLS = 1 - \frac{2|V_{seg} \cap V_{gs}|}{|V_{seg}| + |V_{gs}|}, \quad (2)$$

$$BLS(\partial G, \partial S) = 2\int_{\Delta S} \|q - Z_\partial G(q)\| dq \quad (3)$$

Here, ΔS defines the region between the two contours and $\|q - Z_\partial G(q)\|$. $\Omega \to R^+$ is a distance map with respect to boundary ∂G, that is, $\|q - Z_\partial G(q)\|$ evaluates the distance between point $q \in \Omega$ and the nearest point $Z_\partial G(q)$ on contour ∂G: $\|q - Z_\partial G(q)\|$.

$$L(y, f) = -y \log f - (1-y) \log (1-f) \qquad (4)$$

where y is the inferred probability and f is the corresponding desired output.

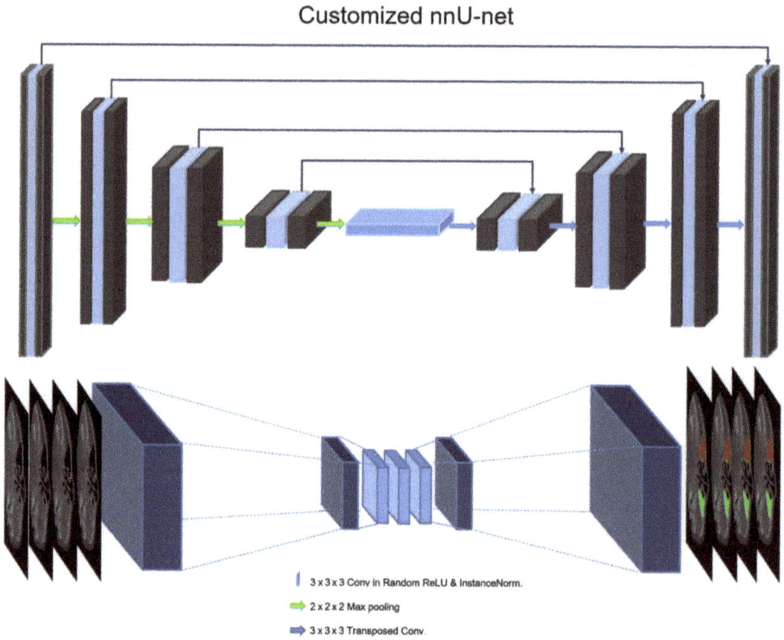

Figure 1. Deep learning architecture of the customized 3D U-Net in the nnU-Net.

2.3. Active Learning

Our active learning framework consists of three steps. This framework adds new volumes per step to improve the performance of the model with limited training datasets, while inferring automatically using the model trained in the previous step.

In the first step, 19 CBCT scans of KUAH were manually labeled by a dentist and an hygienist with more than 7 years of experiences to establish the ground truth. After the labeling process, an oral and maxillofacial surgeon with more than 15 years of experience checked and confirmed all of them. The limited labeled dataset was then initially trained to segment the maxillary sinus on the CBCT of KUAH. After the initial training (first step), the ground truth of the new unlabeled dataset for the next step was acquired for CNN-assisted and post-modified segmentation. In the second step, 19 CBCT scans of KUAH from the first step were reused to train with 30 new datasets, as shown in Figure 2.

After the second step, the CNN-assisted segmentation for the new unlabeled dataset was manually modified for training in the next stage, as performed in the first step. In the final step, 83 scans (49 reused from the second step and 34 new ones) were used to train and improve the model, while the 20 remaining scans (manually labeled in the first step) were used to test each model. The results were evaluated after each step for accurate maxillary sinus segmentation with 20-internal and 20-external scans. The CNN-assisted and post-modified segmentation was conducted using AVIEW Modeler® software, version 1.0.3 (Coreline Software, Seoul, Korea).

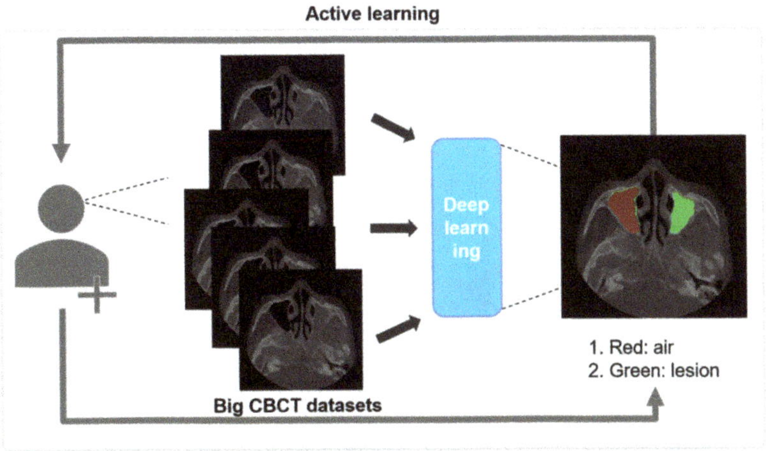

Figure 2. Overall process for the active learning for maxillary sinus segmentation on CBCT.

In 100 slices (KUAH) and 100 slices (KUANH) selected from internal [air-2633 and lesion-3256 slices] and external [air-3266 and lesion-3988 slices], all manual and the inference of deep learning based on active learning for visual scoring were assessed as very accurate (4 grade) to inaccurate (1 grade).

2.4. Experimental Setup

To infer the maxillary sinus on the 3D CBCT volumes of the dental, each axial phase in the volume was inputted sequentially to the model, and multiple 2D segmentation maps were constructed along the z-axis. Only soft tissue lesions such as mucosal thickening or mucosal retention cysts were considered as lesions. The normal soft tissue wall of the maxillary sinus was not considered to be a lesion. The experiment for training and test was conducted on Ubuntu 18.04 with Python 3.6, and used with the TensorFlow 1.15.0 backend with PyTorch 1.4.0 as the deep learning framework. The model was trained on an NVIDIA Titan RTX graphics card (24 GB). To maximize the training speed and optimize the GPU memory, we attempted to use larger input tiles and set the batch size to 6. In the first step, the training saturated approximately after 100 epochs, owing to the small size of the dataset ($n = 19$). The second and last steps required 70 to 100 epochs, owing to the larger datasets ($n = 49$ and $n = 83$). The difference in the overall DSCs between the tuning and test datasets in the final model (step 3) was 2.1. Our model for deep active learning did not overfit for learning with 3D CBCT volumes.

3. Results

We determined the effect of active learning on CBCT volumes of dental with our customized 3D nnU-Net in all three steps. The DSCs between the ground truth and the prediction were analyzed using 20-internal (KUAH) and 20-external (KUANH) datasets out of the 76 scans that were segmented by active learning. Figure 3 shows the worst and best results for the KUAH.

The last step is better than the other steps listed in Table 1. The figures show the maxillary sinus segmentation of 3D volumes on CBCT. As the steps progressed, the segmentation results improved on CBCT and reduced the erroneous areas outside the air. The DSCs at each stage of air were 0.920 ± 0.17, 0.925 ± 0.16, and 0.930 ± 0.16, respectively, as shown in Table 2. The DSCs at each stage of the lesion were 0.770 ± 0.18, 0.750 ± 0.19, and 0.760 ± 0.18, respectively (Table 2).

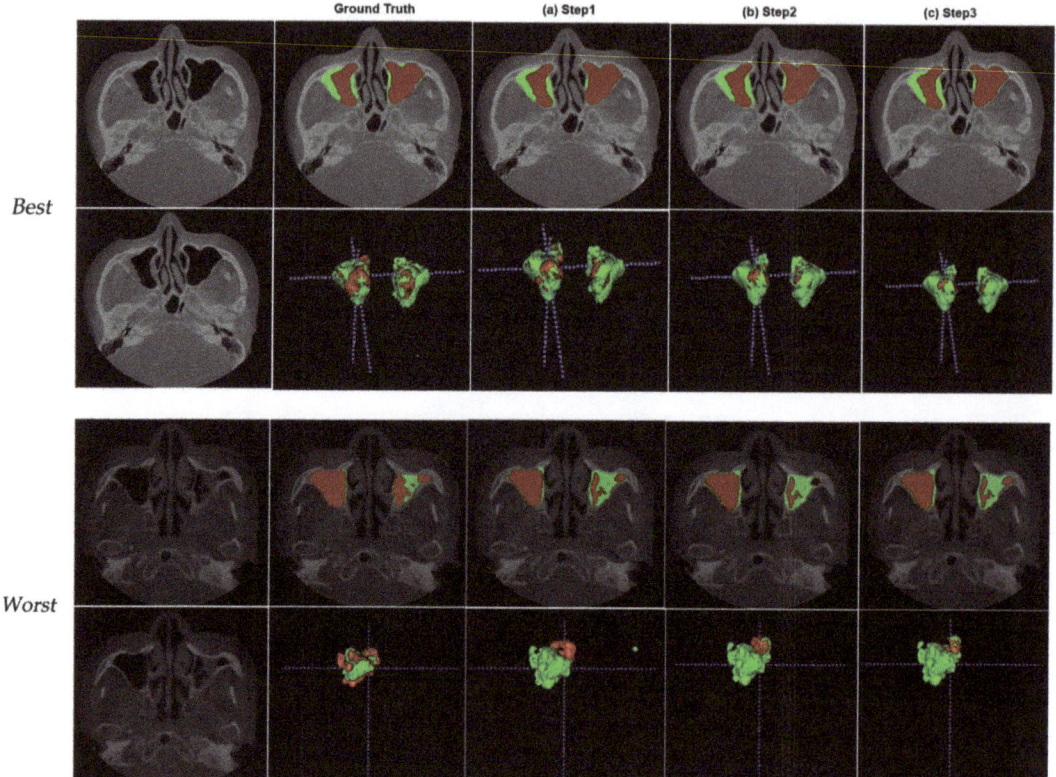

Figure 3. Best (first rows) and worst (second rows) from the test dataset (internal dataset—KUAH) at different analysis points: (**a**) first step, (**b**) second step, and (**c**) last step.

Table 2. DSCs for the first, second, and last steps for the test dataset (20 cases) on KUAH.

Mean ± SD (Range)	First Step	Second Step	Last Step
Air	0.920 ± 0.17 (0.245–0.992)	0.925 ± 0.16 (0.241–0.991)	0.930 ± 0.16 (0.243–0.996)
Lesion	0.770 ± 0.18 (0.208–0.912)	0.750 ± 0.19 (0.205–0.975)	0.760 ± 0.18 (0.208–0.96)

Note: Dice similarity coefficient (DSC); Korea University Anam Hospital (KUAH); Standard deviation (SD).

The average DSCs for maxillary sinus segmentation increased after each step, and the final segmentation in the last step showed the best results (Table 2). Furthermore, we evaluated the obtained inferences in KUANH using the proposed method. The DSCs for maxillary sinus segmentation in KUANH are presented in Table 3. The results of air on KUANH and KUAH were 0.97 ± 0.02 and 0.93 ± 0.16, respectively. Figure 4 shows the worst and best results for KUAH and KUANH.

Table 3. DSCs for the test dataset (20 cases of internal-KUAH and 20 cases of external-KUANH) in Figure 1; 3D-nnU-Net.

Mean ± SD (Range)	Last step (KUAH)	Last step (KUANH)
Air	0.93 ± 0.16 (0.243–0.996)	0.97 ± 0.02 (0.94–0.99)
Lesion	0.76 ± 0.18 (0.208–0.96)	0.54 ± 0.23 (0.12–0.88)

Note: Dice similarity coefficient (DSC); Korea University Anam Hospital (KUAH); Korea University Ansan Hospital (KUANH); Standard deviation (SD).

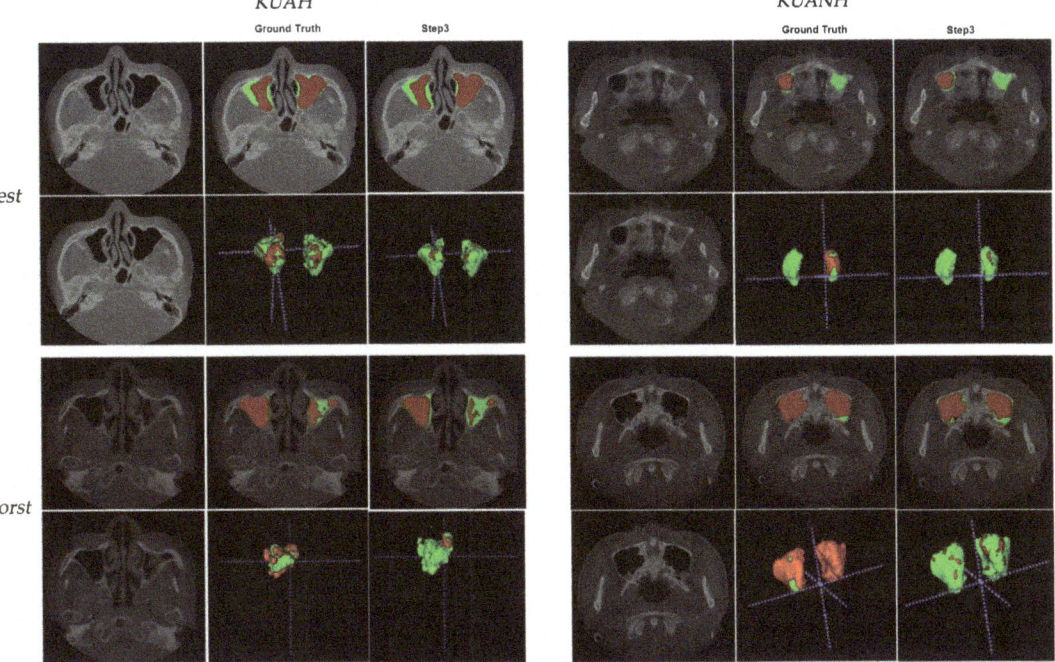

Figure 4. Best (first rows) and worst (second rows) from the test dataset on internal-KUAH and external-KUANH.

Comparisons of the maxillary sinus segmentation times between CNN-assisted and manual segmentation are given in Table 4. The time consumed by the CNN-assisted and manually modified segmentation decreased by approximately 493.2 s for 30 scans in the second step, and by approximately 362.7 s for 76 scans in the last step when compared to that taken in the first step.

Table 4. Comparison of segmentation times between the manual and CNN-assisted and manually modified segmentation approaches.

	First Step	Second Step	Last Step
	Manual segmentation	CNN-assisted and manually modified segmentation	CNN-assisted and manually modified segmentation
Time	1824.0 s	493.2 s	362.7 s

Note: Convolutional neural network (CNN).

Interestingly, the manual and DL segmentations were classified as very accurate to mostly accurate, and there were few inaccurate cases in Table 5. The number of very accurate cases in the DL segmentations was larger than that for manual segmentations (air: 75.7% vs. 91%, lesion 75% vs. 90%) in KUAH. Most of the slices that indicate DL's superior performance are seen in the mistakenly drawn manual segmentations of the maxillary sinus area on CBCT.

Table 5. Qualitative results from visual scoring of automatic maxillary sinus segmentation on CBCT from 100 Randomly Selected slices (internal-KUAH and external-KUANH) *.

Grade	Manual				3D U-Net (Last Step for Active Learning)			
	KUAH		KUANH		KUAH		KUANH	
	Air	Lesion	Air	Lesion	Air	Lesion	Air	Lesion
4—Very accurate	75.7	75	83.7	79.7	91	90	95.3	88
3—Accurate	19.6	16.6	15.3	19.3	8	7.4	4.7	12
2—Mostly accurate	1	3.7	1	1	0	2.3	0	0
1—Inaccurate	3.7	4.7	0	0	0	0.3	0	0

Note: Korea University Anam Hospital (KUAH); Korea University Ansan Hospital (KUANH); * Four-point scale: Three dentists conducted grade (manual vs. deep learning). 4—Very accurate: when the labelled maxillary sinus part completely matches the original sinus (over 95%); 3—Accurate: when the labelled sinus almost completely matches the original maxillary sinus (85–95%); 2—Mostly accurate: when the labelled maxillary sinus part depicts the site of the original maxillary sinus area (over 50%); 1—Inaccurate: when the labelled part depicts outside of the sinus or only matches small area of original maxillary sinus (under 50%).

4. Discussion

In this study, we proposed an active learning framework for maxillary sinus segmentation using a customized 3D nnU-Net on CBCT [16]. The most difficult part of maxillary sinus segmentation was separation, with the opening part that connects with other areas. In particular, the ethmoidal area was difficult because there were many open areas with several small holes. In addition, the part that connects to the nasal cavity is also large, so it is not easy to separate. Discriminating whether it is the maxillary sinus, nasal cavity, or ethmoidal region is a task requiring considerable difficulty even for a specialist. The value of this study lies in the development of a technology that can easily separate maxillary sinus lesions with the help of artificial intelligence.

In addition, the performance of artificial intelligence models has been improved using active learning [20]. As each step was completed, the DSCs increased and exhibited excellent performance. As shown in Table 4, the labeling time for CNN-assisted segmentation is reduced by more than half compared to manual segmentation. Segmentation accuracy increased over the steps, and the overall performance was reasonable compared with other state-of-the-art segmentation networks. 3D segmentation of the maxillary sinus is not an easy task. External validation was performed by dental specialists at both hospitals. No matter how accurately the segmentation was performed, a slight error in the boundary area inevitably occurs when a person performs it manually. CNN segmentation by AI first and modification is more efficient and time-saving compared to manual labeling from scratch. Therefore, it can be concluded that active learning can reduce the labeling effort through CNN-assisted segmentation and increase training efficiency through iterative learning with limited data.

When comparing its performance with other similar studies, 3D U-Net has become one of the most popular methods for pixel-by-pixel semantic segmentation because it shows excellent performance in medical image processing. However, several researchers have further advanced this network by combining detection architectures and cascading methods. Tang et al. proposed a cascade framework consisting of a detection architecture and a segmentation module using the VGG-16 model [21]. Roth et al. also proposed a two-stage FCN model in a cascading manner, with a focus on the target boundary area [22].

Yang et al. proposed a deep active learning framework by combining an FCN with active learning [23]. Lubrano et al. also proposed a similar framework for the segmentation of myelin sheaths in histological data [24]. The authors used Monte Carlo dropout to evaluate the model uncertainty and select samples for labeling. The segmentation performance of this study showed similar or better performance by showing DSC values of 0.92~0.93 in the air layer and 0.75~0.77 in the lesion compared to other studies showing DSC values of 0.66~0.85 [5,25–27]. In addition, unlike other studies, in this study, because the test was performed with multi-center data, it can be said that the generalization of performance was further verified.

In this study, the results of lesion segmentation were inferior to those of air segmentation in this study. Air with a certain radiopacity can be easily separated through threshold adjustment, while the separation of lesions with various radiopacities is difficult. To label the lesion, the entire maxillary sinus area was separated first, and the air layer was excluded. In the process of separating the maxillary sinus, a part of the bone was also included, and errors could also occur in the process of separating it from the adjacent sinuses. In addition, the thickness of the soft tissue wall surrounding the maxillary sinus varies from person to person. In the case of a thin soft tissue wall, a break may occur during the separation process, so the lesion may not be separated neatly.

The limitation of this study is that the segmentation performance of the maxillary sinus appeared to be low when the entire maxillary sinus was filled with inflammatory material. In the case of severe maxillary sinusitis, it can be seen that the inside of the maxillary sinus is hazy, which can be seen as a case where water or inflammatory substances are filled in the maxillary sinus. These artifacts are a factor that makes segmentation difficult. To overcome this, further studies are needed to increase our training dataset and use a better network to address ambiguities to improve segmentation performance. To improve the effectiveness and accuracy of the proposed scheme, further validation with more multi-center datasets and comparisons with other segmented networks, such as cascade networks, should be performed.

As labeling is basic but very labor-intensive, active learning can be considered to be a useful alternative [28,29]. In addition, manual labeling is not always constant in the segmentation process because of differences between people. Active learning frameworks can reduce this uncertainty by improving the accuracy by increasing collaboration with deep-learning algorithms. In addition, it is necessary to study the classification of segmented lesions in the future. This study suggests that, even for organs with complex structures such as the skull, the use of segmentation, lesion analysis, and diagnosis using active learning can be widely used.

5. Conclusions

In conclusion, this study demonstrates that a deep active learning framework (human-in-the-loop) can alleviate annotation efforts and costs by efficiently training limited CBCT datasets.

Author Contributions: Conceptualization, S.-K.J. and H.-K.L.; methodology, Y.C. and I.-S.S.; software, Y.C. and S.L.; validation, S.-K.J.; formal analysis, H.-K.L. and S.L.; investigation, S.-K.J.; resources, I.-S.S. and S.L.; data curation, Y.C.; writing—original draft preparation, S.-K.J. and H.-K.L.; writing—review and editing, I.-S.S. and Y.C.; visualization, S.-K.J.; supervision, H.-K.L.; project administration, I.-S.S.; funding acquisition, I.-S.S. and Y.C. All authors have read and agreed to the published version of the manuscript.

Funding: This research was funded by Korea University Grant (No. K1824471), and the Basic Science Research Program through the National Research Foundation of Korea funded by the Ministry of Education (2020R1I1A01071600).

Institutional Review Board Statement: The study was conducted according to the guidelines of the Declaration of Helsinki and approved by the Institutional Review Board of Korea University

Anam Hospital (2020AN0410, 11/01/2021) and Korea University Ansan Hospital (2021AS0041, 09/02/2021).

Informed Consent Statement: Patient consent was waived because the X-ray image was taken for treatment use, and there was no identifiable patient information.

Data Availability Statement: The data underlying this article will be shared on reasonable request from the corresponding author.

Conflicts of Interest: The authors declare no conflict of interest.

References

1. Shalbaf, A.; Bagherzadeh, S.; Maghsoudi, A. Transfer learning with deep convolutional neural network for automated detection of schizophrenia from EEG signals. *Phys. Eng. Sci. Med.* **2020**, *43*, 1229–1239. [CrossRef] [PubMed]
2. Nogay, H.S.; Adeli, H. Detection of Epileptic Seizure Using Pretrained Deep Convolutional Neural Network and Transfer Learning. *Eur. Neurol.* **2020**, *83*, 602–614. [CrossRef] [PubMed]
3. Kim, T.; Lee, K.; Ham, S.; Park, B.; Lee, S.; Hong, D.; Kim, G.B.; Kyung, Y.S.; Kim, C.-S.; Kim, N. Active learning for accuracy enhancement of semantic segmentation with CNN-corrected label curations: Evaluation on kidney segmentation in abdominal CT. *Sci. Rep.* **2020**, *10*, 1–7. [CrossRef] [PubMed]
4. Lee, K.-S.; Jung, S.-K.; Ryu, J.-J.; Shin, S.-W.; Choi, J. Evaluation of Transfer Learning with Deep Convolutional Neural Networks for Screening Osteoporosis in Dental Panoramic Radiographs. *J. Clin. Med.* **2020**, *9*, 392. [CrossRef] [PubMed]
5. Men, K.; Chen, X.; Zhang, Y.; Zhang, T.; Dai, J.; Yi, J.; Li, Y. Deep Deconvolutional Neural Network for Target Segmentation of Nasopharyngeal Cancer in Planning Computed Tomography Images. *Front. Oncol.* **2017**, *7*, 315. [CrossRef] [PubMed]
6. Samala, R.K.; Chan, H.-P.; Hadjiiski, L.; Helvie, M.A.; Wei, J.; Cha, K. Mass detection in digital breast tomosynthesis: Deep convolutional neural network with transfer learning from mammography. *Med. Phys.* **2016**, *43*, 6654–6666. [CrossRef]
7. Kwak, G.H.; Kwak, E.-J.; Song, J.M.; Park, H.R.; Jung, Y.-H.; Cho, B.-H.; Hui, P.; Hwang, J.J. Automatic mandibular canal detection using a deep convolutional neural network. *Sci. Rep.* **2020**, *10*, 5711. [CrossRef] [PubMed]
8. Jaskari, J.; Sahlsten, J.; Järnstedt, J.; Mehtonen, H.; Karhu, K.; Sundqvist, O.; Hietanen, A.; Varjonen, V.; Mattila, V.; Kaski, K. Deep Learning Method for Mandibular Canal Segmentation in Dental Cone Beam Computed Tomography Volumes. *Sci. Rep.* **2020**, *10*, 1–8. [CrossRef]
9. Lee, K.-S.; Ryu, J.-J.; Jang, H.S.; Lee, D.-Y.; Jung, S.-K. Deep Convolutional Neural Networks Based Analysis of Cephalometric Radiographs for Differential Diagnosis of Orthognathic Surgery Indications. *Appl. Sci.* **2020**, *10*, 2124. [CrossRef]
10. Chang, H.-J.; Lee, S.-J.; Yong, T.-H.; Shin, N.-Y.; Jang, B.-G.; Kim, J.-E.; Huh, K.-H.; Lee, S.-S.; Heo, M.-S.; Choi, S.-C.; et al. Deep Learning Hybrid Method to Automatically Diagnose Periodontal Bone Loss and Stage Periodontitis. *Sci. Rep.* **2020**, *10*, 1–8. [CrossRef]
11. Kim, J.; Lee, H.-S.; Song, I.-S.; Jung, K.-H. DeNTNet: Deep Neural Transfer Network for the detection of periodontal bone loss using panoramic dental radiographs. *Sci. Rep.* **2019**, *9*, 1–9. [CrossRef]
12. Kwon, O.; Yong, T.-H.; Kang, S.-R.; Kim, J.-E.; Huh, K.-H.; Heo, M.-S.; Lee, S.-S.; Choi, S.-C.; Yi, W.-J. Automatic diagnosis for cysts and tumors of both jaws on panoramic radiographs using a deep convolution neural network. *Dentomaxillofacial Radiol.* **2020**, *49*, 20200185. [CrossRef] [PubMed]
13. Kim, H.-G.; Lee, K.M.; Kim, E.J.; Lee, J.S. Improvement diagnostic accuracy of sinusitis recognition in paranasal sinus X-ray using multiple deep learning models. *Quant. Imaging Med. Surg.* **2019**, *9*, 942–951. [CrossRef]
14. Murata, M.; Ariji, Y.; Ohashi, Y.; Kawai, T.; Fukuda, M.; Funakoshi, T.; Kise, Y.; Nozawa, M.; Katsumata, A.; Fujita, H.; et al. Deep-learning classification using convolutional neural network for evaluation of maxillary sinusitis on panoramic radiography. *Oral Radiol.* **2019**, *35*, 301–307. [CrossRef]
15. Qin, Y.; Kamnitsas, K.; Ancha, S.; Nanavati, J.; Cottrell, G.; Criminisi, A.; Nori, A. Autofocus Layer for Semantic Segmentation. *Lect. Notes Comput. Sci.* **2018**, 603–611.
16. Isensee, F.; Jaeger, P.F.; Kohl, S.A.A.; Petersen, J.; Maier-Hein, K.H. nnU-Net: A self-configuring method for deep learning-based biomedical image segmentation. *Nat. Methods* **2021**, *18*, 203–211. [CrossRef]
17. Baid, U.; Talbar, S.; Rane, S.; Gupta, S.; Thakur, M.H.; Moiyadi, A.; Sable, N.; Akolkar, M.; Mahajan, A. A Novel Approach for Fully Automatic Intra-Tumor Segmentation With 3D U-Net Architecture for Gliomas. *Front. Comput. Neurosci.* **2020**, *14*, 10. [CrossRef] [PubMed]
18. *U-GAT-IT: Unsupervised Generative Attentional Networks with Adaptive Layer-Instance Normalization for Image-to-Image Translation*; arXiv:1907.10830 [cs.CV]; Computer Vision and Pattern Recognition (cs.CV); Image and Video Processing (eess.IV); Cornell University: Ithaca, NY, USA, 2019.
19. Kervadec, H.; Bouchtiba, J.; Desrosiers, C.; Granger, E.; Dolz, J.; Ben Ayed, I. Boundary loss for highly unbalanced segmentation. *Med. Image Anal.* **2021**, *67*, 101851. [CrossRef]
20. Sourati, J.; Gholipour, A.; Dy, J.G.; Kurugol, S.; Warfield, S.K. Active Deep learning with fisher information for patch-wise semantic segmentation. *Deep. Learn. Med. Image Anal. Multimodal Learn. Clin. Decis. Support* **2018**, *11045*, 83–91. [CrossRef]

21. Tang, M.; Zhang, Z.; Cobzas, D.; Jagersand, M.; Jaremko, J.L.; Zhang, Z. Segmentation-by-detection: A cascade network for volumetric medical image segmentation. In Proceedings of the 2018 IEEE 15th International Symposium on Biomedical Imaging (ISBI 2018), Washington, DC, USA, 4–7 April 2018; Volume 2, pp. 1356–1359. [CrossRef]
22. Roth, H.R.; Oda, H.; Zhou, X.; Shimizu, N.; Yang, Y.; Hayashi, Y.; Oda, M.; Fujiwara, M.; Misawa, K.; Mori, K. An application of cascaded 3D fully convolutional networks for medical image segmentation. *Comput. Med. Imaging Graph.* **2018**, *66*, 90–99. [CrossRef] [PubMed]
23. Yang, L.; Zhang, Y.; Chen, J.; Zhang, S.; Chen, D.Z. Suggestive Annotation: A Deep Active Learning Framework for Biomedical Image Segmentation. *Evol. Comput. Comb. Optim.* **2017**, *10435*, 399–407.
24. *Deep Active Learning for Axon-Myelin Segmentation on Histology Data*; arXiv:1907.05143 [cs.CV]; Computer Vision and Pattern Recognition (cs.CV); Machine Learning (cs.LG); Cornell University: Ithaca, NY, USA, 2019.
25. Daoud, B.; Morooka, K.; Kurazume, R.; Leila, F.; Mnejja, W.; Daoud, J. 3D segmentation of nasopharyngeal carcinoma from CT images using cascade deep learning. *Comput. Med. Imaging Graph.* **2019**, *77*, 101644. [CrossRef] [PubMed]
26. *Deep Learning for Automatic Tumour Segmentation in PET/CT Images of Patients with Head and Neck Cancers*; arXiv:1908.00841 [eess.IV]; Image and Video Processing (eess.IV); Cornell University: Ithaca, NY, USA, 2019.
27. Ma, Z.; Zhou, S.; Wu, X.; Zhang, H.; Yan, W.; Sun, S.; Zhou, J. Nasopharyngeal carcinoma segmentation based on enhanced convolutional neural networks using multi-modal metric learning. *Phys. Med. Biol.* **2018**, *64*, 025005. [CrossRef] [PubMed]
28. Lentzen, M.-P.; Zirk, M.; Riekert, M.; Buller, J.; Kreppel, M. Anatomical and Volumetric Analysis of the Sphenoid Sinus by Semiautomatic Segmentation of Cone Beam Computed Tomography. *J. Craniofacial Surg.* **2020**. [CrossRef] [PubMed]
29. Descoteaux, M.; Audette, M.A.; Chinzei, K.; Siddiqi, K. Bone enhancement filtering: Application to sinus bone segmentation and simulation of pituitary surgery. *Comput. Aided Surg.* **2006**, *11*, 247–255. [CrossRef] [PubMed]

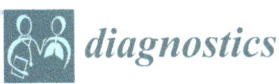

Article

Deep-Learning-Based Detection of Cranio-Spinal Differences between Skeletal Classification Using Cephalometric Radiography

Seung Hyun Jeong [1,†], Jong Pil Yun [1,†], Han-Gyeol Yeom [2], Hwi Kang Kim [3] and Bong Chul Kim [3,*]

1. Safety System Research Group, Korea Institute of Industrial Technology (KITECH), Gyeongsan 38408, Korea; shjeong@kitech.re.kr (S.H.J.); rebirth@kitech.re.kr (J.P.Y.)
2. Department of Oral and Maxillofacial Radiology, Daejeon Dental Hospital, Wonkwang University College of Dentistry, Daejeon 35233, Korea; hangyeol1214@gmail.com
3. Department of Oral and Maxillofacial Surgery, Daejeon Dental Hospital, Wonkwang University College of Dentistry, Daejeon 35233, Korea; hwi1304@naver.com
* Correspondence: bck@wku.ac.kr
† S.H.J. and J.P.Y. contributed equally to this study.

Abstract: The aim of this study was to reveal cranio-spinal differences between skeletal classification using convolutional neural networks (CNNs). Transverse and longitudinal cephalometric images of 832 patients were used for training and testing of CNNs (365 males and 467 females). Labeling was performed such that the jawbone was sufficiently masked, while the parts other than the jawbone were minimally masked. DenseNet was used as the feature extractor. Five random sampling crossvalidations were performed for two datasets. The average and maximum accuracy of the five crossvalidations were 90.43% and 92.54% for test 1 (evaluation of the entire posterior–anterior (PA) and lateral cephalometric images) and 88.17% and 88.70% for test 2 (evaluation of the PA and lateral cephalometric images obscuring the mandible). In this study, we found that even when jawbones of class I (normal mandible), class II (retrognathism), and class III (prognathism) are masked, their identification is possible through deep learning applied only in the cranio-spinal area. This suggests that cranio-spinal differences between each class exist.

Keywords: machine learning; artificial intelligence; malocclusion; diagnostic imaging

1. Introduction

Dentofacial dysmorphosis exhibits various aspects such as prognathism, retrognathism, maxillary hypoplasia, and asymmetry [1,2]. For their treatment, several techniques of orthognathic surgery or orthodontics are applied [2–4]. Meanwhile, the stomatognathic system is composed of static and dynamic structures, and its harmonious functioning is based on the balanced relationship between them [5]. In addition, hard and soft cephalic structures arise, grow, and organize in a mutual balance [6]. Cranio-facial skeletons constantly reflect these influences and their related functional conditions [1,6,7]. Therefore, the genesis of a malocclusion is usually linked to an impairment of some kind to eugnathic growth that involves to various extents the mandible, the maxilla, and the functional matrix (tongue and facial muscles) [5].

Until now, orthodontics and orthognathic surgery have mainly relied on linear and angular measurements for the diagnosis and the planning of the therapeutic procedures [1,3,7–13]. These measurements depend on the identification of several landmarks on cephalometric images, which are then applied to define the aforementioned measurements [1,3,7–13]. It is well recognized that the relation between these metrics varies with the type of bite and therefore is different in skeletal classes I, II, and III [1,7,13]. In addition, most of these landmarks on cephalometric images are concentrated in the maxilla and mandible [7]. However, the authors wondered if the difference between skeletal classes I, II, and III appears only in maxilla and mandible or if not, if is it also revealed in the cranio-spinal area excluding jaw. We also wanted to find a way to intuitively distinguish skeletal classes I, II, and III without linear and angular measurements.

Advances in convolutional neural networks (CNNs) continue [14–17]. They are being applied in a variety of dental and maxillofacial fields. For instance, they are used to assess soft-tissue profiling and extraction difficulty for mandibular third molars [18,19]. In addition, Xiao et al. proposed an end-to-end deep-learning framework to estimate patient-specific reference bony shape models for patients with orthognathic deformities [20]. Moreover, Sin et al. evaluated an automatic segmentation algorithm for pharyngeal airway in cone-beam-computed tomography images [21]. CNNs have proven their applicability to dental and maxillofacial fields through many other studies. However, to the best of our knowledge, CNNs have not been applied yet to clarify cranio-spinal differences between skeletal classification. Therefore, the aim of this study was to reveal cranio-spinal differences between skeletal classification using CNNs.

2. Materials and Methods

2.1. Datasets

In this study, transverse and longitudinal cephalometric images of 832 Korean patients who visited Daejeon Dental Hospital, Wonkwang University between January 2007 and December 2019 complaining about dentofacial dysmorphosis and/or a malocclusion were used for the training and testing of a deep-learning model (365 males and 467 females with a mean age of 18.37 ± 8.06 years). Patients with a congenital deformity, infection, trauma, or tumor history were excluded. The lateral and posterior–anterior (PA) cephalometric images were obtained using a Planmeca Promax (Planmeca OY, Helsinki, Finland), and the images were extracted in JPG format. The original images had a pixel resolution of 2045×1816 with a size of 0.132 mm/pixel.

All radiographic images were annotated by two orthodontists, two oral and maxillofacial surgeons, and one oral and maxillofacial radiologist. Point A–nasion–point B (ANB) and a Wits appraisal were used to diagnose the sagittal skeletal relationship. Jarabak's ratio and Björk's sum were used to determine the vertical skeletal relationship. With consensus of five specialists, patients' skeletal type was determined: class I (n = 272, 111 males and 161 females with a mean age of 17.17 ± 8.28 years); class II (n = 294, 105 males and 189 females with a mean age of 19.47 ± 8.85 years); or class III (n = 266, 149 males and 117 females with a mean age of 18.36 ± 6.61 years).

The purpose of this study was to determine whether there is an additional structural difference that makes it possible to distinguish the skeletal class in the structures of the head and neck other than the jawbone. Thus, labeling was manually performed such that the jawbone was sufficiently masked while the parts other than the jawbone were minimally masked.

The PA cephalometric images were masked with three square markers: a lower large square containing maxilla and mandible (nasal floor and hard palate region~inferior border of mandible) plus right and left small squares containing the condylar process (Figure 1).

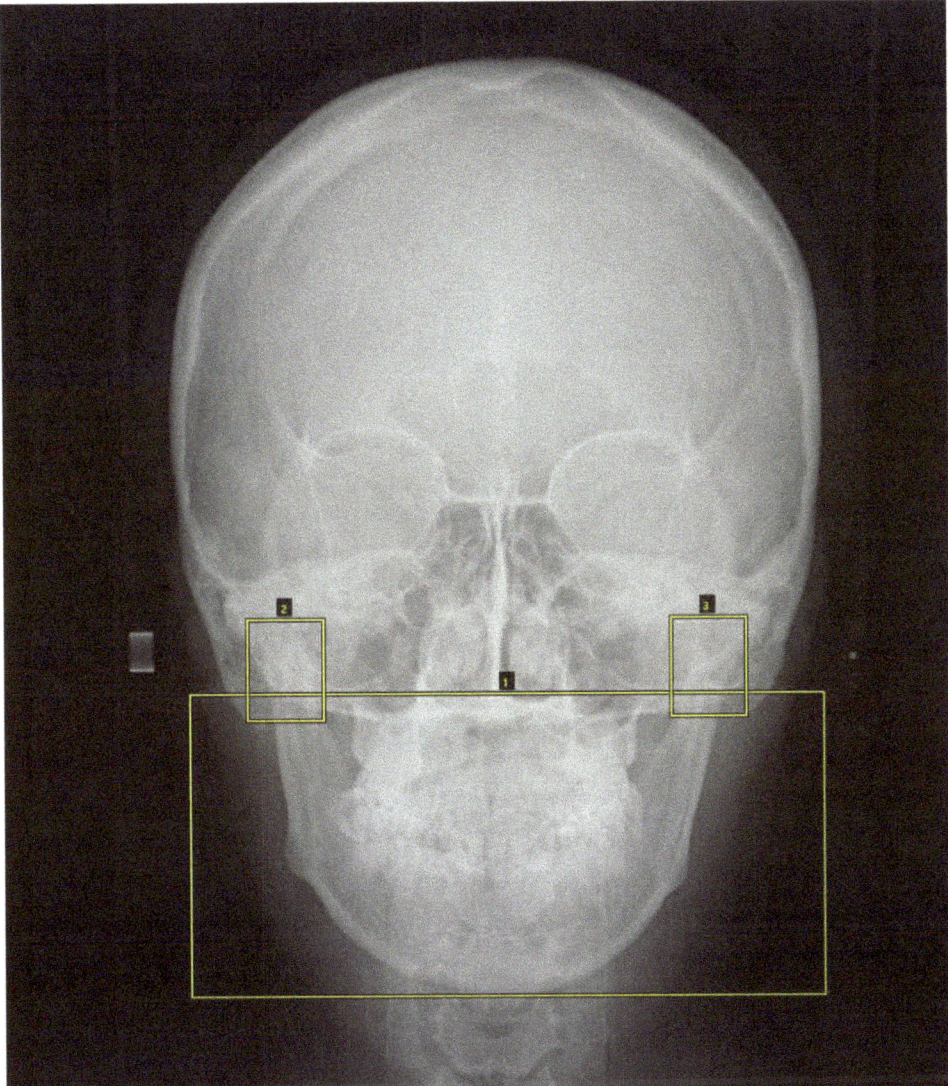

Figure 1. The posterior–anterior (PA) cephalometric images were masked with three square markers: a lower large square containing maxilla and mandible (nasal floor and hard palate region ~ inferior border of mandible) plus right and left small squares containing the condylar process.

The lateral cephalometric images were labeled with two square markers: a left long square containing the condylar process, coronoid process, mandibular ramus, and airway space and a right square containing the dentoalveolar region, maxilla, mandibular body, and lower facial soft tissue (Figure 2).

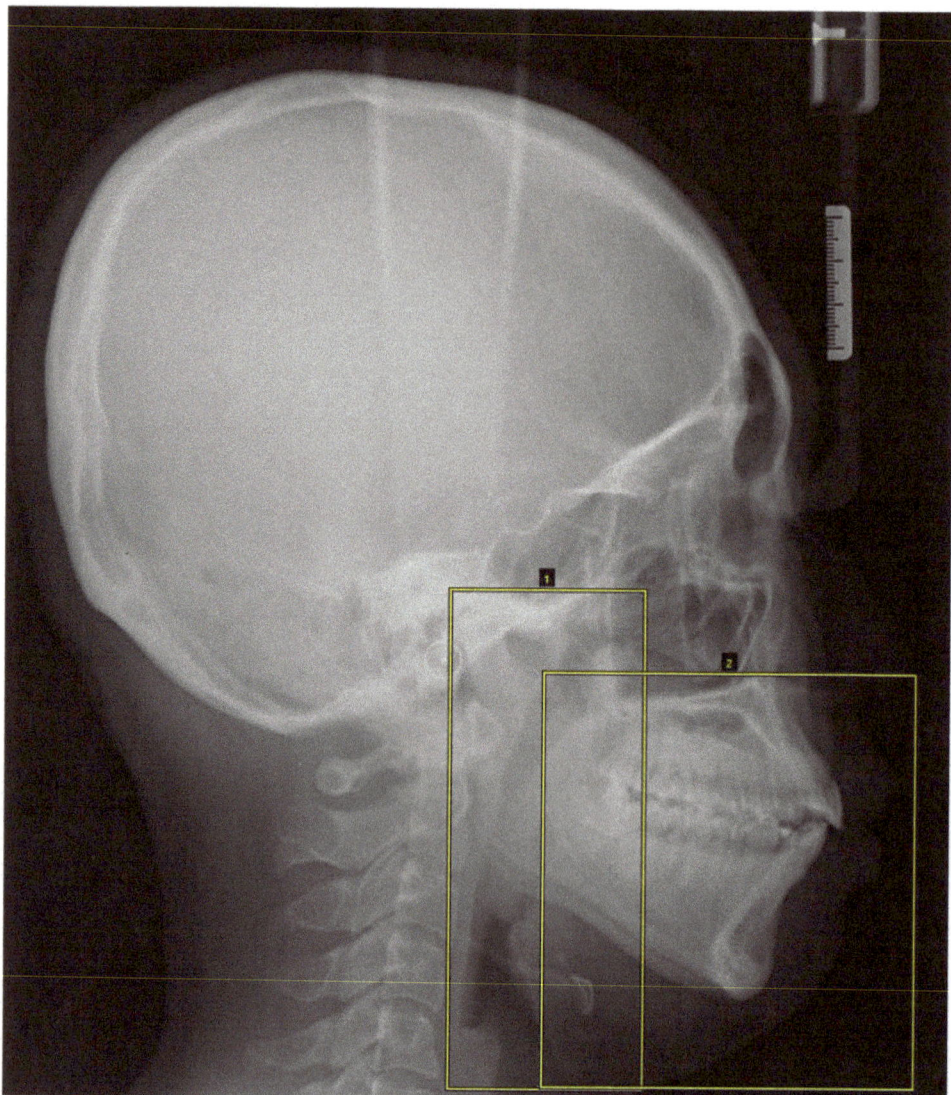

Figure 2. The lateral cephalometric images were masked with two square markers: a left long square containing the condylar process, coronoid process, mandibular ramus, and airway space and a right square containing the dentoalveolar region, maxilla, mandibular body, and lower facial soft tissue.

2.2. Preprocessing and Image Augmentation

Each patient's PA and lateral cephalometric images were preprocessed for training. The acquired data were resized to have the same height and width for training because they were different for each patient. For image resizing, we used OpenCV's API based on interpolation. Given that the skeleton is classified according to a geometric relationship, the height and width were resized at the same ratio. The height of the original cephalometric images was resized to 500, and the corresponding height ratio was applied to the width. After that, the cephalometric images were placed at the middle and zero-padding was performed to obtain 500 × 500 images. Note that the masking process mentioned in the dataset paragraph was applied after image resizing. In addition, data augmentation was performed for the preprocessed images to improve accuracy and prevent overfitting by using Pytorch's color jitter and random horizontal flip. Finally, the data were normalized by using the following equation.

$$p^*_{i,j} = \frac{\frac{p_{i,j}}{255} - mean}{std}. \quad (1)$$

where $p^*_{i,j}$, $p_{i,j}$, mean, and std. are normalized pixel value, original pixel value, mean, and standard deviation, respectively. The values of mean and std. are set to 0.5 and 0.5, respectively.

2.3. Architecture of the Deep CNN

The network structure that classifies into skeletal classes I, II, and III using PA and lateral cephalometric images is shown in Figure 3. The PA and lateral cephalometric images were fed to each feature extractor to obtain the feature map separately. Various backbone networks, such as VGG [22], ResNet [23], and DenseNet [24], can be used as feature extractors, and feature maps of different dimensions can be obtained according to each network's structure. In this study, DenseNet, proposed in 2016, was used as a feature extractor. DenseNet is a network that extracts features by continuously connecting the feature map of the previous layers with the input of the next layer. Figure 4 shows a five-layer dense block with a growth rate $k = 4$. ResNet is a method consisting in adding feature maps, while DenseNet is a structure that concatenates feature maps. Through this structure, the vanishing gradient can be improved, and the feature propagation can be reinforced. The depth of the feature map extracted through DenseNet is determined according to the growth rate and the number of layers of each block, whereas the width and height are determined according to the number of downsamplings. In this study, because pretrained DenseNet121 was used, an input image of 500 × 500 × 3 is converted into a feature map of 15 × 15 × 1024 after passing through the feature extractor. Each feature map output from the PA and lateral cephalometric images is transformed into a vector through global average pooling and merged into one vector through concatenation. The final classification is performed through a dense layer. The proposed network was implemented using Pytorch 1.2.

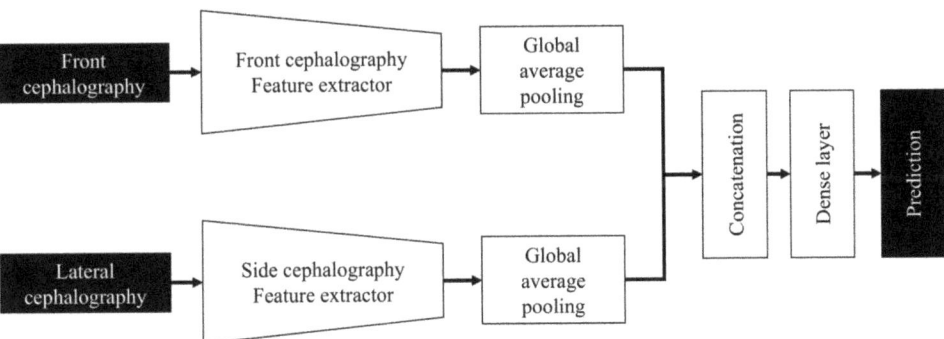

Figure 3. Multiside convolutional neural networks (CNNs) for classification using PA and lateral cephalometric images.

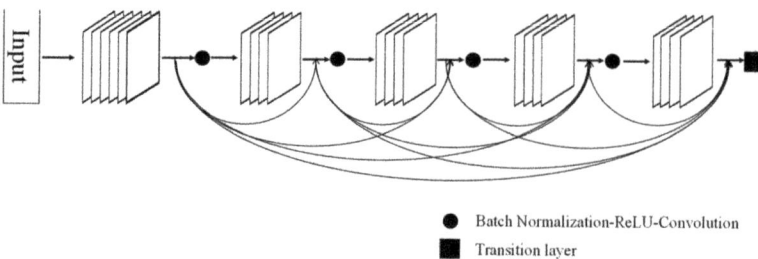

Figure 4. A five-layer dense block with a growth rate $k = 4$.

2.4. Visualization Method

In this study, the feature map was displayed so that the part extracted as a feature of the PA and lateral cephalometric images could be confirmed. The class activation map proposed in 2015 was used as a display method [25]. The class activation map is calculated as the summation of each feature map multiplied by the corresponding weight value of the dense layer, as shown in Figure 5. Through this method, it is possible to check which part of the cephalometric image was activated for classification. The greater the activation, the redder it is; and the greater the inactivation, the bluer it is.

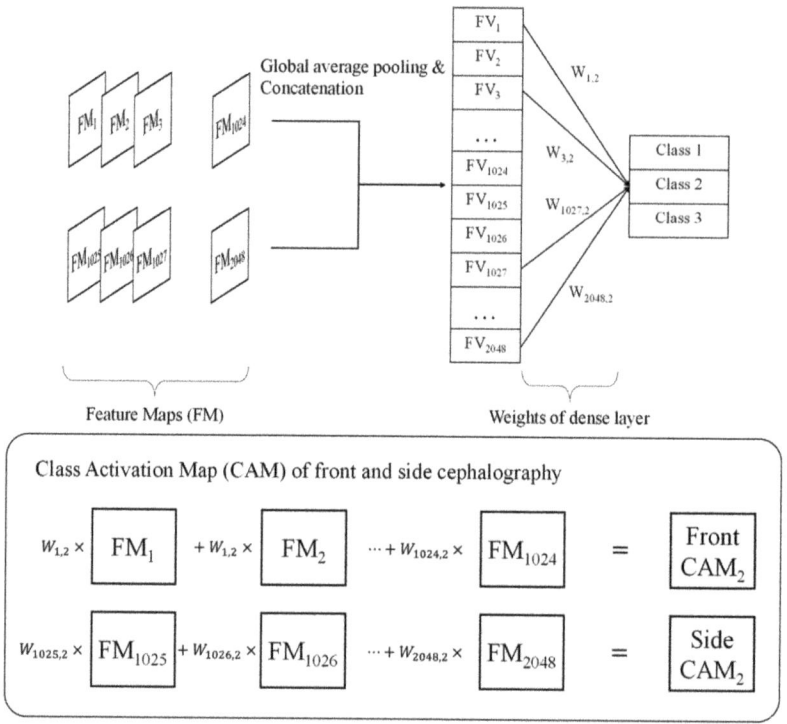

Figure 5. Class activation map (CAM) generation of PA and lateral cephalometric images.

3. Results

The proposed CNNs were trained using the Adam optimizer [26]. The initial learning rate was set to 0.001. The learning rate decay was set to 0.95 and was applied every five epochs. To take into account the randomness of the deep-learning-network training algorithm, five random sampling crossvalidations were performed for two datasets. The average and maximum accuracy of the five crossvalidations were 90.43% and 92.54% for test 1 (evaluation of the entire posterior–anterior (PA) and lateral cephalometric images) and 88.17% and 88.70% for test 2 (evaluation of the PA and lateral cephalometric images obscuring the mandible). A box plot of the accuracy for each test is shown in Figure 6. Table 1 shows the confusion matrix for best accuracy result of each test.

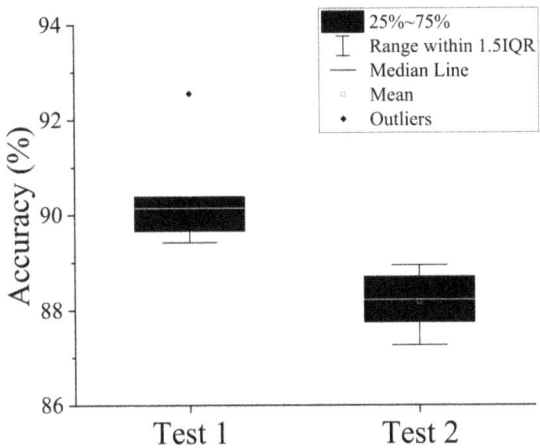

Figure 6. Test accuracies in five random sampling crossvalidations. Test 1: evaluation of the entire PA and lateral cephalometric images. Test 2: evaluation of the PA and lateral cephalometric images obscuring the mandible.

Table 1. Confusion matrices of best accuracy results for (a) test 1 and (b) test 2.

(a)				
			Predictions	
		Class I	Class II	Class III
Ground Truth	Class I	125	9	7
	Class II	11	141	0
	Class III	3	1	119
(b)				
			Predictions	
		Class I	Class II	Class III
Ground Truth	Class I	118	12	8
	Class II	17	136	0
	Class III	8	2	115

Class I: normal mandible; Class II: retrognathism; and Class III: prognathism. Ground truth: actual group of patients classified according to their mandibular class. Prediction: mandibular class predicted by deep learning. Test 1: evaluation of the entire PA and lateral cephalometric images. Test 2: evaluation of the PA and lateral cephalometric images obscuring the mandible.

4. Discussion

The average and maximum accuracies of the five crossvalidations were 90.43% and 92.54% for test 1, and 88.17% and 88.70% for test 2. As expected, the predicted results were more accurate in test 1, in which all cephalometric images could be analyzed without masking the jawbone. However, the difference in accuracy between test 1 and test 2 was within 5%, which is not significant.

At the same time, with the class activation map, it is possible to know where the CNNs focused on the cephalometric images to provide a prediction (Figure 7). As might be expected, test 1 focused on the jawbone, especially on the state of the dentition. However, in test 2, the jawbone and dentition were obscured and could not be analyzed. Therefore, CNNs were forced to identify the remaining uncovered regions, that is, the cranio-spinal area. Figure 7 shows the wide area of the cranio-spinal area excluding the jawbone, which is hidden, marked in red. This reveals that the cranio-spinal area is discernibly different in skeletal classes I, II, and III.

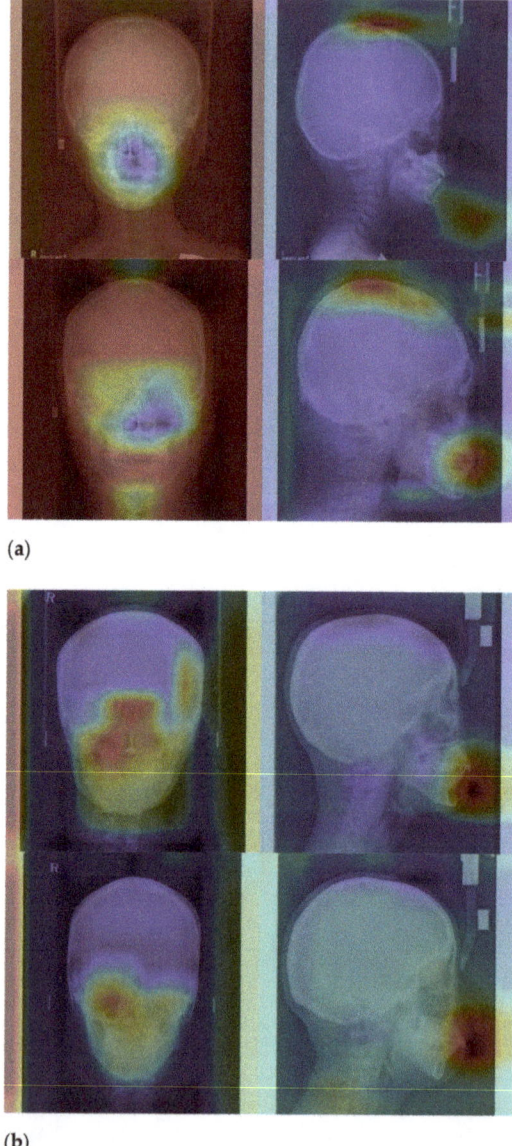

Figure 7. *Cont.*

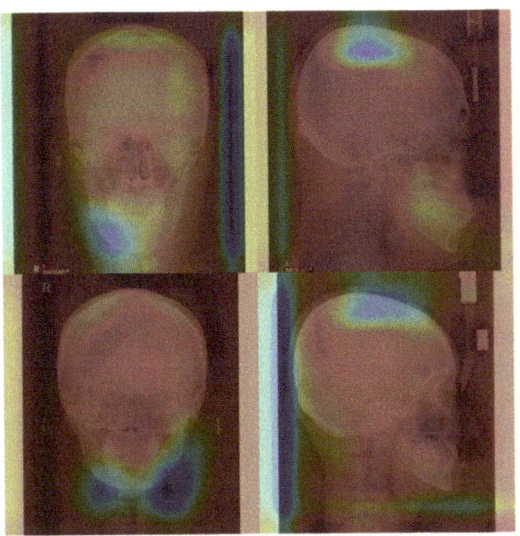

(c)

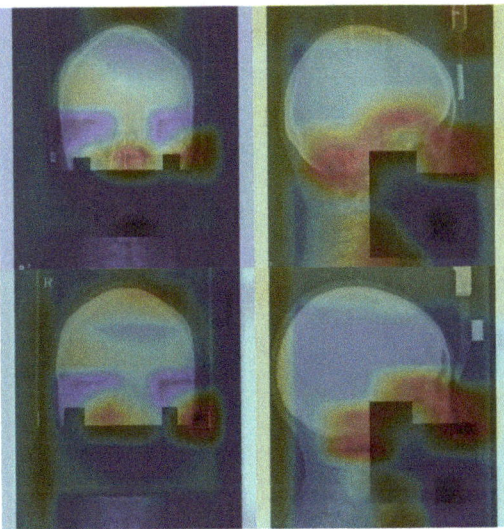

(d)

Figure 7. *Cont.*

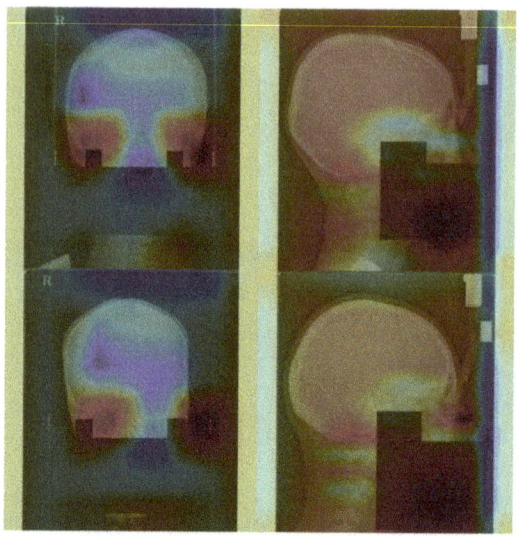

(e)

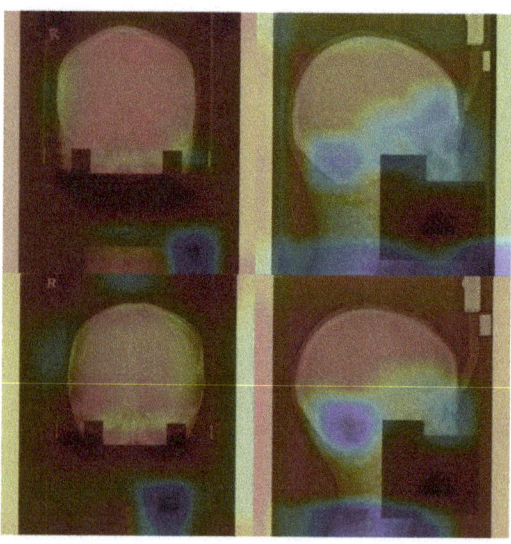

(f)

Figure 7. CAM of PA and lateral cephalometric images for (**a**) Class I of test 1, (**b**) Class II of test 1, (**c**) Class III of test 1, (**d**) Class I of test 2, (**e**) Class II of test 2, and (**f**) Class III of test 2. Class I: normal mandible; Class II: retrognathism; and Class III: prognathism. The greater the activation, the redder it is; the greater inactivation, the bluer it is.

5. Conclusions

In this study, we found that even when the jawbones of skeletal classes I, II, and III are masked, their identification is possible through deep learning applied only in the cranio-spinal area. This suggests that cranio-spinal differences exist between each class. Further research is required about where and how cranio-spinal differences emerge.

Author Contributions: The study was conceived by B.C.K., who also setup the experiments. S.H.J. and J.P.Y. performed the experiments. H.-G.Y., H.K.K., and B.C.K. generated the data. All authors analyzed and interpreted the data. S.H.J., J.P.Y., and B.C.K. wrote the manuscript. All authors have read and agreed to the published version of the manuscript.

Funding: This work was supported by a grant from National Research Foundation of Korea (NRF) funded by the Korean government (MSIT) (No. 2020R1A2C1003792).

Institutional Review Board Statement: This study was performed in accordance with the guidelines of the World Medical Association Helsinki Declaration for Biomedical Research Involving Human Subjects and was approved by the Institutional Review Board of Daejeon Dental Hospital, Wonkwang University (W2007/004-001, July 8 2020).

Informed Consent Statement: Patient consent was waived by the IRBs because of the retrospective nature of this investigation and the use of anonymized patient data.

Data Availability Statement: The datasets generated during and/or analyzed during the current study are available from the corresponding author on reasonable request but is subject to the permission of the Institutional Review Boards of the participating institutions.

Conflicts of Interest: The authors declare no conflict of interest.

References

1. Mun, S.H.; Park, M.; Lee, J.; Lim, H.J.; Kim, B.C. Volumetric characteristics of prognathic mandible revealed by skeletal unit analysis. *Ann. Anat. Anat. Anz.* **2019**, *226*, 3–9. [CrossRef] [PubMed]
2. Lanteri, V.; Cavagnetto, D.; Abate, A.; Mainardi, E.; Gaffuri, F.; Ugolini, A.; Maspero, C. Buccal bone changes around first permanent molars and second primary molars after maxillary expansion with a low compliance ni-ti leaf spring expander. *Int. J. Environ. Res. Public Health* **2020**, *17*, 9104. [CrossRef]
3. Park, J.C.; Lee, J.; Lim, H.J.; Kim, B.C. Rotation tendency of the posteriorly displaced proximal segment after vertical ramus osteotomy. *J. Cranio-Maxillo-Facial Surg.* **2018**, *46*, 2096–2102. [CrossRef]
4. Abate, A.; Cavagnetto, D.; Fama, A.; Matarese, M.; Lucarelli, D.; Assandri, F. Short term effects of rapid maxillary expansion on breathing function assessed with spirometry: A case-control study. *Saudi Dent. J.* **2020**. [CrossRef]
5. Abate, A.; Cavagnetto, D.; Fama, A.; Maspero, C.; Farronato, G. Relationship between breastfeeding and malocclusion: A systematic review of the literature. *Nutrients* **2020**, *12*, 3688. [CrossRef] [PubMed]
6. Delaire, J.; Schendel, S.A.; Tulasne, J.F. An architectural and structural craniofacial analysis: A new lateral cephalometric analysis. *Oral Surg. Oral Med. Oral Pathol.* **1981**, *52*, 226–238. [CrossRef]
7. Lee, S.H.; Kil, T.J.; Park, K.R.; Kim, B.C.; Kim, J.G.; Piao, Z.; Corre, P. Three-dimensional architectural and structural analysis–a transition in concept and design from delaire's cephalometric analysis. *Int. J. Oral Maxillofac. Surg.* **2014**, *43*, 1154–1160. [CrossRef] [PubMed]
8. Shin, H.; Park, M.; Chae, J.M.; Lee, J.; Lim, H.J.; Kim, B.C. Factors affecting forced eruption duration of impacted and labially displaced canines. *Am. J. Orthod. Dentofac. Orthop.* **2019**, *156*, 808–817. [CrossRef] [PubMed]
9. Kim, B.C.; Bertin, H.; Kim, H.J.; Kang, S.H.; Mercier, J.; Perrin, J.P.; Corre, P.; Lee, S.H. Structural comparison of hemifacial microsomia mandible in different age groups by three-dimensional skeletal unit analysis. *J. Cranio-Maxillo-Facial Surg.* **2018**, *46*, 1875–1882. [CrossRef]
10. Kim, H.J.; Kim, B.C.; Kim, J.G.; Zhengguo, P.; Kang, S.H.; Lee, S.H. Construction and validation of the midsagittal reference plane based on the skull base symmetry for three-dimensional cephalometric craniofacial analysis. *J. Craniofacial Surg.* **2014**, *25*, 338–342. [CrossRef]
11. Kim, B.C.; Lee, S.H.; Park, K.R.; Jung, Y.S.; Yi, C.K. Reconstruction of the premaxilla by segmental distraction osteogenesis for maxillary retrusion in cleft lip and palate. *Cleft Palate-Craniofacial J.* **2014**, *51*, 240–245. [CrossRef]
12. Kang, Y.H.; Kim, B.C.; Park, K.R.; Yon, J.Y.; Kim, H.J.; Tak, H.J.; Piao, Z.; Kim, M.K.; Lee, S.H. Visual pathway-related horizontal reference plane for three-dimensional craniofacial analysis. *Orthod. Craniofacial Res.* **2012**, *15*, 245–254. [CrossRef] [PubMed]
13. Park, W.; Kim, B.C.; Yu, H.S.; Yi, C.K.; Lee, S.H. Architectural characteristics of the normal and deformity mandible revealed by three-dimensional functional unit analysis. *Clin. Oral Investig.* **2010**, *14*, 691–698. [CrossRef]
14. Awan, M.J.; Rahim, M.S.M.; Salim, N.; Mohammed, M.A.; Garcia-Zapirain, B.; Abdulkareem, K.H. Efficient detection of knee anterior cruciate ligament from magnetic resonance imaging using deep learning approach. *Diagnostics* **2021**, *11*. [CrossRef]
15. Jeon, Y.; Lee, K.; Sunwoo, L.; Choi, D.; Oh, D.Y.; Lee, K.J.; Kim, Y.; Kim, J.W.; Cho, S.J.; Baik, S.H.; et al. Deep learning for diagnosis of paranasal sinusitis using multi-view radiographs. *Diagnostics* **2021**, *11*, 250. [CrossRef]
16. Kumar Singh, V.; Abdel-Nasser, M.; Pandey, N.; Puig, D. Lunginfseg: Segmenting covid-19 infected regions in lung ct images based on a receptive-field-aware deep learning framework. *Diagnostics* **2021**, *11*, 158. [CrossRef] [PubMed]

17. Singh, G.; Al'Aref, S.J.; Lee, B.C.; Lee, J.K.; Tan, S.Y.; Lin, F.Y.; Chang, H.J.; Shaw, L.J.; Baskaran, L.; On Behalf Of The, C.; et al. End-to-end, pixel-wise vessel-specific coronary and aortic calcium detection and scoring using deep learning. *Diagnostics* **2021**, *11*, 215. [CrossRef] [PubMed]
18. Jeong, S.H.; Yun, J.P.; Yeom, H.G.; Lim, H.J.; Lee, J.; Kim, B.C. Deep learning based discrimination of soft tissue profiles requiring orthognathic surgery by facial photographs. *Sci. Rep.* **2020**, *10*, 16235. [CrossRef] [PubMed]
19. Yoo, J.H.; Yeom, H.G.; Shin, W.; Yun, J.P.; Lee, J.H.; Jeong, S.H.; Lim, H.J.; Lee, J.; Kim, B.C. Deep learning based prediction of extraction difficulty for mandibular third molars. *Sci. Rep.* **2021**, *11*, 1954. [CrossRef]
20. Xiao, D.; Lian, C.; Deng, H.; Kuang, T.; Liu, Q.; Ma, L.; Kim, D.; Lang, Y.; Chen, X.; Gateno, J.; et al. Estimating reference bony shape models for orthognathic surgical planning using 3d point-cloud deep learning. *IEEE J. Biomed. Health Inform.* **2021**. [CrossRef]
21. Sin, Ç.; Akkaya, N.; Aksoy, S.; Orhan, K.; Öz, U. A deep learning algorithm proposal to automatic pharyngeal airway detection and segmentation on cbct images. *Orthod. Craniofacial Res.* **2021**. [CrossRef] [PubMed]
22. Simonyan, K.; Zisserman, A. Very deep convolutional networks for large-scale image recognition. In Proceedings of the The International Conference on Learning Representations, San Diego, CA, USA, 7–9 May 2015.
23. He, K.; Zhang, X.; Ren, S.; Sun, J. Deep residual learning for image recognition. In Proceedings of the IEEE Conference on Computer Vision and Pattern Recognition (CVPR), Las Vegas, NV, USA, 27–30 June 2016; pp. 770–778.
24. Huang, G.; Liu, Z.; Maaten, L.v.d.; Weinberger, K.Q. Densely connected convolutional networks. In Proceedings of the IEEE Conference on Computer Vision and Pattern Recognition, Honolulu, HI, USA, 21–26 July 2017.
25. Zhou, B.; Khosla, A.; Lapedriza, A.; Oliva, A.; Torralba, A. Learning deep features for discriminative localization. In Proceedings of the IEEE Conference on Computer Vision and Pattern Recognition (CVPR), Las Vegas, NV, USA, 27–30 June 2016.
26. Kingma, D.P.; Ba, J. Adam: A method for stochastic optimization. *arXiv* **2014**, arXiv:1412.6980.

MDPI
St. Alban-Anlage 66
4052 Basel
Switzerland
Tel. +41 61 683 77 34
Fax +41 61 302 89 18
www.mdpi.com

Diagnostics Editorial Office
E-mail: diagnostics@mdpi.com
www.mdpi.com/journal/diagnostics

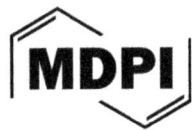

www.ingramcontent.com/pod-product-compliance
Lightning Source LLC
LaVergne TN
LVHW070710100526
838202LV00013B/1064